D1572425

Behind the Mask

Behind the Mask

Vernacular Culture in the Time of COVID

Edited by
Ben Bridges
Ross Brillhart
Diane E. Goldstein

Utah State University Press
Logan

© 2023 by University Press of Colorado

Published by Utah State University Press
An imprint of University Press of Colorado
1580 North Logan Street, Suite 660
PMB 39883
Denver, Colorado 80203-1942

All rights reserved
Printed in the United States of America

 The University Press of Colorado is a proud member of
the Association of University Presses.

The University Press of Colorado is a cooperative publishing enterprise supported, in part, by Adams State University, Colorado State University, Fort Lewis College, Metropolitan State University of Denver, University of Alaska Fairbanks, University of Colorado, University of Denver, University of Northern Colorado, University of Wyoming, Utah State University, and Western Colorado University.

∞ This paper meets the requirements of the ANSI/NISO Z39.48-1992 (Permanence of Paper).

ISBN: 978-1-64642-479-5 (hardcover)
ISBN: 978-1-64642-480-1 (paperback)
ISBN: 978-1-64642-481-8 (ebook)
https://doi.org/10.7330/9781646424818

Library of Congress Cataloging-in-Publication Data

Names: Bridges, Ben, editor. | Brillhart, Ross, editor. | Goldstein, Diane E., editor.
Title: Behind the mask : vernacular culture in the time of COVID / edited by Ben Bridges, Ross Brillhart, Diane E. Goldstein.
Description: Logan : Utah State University Press, [2023] | Includes bibliographical references and index.
Identifiers: LCCN 2023015910 (print) | LCCN 2023015911 (ebook) | ISBN 9781646424795 (hardcover) | ISBN 9781646424801 (paperback) | ISBN 9781646424818 (ebook)
Subjects: LCSH: COVID-19 Pandemic, 2020—Influence. | COVID-19 Pandemic, 2020—Social aspects. | Epidemics in mass media. | Language and culture. | Communication and culture.
Classification: LCC RA644.C67 B426 2023 (print) | LCC RA644.C67 (ebook) | DDC 362.1962/4144—dc23/eng/20230705
LC record available at https://lccn.loc.gov/2023015910
LC ebook record available at https://lccn.loc.gov/2023015911

This work was partially funded by Indiana University Research through the Faculty Grant-in-Aid Program.

Front-cover illustrations: © Blanscape/Shutterstock (*top right*), © Charlie Waradee / Shutterstock (*middle*), © Bill Roque / Shutterstock (*bottom left*), © Andrew Rodgers (*bottom right*)

Contents

Figures

Acknowledgments

THIS VOLUME GREW OUT OF A COVID-19 INTEREST group in the Department of Folklore and Ethnomusicology at Indiana University that began with biweekly meetings on Zoom during the early days of the pandemic lockdown. We are grateful for the inspiration, thoughtfulness, and support of our fellow group members, some, but not all, of whom are represented in these pages. We would also like to thank the contributors that joined us at a later stage in the process. Your contributions helped us achieve a volume that came very close to what we imagined in the early excited days of planning. The manuscript reviewers and the directors, editors, and staff at Utah State University Press, including Rachael Levay, Laura Furney, Dan Pratt, Chiquita Taborn, and Darrin Pratt, understood the time sensitivity of our topic and helped us achieve publication while the experience of COVID was still very much in all our hearts and minds. This work was partially funded by Indiana University Research through the Faculty Grant-in-Aid Program. We also thank Bridgette, Jesse, Lexi, and Mia for all their support. Most of all, we would like to thank the people all over the world who came forward during the darkest days of the pandemic to make life just a little bit easier, more creative, and less isolating for their communities. We hope this volume documents even just a part of the power of the vernacular that helped us all get through some very challenging times.

Behind the Mask

Introduction

Ben Bridges, Ross Brillhart, and Diane E. Goldstein

YOU COULD ONLY DESCRIBE HALLOWEEN 2020 IN THE United States as strange. In Indianapolis, parents drove their children past the jail downtown where deputies wearing gloves handed out sanitized candy packages to kids in costumes who remained locked in cars, looking on at the waving officers. Just Born Quality Confections in Pennsylvania, which makes "peeps," the popular Halloween marshmallow treats that come in the shape of birds and ghosts, suspended production until it could put protocols in place to protect employees. The Centers for Disease Control recommended avoiding high-risk activities—no traditional trick-or-treating, no hayrides, no haunted house walks. Thirty-seven states in 2020 canceled Halloween events. And where there was Halloween dress-up, in addition to the ever-present princess costumes and characters from movies, some of the most popular costumes of 2020 were frontline healthcare workers, Dr. Anthony Fauci—lead scientist on the Whitehouse Coronavirus Task Force—and the anachronistic long-beaked, heavily costumed plague doctor. All of them were masked. Halloween is one of the very few places where masks don't bother us. Normally a special association with costume and carnival, masks for us have generally been "othered"—we associate them with global diseases affecting countries halfway around the world, with the work of surgeons and other medical professionals, or with crime and violence. But in 2020 we were asked to own them, to protect ourselves and the world around us by donning a mask.

The iconic heavily masked plague doctor traces back to 1619. The costume was first described by Charles de Lorme, who served as the royal physician to King Louis XIII of France. Plague doctors were sometimes physicians, but just as frequently they were laypeople who treated patients at a time when there were no antibiotics and only a very basic concept of immunity. They treated plague patients with leeches and cupping and herbs, but they more often laid out the dead, witnessed wills, kept track of deaths, and performed body removals. The plague doctors' costume consisted of a waxed ankle-length overcoat, gloves, boots, a wide-brimmed hat,

https://doi.org/10.7330/9781646424818.c000

and a wooden walking stick used to examine patients without getting too close—it was a sort of seventeenth-century hazmat suit. The truly notable part of the uniform was the mask, which was tight fitting and birdlike, with glass eyes and a long beak with slits or holes on either side. The beak, which startled everyone, measured at least six inches long and contained a chamber for herbs, flowers or other aromatics, or vinegar-soaked sponges. It was thought to prevent the wearer from suffering *miasmas* from breathing diseased air.

Writing about pranksters dressed as plague doctors in England in May 2020, Greg Kelley (2020) argues:

> I would submit that by donning the garb of plague doctors who centuries before tended to victims of the pestilence, these pranksters are, in a sense, staging a legendary past in the present. This is performed anachronism, and the plague doctor *habiliment* brings with it a cluster of associations of the bad old days before vaccines and germ theory—associations that, although outdated, feel uncannily relevant to the contemporary circumstances of the COVID-19 pandemic. Pointing the way for us, these present-day pranksters conjure and embody a complex of age-old legends around early modern medical procedures, folk curatives and prophylactics, mysterious immunities, and eerily preternatural practitioners. (48–49)

Kelley ends by noting, "In reality, the plague doctor's protective gear, for all its orphic allure . . . had little preventative effect during the great plagues in Europe. But the mythos around them was persistent, providing perhaps some thread of hope amid dreadful circumstances" (66).

If we jump forward a few centuries to the Spanish flu of 1918, masks again appear, this time closer to the cloth or paper surgical mask to which we are now accustomed, sometimes recommended or even legislated for the general population. Just as today, there was mask resistance. Some people snipped holes in their masks to smoke cigars. Others argued they were symbols of government overreach. There were fines and jail terms and fights, people who hung the mask around their necks, and there was even—in parts of the US—an anti-mask league. Suffragettes felt the masks hurt their necessary visibility and barbers complained of lost business. Masks were multivocal and multivalent, as were the pandemics that initiated their use.

Really understanding the terrifying image of the plague doctor or the complicated Spanish flu mask fights meant seeing behind the mask to the vernacular understandings and meanings invoked there. How were people living in the face of a pandemic? What were they really doing to keep themselves healthy or to treat themselves if sick? How were they finding supplies?

What were they talking about and how were they passing pandemic time? With both the plague and the Spanish flu, we actually know very little about the vernacular responses of regular people. Now, with COVID-19, we offer a look behind the mask at the vernacular culture affected or inspired by this pandemic.

COVID VERNACULARS

Arising initially out of a coronavirus interest group at Indiana University, this volume explores the nature and shape of vernacular responses to the public health crisis. Although the current volume originates from this core group, we have branched out to include folklorists and other scholars from the US and Western Europe. While this group is more expansive than our original base, we recognize our inability to provide a global view. Nevertheless, we have tried where possible to place observations and discussions in conversation with other vernaculars internationally. For the purposes of this collection, we define the vernacular as a broad category of local knowledge production and action that is reflective of a particular group or region and focused on community-based forms of expression. As Margaret Lantis (1960) notes, the vernacular is "culture as-it-is-lived appropriate to well-defined places and situations" (203). Based on Leonard Primiano's work, we also highlight in the vernacular the "personal, aesthetic, cultural, and social investment [of an individual] . . . as well as the way individuals privately and creatively adapt [culture] to their specific life needs" (1995, 43). As such, vernacular culture can be flexible, dynamic, multi-sourced, and global.

While vernacular culture may or may not run against the grain of prevailing discourses—incorporating concepts and ideological content derivative of hegemonic forms; borrowing, appropriating, or commodifying—it makes its fullest sense out of the cultural context in which it arises. Despite its potential nod to dominant or external culture, it is its strong connection to the local that helps ground the vernacular within the experiential context that it occupies. Locked down in our homes and separated from the normal ebb and flow of life, our experience of COVID-19 highlights community and creativity, adaptation and flexibility, traditional knowledge, emergence, resistance, and dynamism. In its removal from assumed norms and dailiness, the pandemic provides a moment of insight into the nature of vernacular culture as it is used, abused, celebrated, critiqued, and discarded. It is this insight that our volume documents, ranging from bread competitions and sidewalk chalk rainbows to the exacerbation of racism and economic precarity caused or suggested by COVID.

Three themes crisscross through contributions to this volume despite the individual focus of each chapter on different COVID-related issues and practices.

The Vernacular to the Rescue: Community, Creativity, and Coping with COVID-19. In section I of this volume, we investigate the ways in which individuals and communities have used the vernacular to deal with the public health crisis as some found themselves suddenly experiencing strains on budget and supply chains, sheltering in place with inadequate resources, or missing community connections. As is so often the case, people found creative means of coping with the challenges presented to communities through vernacular culture. Within this context we explore vernacular creativity, including such topics as scavenger hunts, the creation of vernacular education opportunities for children, COVID cooking, sustainable living, and folk artistry.

The Failure of Experts and the Rise of Vernacular Expertise. In section II of this volume, we explore the places where governmental and organizational cultures were unwilling or unable to adequately address concerns of different groups. Our interest here is not only in the failure of experts within these contexts but also in the way vernacular culture expanded to fill the needs of communities. Within this context, COVID-19 existed alongside social justice issues including Black Lives Matter, a contentious election, the events of January 6, 2021, product shortages, and economic challenges. The pandemic did not happen in a vacuum; it dovetails with a variety of other social and political phenomena. We discuss lay health theories, the creation of rumor and conspiracy theory to fill the information vacuum, and local responses to xenophobia and hate.

When Vernaculars Meet. In the third section, we address how the rules that evolved in the face of the pandemic suggest numerous areas of incongruity. The term *social*, for example, would appear inconsistent with "social distancing." Likewise, masks, which have traditionally been markers of chaos and crime (within the US context), are meant to acquire meanings of safety and trust. *Home* typically suggests comfort and warmth, but this was not necessarily the case for those following "stay-at-home orders"—some found themselves shut in or shut out of desired contexts, such as individuals experiencing homelessness or people experiencing domestic abuse. In this section we explore emergent notions of community, understanding that the dynamic of the pandemic requires exploring preexisting and emergent vernacular forms.

For many of us, COVID-19 and its changing dynamics have made our experience feel as though we have recently lived through three or four epidemics, not one. Quarantining our mail and groceries, searching for toilet paper and diapers, baking banana bread, and participating in scavenger hunts to find slogans or symbols left out for neighbors to see—these activities seem to have occurred years ago, and yet just yesterday. The events of the pandemic seem to have operated outside of time, in a unique dimension—in what we might want to refer to as "COVID time." The corona crisis has shaken up our rhythms with work, childcare, schooling, eating, and sleeping, all of which seem to have been rearranged. Curfews and lockdowns have affected our natural patterns, social time has broken down, and past, present, and future feel like they have become confused. Clear separations between work and time at home are challenged. Days and weeks are disordered, even indistinguishable.

As German memory scholar Astrid Erll noted after asking what COVID-19 has done to time, the "new rhythms of everyday life may almost seem medieval, pointing back to a time when workplace (the bakery, the pottery, the blacksmith's forge) was part of the home, and working rhythms were weaved together with domestic rhythms" (2020, 862). While the rapidity of the spread of the virus is mind-boggling, for some, the slowness of COVID time was a relief from our otherwise accelerated lives—like a school snow day for children or a sick day off work. Of course, for physicians, medical researchers, and caregivers, as they strain under the burden of rising cases and unimaginable death rates, the reverse is true: COVID time is a speeding train, threatening at any moment to go off its rails. An existential puzzle extraordinaire, COVID is both a digital marvel—moving information, interventions, and science rapidly across the world and providing in digital social media new and better ways to pretend we are together (see Brooke, this volume)—and yet at the same time it is an almost old-fashioned return to ways of coming together in vernacular practices like baking and singing across balconies (see Eriksen and Kverndokk; Inserra, this volume). And lest we lean too far into romanticizing COVID time, countries responded differently to the COVID experience, based on the nearness in recent memory of other related traumas, such as the epidemic of Ebola in West Africa, wildfires in Australia, Brexit in the United Kingdom, or the rise of authoritarian governance and threats to democracy in the United States, Brazil, Hungary, and elsewhere. Our concerns about the slowness and speed of time were completely intertwined with our fear of and desire for change.

This simultaneous break in and coexistence of temporal experience compelled a sort of liminality throughout the pandemic, a variable van Gennepian period of social limbo.[1] However, people did not initially intend to engage in any sort of ritual reemergence or reidentification. The resulting moments of "betwixt and between" often seemed to move at a molasses-like pace because we were compelled to exist temporally between the timelines of pre-pandemic status quo and the eventuality of a "new normal." The progress of science, medicine, and the vernacular was swift, perhaps faster than many people had previously experienced. However, the new normal many strove to find connoted a new system, a new whole, some sort of finality. The slowness of COVID time, then, was perhaps experienced, and felt, in light of that daunting task of a reintegration, or incorporation, that was widely contested. This light at the end of the tunnel barely flickered as people and their communities around the globe constructed ways to understand this different experience of time and sociality. The once-normal bustle of everyday life was replicated by some in the realm of the online; however, others found that embodied being and the collapsing of social space could be understood, or could become more familiar, in the words and practices of previous generations, what many imagine as "simpler times" that, perhaps, also moved slowly. And so, we should not be surprised that COVID time over the two plus years of the pandemic seems to require the rehearsal of a timeline to remind us of where we are and where we have been.

DAYS LIKE NO OTHER

December 1, 2019 was, for many of us, a day like any other. We went about our business, attended school or work, stopped at the gym, the post office, the grocery store, or a friend's house on our way home, ate a quick dinner, and then perhaps went out again. Little did we know that a few months later all of that would become impossible.

On January 9, 2020, the World Health Organization announced a mysterious coronavirus pneumonia reported from Wuhan, China. By January 21, the Centers for Disease Control confirmed the first American case of the novel coronavirus, diagnosed in a Washington State resident who had returned one week earlier from a trip to Wuhan (Centers for Disease Control and Prevention 2020). Europe began to face several major outbreaks by the end of February, beginning in Italy, and the first Latin American case was reported that same month. On March 11, the World Health Organization declared COVID-19 a pandemic. In the United States later that week, California became the first state to issue a stay-at-home order mandating that all residents remain in their dwellings, venturing out only to engage in essential tasks. As hospitals became overwhelmed and case numbers skyrocketed, more and more states followed suit, suggesting or mandating that their residents stay home. By the end of March, most of the United States was in lockdown and gatherings of all kinds were canceled or moved online, including weddings, parades, and conferences. There was a run on grocery stores, which quickly sold out of hand sanitizer, detergents and, inexplicably, toilet paper. Public health officials stressed the need for mask wearing and "social distancing" at the same time as there was a nationwide shortage of personal protective equipment (PPE) needed by healthcare workers. Countries around the world sealed their borders, sports teams canceled their seasons, schools closed, and employees increasingly were laid off or instructed to work from home. By April 2, more than 1 million people in 171 countries across six continents had gotten COVID and fifty-one thousand deaths had been reported. By May 28, the CDC reported US deaths in excess of one hundred thousand, and by November 8, the number of US cases surpassed 10 million (AJMC Staff, 2021). At the end of December 2020, cumulative global numbers stood at 79 million reported cases, with 1.7 million deaths (World Health Organization 2020), and by March 1, 2022, the virus had infected almost 390 million people worldwide and deaths had reached 5.96 million (Ritchie et al. 2022). The most severely affected countries included the US, India, Brazil, Russia, and the United Kingdom (Taylor 2021).

In December 2020, the FDA granted emergency use authorization to Pfizer and Moderna, indicating that both mRNA two-dose vaccines were shown to be safe and effective against COVID-19. The Johnson and Johnson single-shot vaccine was approved in February. By the end of December, the UK approved emergency authorization for the AstraZeneca and Oxford AZD1222 vaccines. As the year closed, the approved vaccines started to roll out, first to healthcare providers and first responders, then to the elderly and the immunocompromised, and finally to the general population. China, Brazil, India, and Russia were producing and manufacturing vaccines at scale, and by June 30, 2021, more than a dozen vaccines had been approved around the world. Residents of the US, Europe, Canada, and a few other wealthy countries had access to a vaccine, while those who lived in lower-income countries, particularly in sub-Saharan Africa, would likely have to wait until 2023. Later in summer 2021, more than 3 billion doses of vaccines had been administered worldwide. Several countries, including Bahrain, Israel, and the United States, had made significant progress in immunizing their citizens. Other countries had no access to vaccines and had yet to start. By the end of summer 2021, as the Delta variant continued to rapidly spread, only 1 percent of Africans had been immunized. Today, as finances, logistics, and politics affect global access to the vaccines, COVID-19 continues to mutate, with scientists anxiously watching new variants emerge wherever the spread of infection has not been significantly curtailed (Taylor 2021; Terry 2021). In November 2021 a new variant, Omicron, was discovered, which had far greater transmissibility, creating a new significant wave of infections in the months that followed.

Politics and economics always play a critical role in health policy and care. Healthcare is gendered and racialized, different for the poor, the marginalized, and the isolated than it is for those who inhabit spaces of dominance. Minorities and the poor were particularly affected by COVID-19, experiencing discrimination in access and service availability; disproportionate representation in occupations and geographical areas with greater exposure to COVID; educational, income, and wealth inequalities; and housing conditions that rendered prevention strategies more difficult to implement (Bonotti and Zech 2021, 3). Rising unemployment, food insecurity, a housing crisis, overfull hospitals, and diminished access to services all were byproducts of the pandemic and lockdown, which aggravated preexisting inequities. Food lines were long, eviction notices became plentiful, and lack of childcare and transportation made work impossible even for those whose places of employment were open. Lockdowns exaggerated the situations of those who were housing insecure, those who faced heat shortages, and those who shared their homes with domestic abusers. A shortage of PPE—including masks and gloves—placed caregivers in danger, made factories petri dishes for closely placed workers, and added to the isolation and loneliness of the elderly or vulnerable.

Throughout the pandemic, social distancing and more time at home compelled by lockdowns and community expectations resulted in a meteoric rise of media consumption, particularly in places where such was already commonplace. Media—social, news, fake, mainstream, online, radio, streaming, videos, signs, discussion boards, games—solidified its existence as a buzzword and, for some, a way of extending and negotiating one's identity and continuing with life. During our collective pandemicking, the role of the virtual and of media in general cannot be overstated, and some contributors in this volume thoroughly explain some of the particularities of people's interactions, understandings, and negotiations with it (see Graper; Brooke; Inserra). On a larger scale, according to a Nielsen report examining media consumption during the early stages of the pandemic (spring 2020), the amount of time television was consumed (in multiple formats, including streaming) went up nearly 75 percent in this quarter alone (Adgate 2020). Similar trends can be seen across various spectrums of media, including an over 50 percent rise in hours watched on the popular platform Twitch.tv.[2] It is intuitive that, given the nature of the initial lockdowns and uncertainty compelled by a global pandemic, many would turn to their televisions and various media outlets to stay up to date with events and even stay in touch with their communities, while others searched for new forms of entertainment.

According to the same Nielsen report, some respondents even described their radio programming as their "comfort food." Juxtaposing the molasses-like tempo of "COVID time" detailed above, the ability of the internet and media to "small up" the world at a pre-pandemic pace was profound, as new identities were formed and ideologies were negotiated, constructed, and spread between disparate geographies. On the one hand, media was one avenue by which people could continue to form and interact with community. Social media platforms such as Facebook and Instagram provided sites for imagined and once-embodied communities to share their efforts and creativity amid lockdowns and social distancing, among other things, while other platforms such as Zoom and Teams gained widespread acceptance as alternatives to the socially embodied, brick-and-mortar workplace. On the other hand, and certainly not completely separated, media in all forms was used to attempt to understand the pandemic. This can be seen and heard in the politicization of pandemic performances and practices, which were swiftly negotiated via social media and disseminated through multiple channels, including "news" organizations both online and on television (see Bock; Graper, this volume).

But the COVID-19 picture was also interwoven with and complicated by a series of ongoing political and social issues in the United States and globally. As the pandemic spread, the Trump administration continually underestimated, minimized, misunderstood, and ignored the nature of the threat presented by COVID-19; damaged efforts to prepare for testing, treatment, and prevention; sabotaged work to slow the spread of the disease and to speed care; engaged in disinformation and the stigmatization of groups and individuals; and diminished the importance of mask wearing and social distancing. These actions continually politicized the virus, most particularly as it related to mask wearing and ultimately vaccine use—themes that became central to a partisan fight—with anti-mask, anti–social distancing and anti-vaccination positions becoming the stance of many lawmakers and politicians on the right (see Kitta, this volume). Outside of the United States, the same politicization was reflected in the COVID attitudes and policies of populist right-wing leaders including, among others, British prime minister Boris Johnson and president of Brazil Jair Bolsonaro. Not only in the US but globally, COVID-19 became entangled with right-wing agendas, especially in terms of anti-immigration sentiment, anti-China sentiment, and technophobic conspiracy theories.[3]

While COVID-19 raged, other cultural issues and moments of import swirled around the pandemic in the United States (and elsewhere), making the situation even more complicated. In the background to the anti-mask, anti-distancing, anti-vax movements, numerous political campaigns were underway, including a contentious battle for president of the United States that ultimately came down to a contest between incumbent Republican Donald Trump and Democrat Joseph Biden. Due to the pandemic, new, untried campaign events and tactics occurred daily, testing the limits of safeguards between political activities and prohibitions on using the White House or the executive branch for political purposes (prohibited by the Hatch Act.)[4] The pandemic also tested the limitations on the use of video and other technology to replace campaign events, even the Republican and Democratic National Conventions. In an effort to allow socially distanced voting, numerous states tried to ease the burden at the polls by instituting mail-in voting, drop boxes, drive-through polls, early voting, and longer polling location hours. These efforts (particularly mail-in voting) created a GOP backlash alleging election fraud and ultimately leading to a Stop the Steal campaign instituted by Trump and his followers. That campaign resulted in the so-called insurrection—on January 6, 2021, a mob of Trump supporters attacked the United States Capitol in an attempt to disrupt the counting of electoral votes that would formalize Joe Biden's win in the 2020 presidential election. On January 13, 2021, one week before his term expired, Donald Trump was impeached (for a second time) for "incitement of insurrection."

Sometimes referred to as the double pandemic, COVID-19 also intersected with a wave of anti-Black and anti-Asian racism and antisemitism in 2020 and 2021. While notions of the "Chinese virus" stoked anti-Asian and anti-immigrant tensions that had been simmering just under the surface, public health closures, mask mandates, and eventual vaccine mandates incited white nationalists to protest the infringement of American "civil liberties." White supremacists and nationalist extremists saw COVID-19 as an opportunity to push their agenda and recruit, spreading pandemic disinformation and promoting their ideas on social media to inspire and fuel protests around the country. Extremists dismissed COVID as a hoax, a result of Jewish-run conspiracies, or a disease spread by immigrants.

While white supremacy flourished in response to COVID, so too did social justice movements such as Stop Asian Hate and Black Lives Matter.[5] One of the most significant intersections with our experience of COVID-19 was a contemporaneous societal reckoning with police brutality against people of color in the United States (and elsewhere) as well as a response to the structural violence that limits the opportunities of Black and Brown communities and causes health disparities. The murder of George Floyd at the hands of white Minneapolis police officers on May 25, 2020 reenergized the Black Lives Matter movement, which began in 2013 after the acquittal of George Zimmerman in the shooting death of Trayvon Martin. During 2020, an estimated 15 to 26 million people participated in Black Lives Matter protests in the United States, making it one of the largest political movements in US history (Buchanan et al. 2020). Activists around the world also engaged in Black Lives Matter efforts to reform global Black discrimination, marginalization, and state violence in their respective countries. COVID-19 intersected with BLM in multiple ways, creating large social protest gatherings that challenged public health measures known to exacerbate inequities (including increased unemployment and financial inequity experienced through pandemic-related job losses and economic threats), amplify health disparities through higher rates of COVID infection and death in Black communities, and induce a resurgence of historical mistrust of medical research and care stemming from both the abuse of Black bodies in Tuskegee-like experiments throughout American history as well as maltreatment in healthcare settings and situations. COVID-19 amplified virtually every social and political issue facing the population.

The pandemic also amplified the performance and understanding of "health" broadly understood. Almost overnight, people across the globe were compelled to renegotiate how they participated and performed in their worlds with a new awareness of the ramifications for those around them. Before the pandemic, one could have thought of health in many cases as a silo of practice, or a practice that silos particular spaces, performances, practitioners, and ideologies, among other things (even if this was not actually the case then). However, the pandemic shone a light on the ubiquity of health and the far-reaching effects that its recognition can have on our lives. The customary embodied practice of a handshake, for example, was immediately utilized as a model for unhealthy behavior—a compromise of social distancing. A common form of social networking emerged in the form of "bubbles" or "pods," a creative adaptation to interactional restrictions in which small groups of individuals agreed to limit in-person contact exclusively to one another. With the assumption that everyone committed to an identical social bubble, all participants would presumably remain healthy or—if an infection were to occur—limit its spread to a single network of people. Such methods were even promoted as part of lockdown exit strategies in the UK, New Zealand, and Germany (Leng et al. 2020). Yet for many, such circles were more imagined networks of exclusivity than rigorous health code abidance (Gutman 2020). Differing social expectations and perceptions of COVID could be enough to burst a bubble, leaving individuals left to negotiate new means of maintaining relationships in pandemic contexts. While the global ubiquity of a particular strain of health behavior is fairly unprecedented in living experience, the ways that health is amplified and creatively expressed in response to the unknown, the social, and the political is hardly novel and can thus be traced through other pandemics, epidemics, and crises.

SPIT SPREADS DEATH: REMEMBERING (AND FORGETTING) PANDEMICS

As we struggle to reflect on or even remember the absurdity of the timeline we have just lived through and are still experiencing, numerous authors have inspired a revitalization of reflections on that other devastating flu, the Spanish flu of 1918–19, caused by the H1N1 influenza A virus. It is believed that the 1918 pandemic killed between 50 million and 100 million people, representing 5 percent of the world's population at the time, and possibly exceeding the death toll of both world wars. Half a billion people were infected. Although it has been referred to as "the greatest disaster of the twentieth century, possibly any century" (Spinney 2018, 171) and "the mother of all pandemics" (Erll 2020, 864), there is, oddly, very little information about the Spanish flu that has survived the century since its ravages. Historian Guy Beiner notes: "Considering the sheer magnitude of the phenomenon, there is a relatively slim body of literature on the topic, a dearth which stands out in comparison to the voluminous historiography on the First World War. Overall, the Great Flu remains a remarkably under-studied field in modern history" (2006, 503). According to Beiner, it took eighty years until the first conference on the subject was convened, in Cape Town, and no cultural history of the pandemic has been written to date (503). Erll observes, "There are no major contemporaneous (or later) memoirs, paintings, novels, or films dedicated to the Spanish Flu" (865). And to date, there are no monuments or memorials to the pandemic. Beiner and others call the 1918 flu the "forgotten pandemic," and Pete Davies (1999) refers to it as the "forgotten Tragedy." COVID has created a new wave of Spanish flu historiography, as well as new fiction, film, and museum exhibitions reflecting back on the 1918 influenza pandemic.

The suggested reasons for the "collective forgetting" associated with the 1918 flu are multiple, and perhaps all the suggestions have some merit.[6] Beiner posits that it was difficult to associate meaning with an illness that came so fast and killed so quickly, extensively, and incomprehensively. "In all patterns of remembrance," he argues, "what matters is that individuals acted in certain ways to the past—that they had choices . . . For many, such was the fate of the influenza pandemic of 1918–19, one of those moments difficult to fit into narratives of meaning . . . Out of social agency," says Beiner, "out of mind" (2021, xxvi). Erll argues that there was a question of the discreteness of historical events, that the flu was deeply entangled with other rampant illnesses, war, and other entrenched events (2020, 865). Ryan Davis (2013) argues that the mundaneness of the notion of "flu" worked against it being marked or remembered—that there was a certain embarrassment about something as simple as the flu having such an effect. Erll appears to agree, writing that the flu "lacked tellability: Harrowing as they were, flu deaths were less tellable (i.e.: less noteworthy, they had less of a 'point') than stories of heroic deaths on the battlefields of the First World War" (865). And yet there are areas where extant information on the pandemic *can* be found—including the reconfiguration of the virological and genomic data preserved from the illness, traces of information depicted in the arts, and what remains in family history and in the attics and garages of later generations (Beiner 2006).

One wonders what from the Great Flu might have been useful to our current experience had we greater access to those memories. What might we have come to understand about quarantines or masking or resistances? Stories of epidemics do not only describe illnesses, they also create illness realities.[7] While Beiner highlights for us the residual information that the arts or family history might have provided about the 1918 epidemic, the suggested usefulness of both of these categories of information stands as a reminder of the ways that vernacular forms encode experience and memory for the future.

It is worthwhile to think about pandemic memory as embodied—not just in the sense of the ways the disease itself interfered with bodily function, but in terms of how we all experienced the pandemic through our bodies. What did it mean to have and be a body during COVID? How did our bodies work together while not in physical proximity? How did we co-create socially distant space? How did smell, sound, or sight change in bustling spaces that were now empty? How did "the inactivity and immobility of doing nothing, do something?" (Vallee, 2020). Such stillness induced a sense of stagnation or even tranquility for some people, but it also compelled many others into creative action.

COVID CREATIVITY AND PANDEMIC *BRICOLEURS*

It is Friday afternoon at Linda's house. She is going through old fabric scraps looking for ones that might make suitable masks. Her husband is at the bar they own, which is closed down, all the employees furloughed.

He's trying to learn how to make hand sanitizer out of the alcohol on the bar shelves. Linda's two children are online finding clues that will help them later during the family walk as they locate painted and molded unicorns hidden by their neighbors, who created scavenger hunts to entertain the families confined to home. Linda and her husband, and even their children, have become pandemic *bricoleurs*, applying combinations of the resources at hand to solve the new problems created by COVID.[8]

Locked down in our homes, with public gatherings prohibited, businesses and schools closed, restricted access to stores and restaurants, and with museums, theaters, and sporting events curtailed, we were all forced to turn to forms of work, creativity, and social interaction that were different from our regular norms of production and entertainment. Whether exercised to cope with, escape from, think through, or endure the hardships wrought by COVID, the revived and introduced traditions served as tools for living through the pandemic.

The creative forms prompted by or produced during COVID performed a variety of functions, ranging from personal protection to means of social engagement. Homemade hazmat suits and face masks modeled vernacular interpretations of medical advice, as did the balloon hats that comically extended in six-foot circles to promote social distancing. Graduations and birthday parties happened from the comfort of one's own car, and friends could congregate around their own computers for a synchronized watch party of shows and movies. Domestic artistic traditions, such as baking, gardening, or sewing, surged in households as individuals preoccupied themselves with indoor activities. Board and video game sales spiked in 2020 for similar reasons (Wannigamage et al. 2020), and daily walks became regular rituals for folks seeking to get outside (Anderson 2020). Even museums and galleries became available to visit virtually, with content becoming readily and often freely accessible to spectators (King et al. 2021).

The renewed investment in artistic creativity, coupled with public health concerns and access to online shopping, spurred a demand economy for homemade masks and other art, which was readily supplied by artists using virtual storefronts such as Etsy, Shopify, and Instagram. Although more than 12 million masks had been sold on Etsy by April 2020, mask sales ultimately accounted for only 10 percent of gross merchandise sold on the platform during its highly successful year, indicating a proliferation in homemade art sales overall during COVID (Richter 2020). Blogs and videos of DIY mask making emerged for those who wanted to try the craft at home, as did resources for home construction and landscaping projects. Instagram's Checkout feature, rolled out a year earlier, catalyzed the art-making and selling capabilities for many artists during COVID, too. With an invigorated public interest in buying from Black- and Indigenous-owned businesses on the heels of the aforementioned social movements, marketplaces dedicated to such companies and individuals sprung up, such as From the People, Collective49, and Miiriya.

People also sought ways to connect with others outside the home while working within the recommended or enforced restrictions imposed on social interactions. "Zoom" entered the lexicon of computer owners, the video networking software quickly becoming a verb among colleagues, friends, and family members who wanted to chat with each other remotely. Many neighborhoods started scavenger hunts or sidewalk chalk galleries that allowed adults and children alike to interact with their neighbors from safe distances (Anderson 2020). Some people entered trade networks with friends, taking turns shopping for groceries or running errands, thus limiting cumulative public interaction. Workers rearranged their living rooms into offices, students into classrooms, and musicians into concert halls to accommodate the online space, some even turning to virtual backgrounds to be simultaneously at and away from home.

Many people assumed the bricoleur role that Linda and her family aptly embodied. The creative manipulation of materials found at home, online, and in socially distanced public spaces allowed people to express themselves and connect with others while operating within appropriate public health guidelines. For these bricoleurs, COVID presented an opportunity to kindle relationships with close friends and family through shared adaptations to imposed limits. Even strangers could build upon one another's creations in collective settings, such as collaborative chalk murals or TikTok memes, akin to Lynne McNeill's (2007) concept of serial collaboration. Notwithstanding the hardships wrought by COVID, the defining characteristics of 2020—lockdowns and social distancing—often fueled moments of artistic creation and community building that helped many people navigate through the pandemic's troubling times (see Geist et al.; Long and Vaughan, this volume).

STORIES LIKE SO MANY OTHERS

In his book *An Epidemic of Rumors: How Stories Shape Our Perception of Disease*, Jon D. Lee wrote:

> In 2003, for a frantic few months, a virus assaulted humanity with a fury that seemed apocalyptic. This novel disease came from China but quickly

slipped that country's boundaries to bound halfway around the world in a matter of hours. Its speed left doctors and researchers gasping in the wake, struggling to erect walls both physical and intellectual against the onslaught. But their reactions were nothing compared to the fear that gripped the nations of the world as they suddenly confronted a strange, invisible, and unexplained foe that killed one out of every five people it touched. Panic ensued. Thousands of people were involuntarily quarantined. Thousands more simply chose to stay home rather than risk catching the new virus from a coworker or stranger. The tourism industry ground to a halt. Airlines, theaters, restaurants, hotels, and other businesses showed record losses. Chinatowns all over North America virtually emptied. And people were dying, not only laypersons, but doctors and nurses too, cut down by the very disease they were struggling to understand . . . And then almost as suddenly as it had arrived, the virus disappeared. (2014, 4–5)

Although this description refers to the 2003 SARS epidemic, Lee continues: "Change the date to 2009, the word China to Mexico, and the name of the disease from SARS to H1N1, and with little further effort we have a new etiological narrative that still proves surprisingly accurate in describing the H1N1 pandemic. With just a few more changes, we could have a series of paragraphs describing the origins of avian flu, Ebola or AIDS" (5). Lee's focus is on the narratives in circulation at the time pertaining to SARS, but, he argues, "These same processes—akin to using a word processor's find and replace tool on a series of oral narratives, are the very ones that appear over and over in actual disease epidemics." Indeed, the narratives that arose during the SARS epidemic resembled those that emerged during Ebola, the H1N1 epidemic, and the AIDS epidemic.

Shortly after the beginning of the COVID-19 pandemic in 2020, COVID-19 started to be referred to by some (including then President Trump) as the China or Wuhan virus. The adoption of a disease nickname associated with a country or a group of people is, of course, not uncommon. In fact, in May 2015, the World Health Organization (WHO) issued a policy paper on the best practices for the naming of new human infectious diseases, suggesting that diseases *not* be named after geographic locations (cities, countries, regions, or continents); people's names; species or class of animal or food; cultural, population, industry, or occupational references; or terms that incite undue fear (World Health Organization 2015). The tendency to resort to disease name-calling, however, runs throughout history. The 1918 flu epidemic popularly known as the "the Spanish flu" most likely did not originate in Spain. In Spain it was referred to as "the French flu," in Brazil it was the "German Flu," in Poland it was called "the Bolshevik disease," and in Senegal it was "the Brazilian Flu" (Cohut 2020). It is not new to name a disease after a political opponent, nor is it new to associate the disease with beliefs about germ warfare. Throughout Europe, the Spanish flu was linked in the newspapers to German sub boats that were said to have brought the disease to the shores of Spain. In the US, the story spread that a camouflaged German ship infiltrated Boston Harbor and "released the germs that seeded the city" (Aderet 2020). In 2020, the story began to spread that the coronavirus was a genetically engineered bioweapon that escaped from a high-level lab in Wuhan, China. Chinese officials at the same time claimed that the US Army had introduced the virus to China. Matteo Salvini, the leader of Italy's anti-migrant League Party, contended that the outbreak of the virus was a result of the Chinese deliberately cultivating a "lung supervirus" from "bats and rats" (see Graper, this volume). And on social media, people shared speculations that Bill Gates, on behalf of Big Pharma, was behind the emergence of COVID-19. As the coronavirus became a global pandemic and posed a major challenge to health systems, numerous rumors, stories, and hoaxes spread regarding causes, transmission, prevention, and cures of the disease.

Rumors included suggestions that wearing masks will make you sick; that COVID is transmitted through 5G networks; that the vaccines contain a microchip designed to track your movements; that certain foods and drink were effective against COVID, including lukewarm water, alcohol, onion, ginger, sea lettuce, and bleach; and that one should avoid spicy foods and drink cows' urine. Other rumors suggested it was unsafe to receive packages from China, that you could get COVID from eating in Chinese restaurants, and that the origin of COVID was Chinese people eating bat soup. There were stories of numerous individuals who were deliberate infectors, such as those who spat or coughed on produce in the grocery store (see Bock, this volume) or "superspreaders," such as the woman in Korea referred to as Patient 31 who was believed to have infected thirty-seven people.

Such rumors are not without consequence. Stories, for example, that indicated hand sanitizer could protect those who drank it from contracting COVID resulted in 5,900 hospitalizations, eight hundred deaths, and sixty cases of blindness (Doheny 2020). But these rumors and narratives are neither new, unpredictable, nor surprising. A look at the recycled stories of epidemics demonstrates the patterns that stories of disease replicate and how they illustrate lay perceptions of risk.

Although legend analysis demands that we recognize changes in narratives over time and space, legend scholars have simultaneously paid attention to historical consistencies in narrative plots and motifs, sometimes tracing them back hundreds of years. The repetition of narratives that have remained culturally viable and that resurface—albeit in new clothing—centuries later underscores the cyclical nature of cultural attitudes and the centrality of narrative articulations of pervasive concerns. Although HIV/AIDS, for example, was a relatively new disease, its legends were often reformulations of narratives that circulated in response to smallpox, leprosy, bubonic plague, syphilis, and numerous other historical epidemics. The precursors of current popular health legends are bone-chilling in their suggestion that hundreds of years of modern medical advancements have made little difference in our gut reactions to illness and disease.

By way of example, one of the most widely disseminated and frequently told HIV/AIDS legends involves a man who meets a woman in a bar, takes her to a hotel or back to his apartment, and sleeps with her. In the morning when he wakes up, the woman is gone. He gets out of bed and walks into the bathroom, where he finds a message written on the mirror in lipstick: "Welcome to the World of AIDS." Often the narrative also contains a coda in the message: "I am going to die, and so are you." Daniel Defoe's *Journal of the Plague Year*, set in London in 1665, provides an early analogue to the "Welcome to the World of AIDS" narrative.

> A poor unhappy gentlewoman, a substantial citizen's wife, was (if the story be true) murdered by one of these creatures in Aldersgate Street, or that way. He was going along the street, raving mad, to be sure, and singing; the people only said he was drunk, but he himself said he had the plague upon him, which, it seems, was true; and meeting this gentlewoman, he would kiss her. She was terribly frightened, as he was only a rude fellow, and she ran from him, but the street being very thin of people, there was nobody near enough to help her. When she saw he would overtake her, she turned and gave him a thrust so forcibly, he being but weak, and pushed him backward. But very unhappily, she being so near, he caught hold of her, and pulled her down also, and getting up first, mastered her, and kissed her; and which was worst of all, when he had done, told her he had the plague, and why should not she have it as well as he? (Smith 1990, 129–30)

There are numerous antecedents to the "Welcome to the World of AIDS" tale told about herpes, gonorrhea, and syphilis. The narratives share the notion of a deliberate infector who, upon finding out about his or her own condition, seeks revenge by transmitting the disease. The longevity of this narrative, continually resurfacing with new diseases and new health concerns, suggests the diachronic persistence of concepts such as the infected body as weapon, the personification of disease, and the evil contaminated "other" seeking revenge.

Over the last decade and a half, folklorists have come to refer to the "Welcome to the World of AIDS" story as "AIDS Mary" (or "AIDS Harry" when the antagonist is male). The reference alludes to the story of "Typhoid Mary," an Irish American cook who spread typhoid to some fifty people in the early 1900s (Brunvand 1989, 197). Typhoid Mary supposedly knew of her "carrier" status and yet continued to spread the disease for eight years after her discovery of the risk. Fast-forward to this century and we find a news story relating that Thomas Duncan, a man who came from West Africa to visit family, died of Ebola in a Dallas, Texas hospital in 2014. The headline, just one among many, notes a Typhoid Mary connection: "21st Century Typhoid Mary: Ebola Tom, the Liberian Medical Moocher, Traveled to US for First-World Healthcare." Numerous news stories have been printed discussing "COVID-19's Typhoid Mary or Patient Zero" (see, for example, Ahuja 2022). In March 2020, a single individual, dubbed "Patient 31," was blamed for a massive rise in South Korean cases of COVID (Kasulis 2020). Legal cases are just beginning to be prosecuted for deliberate transmission of COVID-19. In 2021, Christopher Charles Perez was sentenced to fifteen months in jail for posting on Facebook that he had paid someone with COVID to lick items at a grocery store in San Antonio (see O'Kane 2021). The stories go on, casting blame and creating scapegoats.

The 2014–15 outbreak of Ebola in Liberia, Sierra Leone, and Guinea created the same rumor panic we are accustomed to seeing in epidemics and highlights the traditional nature of epidemic legends and rumors. In Atlanta, following the transport of two patients from Liberia to Emory University hospital, there was a rumor of a massive outbreak of 145 cases in the city. Later in the fall, a Facebook rumor stated that seven Kansas third graders had been infected with Ebola by their substitute teacher, and in Wortham, Texas, seventeen kindergarteners were rumored to have contracted the disease from an exchange student. We heard that the US government had issued a travel advisory after a family of five in Texas had been diagnosed with the disease, that U2 singer Bono had contracted Ebola while caring for a man in Liberia, and that three workers in a Doritos factory had died of the disease. We heard that Ebola was airborne, that it could only be destroyed by nuclear warheads, that the US government was planning to build death camps to intern the millions of victims who were inevitably going to come down with the disease, that Ebola was a biowarfare weapon created by the US, that the iPhone 6 was contaminated by Ebola, that the US government was planning mandatory vaccination, and that the CDC had created Ebola and obtained a patent for it to profit from the development of a vaccine.

Much of this should sound familiar. The rumors address issues that surface in every epidemic—contamination, conspiracy, and stigma. Focusing more closely, we can divide many recycled epidemic legends and rumors up into topical areas that lend themselves to rumor and legend: contaminated food (see Graper, this volume), contaminated spaces, and contaminated people (see Kitta; Bock, this volume). The rumors address gulfs between medical and governmental institutions and the populace, topics of distrust of medicine, greed and Big Pharma, lack of transparency and communication, and medical inequities and incompetence—all red flags of lay concern (see Hiiemäe et al. 2021).

It is also clear that public health and the media are tradition bearers in the disease legendary process. They help mediate these narratives, providing a template for what becomes legend. What's more, public health creates epidemiological trajectories with interstitial gaps—in other words, spaces for legend to intervene. Contact tracing, just as an example, inadvertently personifies epidemics and creates a profile of the disease carrier, shaping public perceptions of vulnerability, rates of infection, and geographic and ethnic associations with a disease.[9] Further, the disease itself becomes a character, imbued with disregard for morality or borders. The notion of contaminated foods, spaces, and people, continually recycled in the narrative traditions of laypeople, the media, and public health, makes it clear that the vernacular, popular, and scientific constructions of disease all fall predictably along the lines of home and away, familiar and foreign, civilized and uncivilized, moral and immoral.

CONSPIRACY NARRATIVES AND CONSPIRACY THINKING

Over the weekend of January 22–23, 2022, flyers linking Jewish government officials to COVID were left on the doorstep of hundreds of homes in Miami Beach. The flyers featured a Jewish Star, a pentagram, and the names of fourteen people working for the CDC, the Department of Health and Human Services, and vaccine companies Pfizer and Moderna. At the top of the flyer, it read, "Every single aspect of the COVID agenda is Jewish." The statement is just one in what has become a common conspiratorial linkage of the COVID virus with Judaism. During the COVID years, Jews were frequently blamed on far-right platforms for creating, causing, or spreading the virus. Common antisemitic COVID tropes include Jews developing the virus in a laboratory to create a "superelite designer world," Jews exploiting the virus to get rich, unsanitary Jews spreading the infection, Zionists developing a deadlier strain of the virus to use against Iran, and Jewish American democratic financier George Soros working with Big Pharma to spread the virus.

Such stories are not new. During the bubonic plague, Jews were accused of poisoning the wells, resulting in a massive massacre of the Jewish community. Antisemitic conspiracy narratives are recycled around the world with nearly every public health crisis. The classic motifs tend to be variations on two ideas—the "poisoning of gentiles" modern mutation of the blood libel story or the "Jews want to control the world" motif. Freeman et al. (2022), in a survey of coronavirus conspiracy beliefs in England, found that almost half of their 2,501 participants endorsed to some degree the idea that "coronavirus is a bioweapon developed by China to destroy the West" and around one-fifth endorsed to some degree the idea that Jews have created the virus to collapse the economy for financial gain.

While conspiracy theories evolve around every major disease, COVID-19 is arguably the most conspiracy-laden disease ever experienced. In the summer of 2020, the Pew Research Center found that 71 percent of Americans had heard the widely circulating conspiracy theory alleging that powerful people intentionally planned the coronavirus, and 25 percent believed the theory to be true (Schaeffer 2020). The YouGov-Cambridge Globalism Project, a survey of about twenty-six thousand people in twenty-five countries designed in collaboration with the *Guardian*, found widespread conspiracy-related skepticism concerning COVID. Among the most widespread of those theories was that COVID death rates had been deliberately and greatly exaggerated. Nearly 60 percent of respondents in Nigeria believed this to be true, along with 40 percent in Greece, South Africa, Poland, and Mexico and 38 percent of Hungarians, Italians, Germans, and Americans. Across nineteen different countries, 20 percent or more of respondents said they gave at least some credibility to the view that "the truth about the harmful effects of vaccines is being deliberately hidden from the public," including 57 percent of South Africans, 48 percent of Turks, 38 percent of French people, 33 percent of Americans, 31 percent of Germans, and 26 percent of Swedes (Henley and McIntyre 2020). A December 2020 NPR IPSOS poll found that more than one in three Americans believe in the existence of a "deep state" (Newall 2020).[10]

The extensive belief in COVID conspiracy theories is likely tied to a wave of disinformation from science deniers, the political/governmental manipulation of COVID information and efforts, and the general rise of social media (Shahsavari et al. 2020). Arising out of waves of politically centered disinformation and the fake news debates (see Mould 2018) centered in the Trump White House, COVID conspiracies found an easy niche.

Perhaps best understood as existing on a continuum of more extreme and less extreme conspiratorial beliefs, conspiracy theories can vary greatly. At the more extreme pole, some COVID conspiracy theories find their inspiration in QAnon, a conspiratorial group that emerged on October 28, 2017, on 4chan, an image-based anonymous internet bulletin board. With origins in the Pizzagate[11] conspiracy a year earlier, QAnon primarily held to the theory that President Trump was waging a secret war against a pedophilic ring of "deep-state" elites linked to the Democratic Party (see Bodner et al. 2021, 143–63). Starting as an American phenomenon, QAnon moved quickly to Europe, creating hotspots in Germany, Britain, the Netherlands, France, Italy, and Spain. QAnon was tied to anti-masking and anti-vaccine theories, claiming that 5G mobile networks created the pandemic, that the pandemic was created to control the masses through lockdowns and vaccines, and that vaccines were useless or harmful medicines devised by pharmaceutical giants with the help of corrupt Democrats. The results of the popular spread of QAnon theories have been dangerous, leading to mask and vaccine resistance, violence against those seen as deep-state actors or defenders, and threatening real-world responses to the narrative. At the end of 2020, for example, Anthony Quinn Walker planted a bomb in downtown Nashville that destroyed several city blocks. Warner's target was an AT&T building, which provided what he believed was the COVID-causing 5G network.

But not all conspiracy theories are as extreme as those pushed by QAnon. Numerous studies show that conspiracy theories have been a staple of American political and public health culture long before COVID. Oliver and Wood (2014) note that a number of national surveys sampled between 2006 and 2011 found that half of the American public endorse at least one conspiracy theory. Anna Merlan defines conspiracy theories as ideas that, in their most fundamental sense, seek to explain upsetting events by identifying a supposed secret group of evildoers who must be opposed in order to bring the world back into a state of calm and order (in Bodner et al. 2021, 2). Anika Wilson suggests a definition that presents a more sympathetic view of conspiracy theories, cognizant perhaps of another, less extreme pole of conspiracy believers. She notes, "As theories based in observation and the authoritative weight of past traditional narratives of suspicion, conspiracy rumors often posit compelling interpretations of real events" (2013, 58). Indeed, some conspiracy theories are based heavily on real events that have indicated a reasonable need for distrust. The forty-year Tuskegee experiment that was intent on observing the course of untreated syphilis in African American males, thereby withholding treatment, had lasting effects on public confidence in medical research, public health, and the American government, within but also outside Black communities. The long history of involuntary or coerced sterilization of Latinas in the United States has had a similar impact. In each of these cases, health conspiracy theories are based on a sound and appropriate distrust of our medical systems. The perceived threat of "vaccine passports" and other digital and bureaucratic tracking technologies (Rouhier-Willoughby 2020, iv) and the belief in medical experimentation of COVID treatments on minorities are both old traditions, and ones that may not seem at all inconsistent with the prior horrors of inhumane medical research and care. Conspiracy theories existing at the opposite pole from QAnon-type beliefs may be collective narratives or beliefs that are based on community experiences that demonstrate the foolhardiness of placing trust in the medical establishment. While conspiracy theories may seem highly implausible, they are best understood when placed within the larger discursive, social, and political context (Briggs 2004) affecting community and individual concerns about the COVID epidemic and healthcare. Conspiratorial thinking thrives in environments of low confidence and low trust (Shahsavari et al. 2020, 279) and as such, they are informative. They can point to areas of vernacular concern, identify inequalities in the system, and highlight areas where there are clashes in medical worldviews (Goldstein 2004, 53).

NOT THAT, THIS: COVID-INSPIRED FUTURES

Necessity, we remembered so well during COVID, is the mother of invention. As goods and service distribution pipelines became stressed by COVID, a new tradition began that some have called "Not that, this." The idea was that we have, by necessity, become more flexible about substitutions for products we once embraced with fierce dedication. "Not that, this" became a gift for friends, made up of items that we were once forced to use as a substitute but that we now found superior to the original. Just as COVID made the world fearful and bleaker, it also provided suggestions for a better future. As COVID has dragged on, it has become commonplace to see news pieces on the parts of COVID life that will be with us for some time to come—remote work, curbside delivery, Zoom education. Some of those things sadden us, tied to the impersonality of modernity or suspicions that they will increase the work or school week. Yet "Not that, this" reminds us that a part of COVID vernacular culture is not just what we are forced to do now, but also things that will become a more permanent part of our traditions, things that have drawn us in and improved our lives. And in some cases, the vernacular has even inspired more official changes.

We have seen this before as well. Between 1873 and 1945, Dr. Edward Livingston Trudeau ran a center for the treatment of tuberculosis in Saranac Lake, New York. Inspired by reading about Prussian success treating tuberculosis with the "rest cure" in cold mountain air, Trudeau began his own world-renowned sanatorium dedicated to "the fresh air cure." Trudeau's sanatorium was based on the notion that the best way to cure tuberculosis was fresh air and complete bed rest. To facilitate both treatments, Trudeau created what he called "cure cottages"—houses with several porches, balconies, and sunrooms that could accommodate outdoor exposure for multiple patients on cots. Many of the cure cottages had sliding glass walls that could open up a room to the outside. Patients spent at least eight hours a day on the cure cottage porches. As the treatment got more popular, architects collaborated with the doctors to develop better ways to accommodate patients' fresh air needs while protecting them from the elements (Baldwin 1932; Woodward 1994). One of Trudeau's staff physicians subsequently designed a "cure chair," now known as the Adirondack recliner, that had a slightly reclining back, wheels, and wide arms. Both the architecture of the cure cottages and the design of the Adirondack chair became popular and remained sought after long after the fresh air cure was no longer needed for tuberculosis. Many of us today have cure cottage–inspired porches on our homes or Adirondack chairs on our decks.

Just as tuberculosis created designs that reflected new values in living, so too, it appears, has COVID. Balcony singing, eating, and visiting during COVID have led to an international reappraisal of the balcony as a part of home architecture (see, for example, Emekci 2021; Sepe 2021), even in those places where they are not currently used. Once seen as a way to dress up building facades or to create a few square feet of fresh air, balconies during COVID suddenly became important places to share experience and demonstrate national solidarity. Not only were balconies a part of public life under confinement, they also became a part of the reappraisal of the juncture between urban design and disease, as well as notions of lifestyle, sociability, and architecture. Numerous architectural design articles have been published since 2020 suggesting that homes require greater outdoor transitional spaces, including porches, decks, and balconies.

COVID has also changed attitudes toward cooking and eating, at least for the near future. A survey by Hunter, a consumer market research firm, found that 71 percent of people in the US indicate they will continue to cook at home more following their COVID experience. In a survey reported in *Food Dive* magazine, sales and marketing agency Acosta found that 35 percent of those surveyed indicated a post-COVID newfound passion for cooking (Devenyns 2021). Just as COVID provided inspiration for home cooking and eating, it also engendered experimentation with bread making and sustainable gardening that are likely to be seen as positive future commitments. Family and community regular events like game nights and scavenger hunts are also likely to remain an ongoing part of the post-COVID picture, at least for some. The slower lifestyle and appreciation of those around us may be a part of "Not that, this" for some time to come, and the vernacular traditions that helped us survive "behind the mask" just might carry on.

NOTES

1. Victor Turner (1974) refers to plague transitioning to periods of community health in his reading of van Gennep and discussion of liminality.

2. https://blog.streamelements.com/state-of-the-stream-june-q2-2020-livestreaming-is-getting-much-larger-and-more-global-8acfc3fadbba Accessed February 20, 2022

3. According to surveys, Republicans believe twice as often as Democrats that Chinese scientists engineered the coronavirus and that Bill Gates wants to use a mass vaccination campaign against COVID-19 to implant microchips in people to track them with a digital ID. See Sanders 2020.

4. The Hatch Act of 1939 banned the use of federal funds for electoral purposes and forbade federal officials to coerce political support with the promise of public jobs or funds. The act prohibits federal employees below the policy-making level from taking "any active part" in political campaigns, such as running for office in partisan political campaigns, giving speeches on behalf of partisan political candidates, or soliciting money for such candidates (Asp 2021).

5. Stop Asian Hate is the slogan promoted by Stop AAPI Hate (Asian Americans and Pacific Islanders), which is the organization that tracks related hate statistics. Black Lives Matter is the name of both the slogan and the decentralized confederation of groups advocating for justice, healing, and freedom for Black people.

6. Contrast this with the polio epidemic. Polio was visible for a long time in the population among those who survived the disease but required lifelong access to a wheelchair, crutches, or leg braces, or who retained a limp. Franklin D. Roosevelt contracted polio twelve years before becoming president and despite trying to conceal the extent of its impact, he acknowledged having contracted it. His presidency put polio front and center in the US. Even once a vaccine severely limited the number of cases in the Western Hemisphere (and internationally until 2003, when a break in international vaccination reinstated the disease in developing countries that had previously eliminated polio), the visual remnants of the disease remained. This was especially the case because of post-polio syndrome—potentially disabling symptoms that can appear decades after the initial illness. Polio's hypervisibility kept it in the public imagination; it was (and is) the subject of numerous histories, literature (including children's literature), artwork, and works on public health, virology, and vaccine development.

7. This is shown over and over in the work of folklorists writing on epidemics (see, for example, Turner 1993; Briggs and Mantini-Briggs 2003; Goldstein 2004; Bennett 2005; Wilson 2013; Lee 2014; Kitta 2012, 2019).

8. Claude Lévi-Strauss (1966) theorized the *bricoleur* (bricklayer) as a person who uses their surrounding resources to create something new.

9. Or, as is seen in Julianne Graper's contribution to this volume, various agents, institutions, and ideologies, political or otherwise, can compel the personification of disease in terms of race, ethnicity, or other characteristics to provide profiles and personifications of a scapegoat for crises.

10. While the ISPOS poll does not define "deep state," according to Merriam-Webster, the term refers to "an alleged secret network of especially nonelected government officials and sometimes private entities (as in the financial services and defense industries) operating extralegally to influence and enact government policy" (https://www.merriam-webster.com/dictionary/deep%20state).

11. QAnon alleged that coded words and satanic symbolism purportedly apparent in John Podesta's emails, hacked during his tenure as chair of Hillary Clinton's 2016 US presidential campaign, point to a secret child sex-trafficking ring at a pizza restaurant in Washington, DC, called Comet Ping Pong. QAnon originated out of the Pizzagate conspiracy theory and maintains the central belief that a covert cabal of powerful elites controls the world, using their power to abuse children.

REFERENCES

Aderet, Ofer. 2020. "A Spanish New Weapon of War: The Spanish Flu Had Its Own Share of Conspiracy Theories." *Haaretz*, March 26. https://www.haaretz.com/israel-news/.premium-the-spanish-flu-had-its-own-share-of-conspiracy-theories-1.8713448.

Adgate, Brad. 2020. "Nielsen: How the Pandemic Changed At-Home Media Consumption." *Forbes*, August 21. https://www.forbes.com/sites/bradadgate/2020/08/21/nielsen-how-the-pandemic-changed-at-home-media-consumption/?sh=55540a8c5a28.

Ahuja, Anjana. 2022. "To Beat COVID-19, Find Today's Superspreading 'Typhoid Mary's.'" *Financial Times*, February 23. https://www.ft.com/content/121c2f30-9f69-11ea-ba68-3d5500196c30.

AJMC Staff. 2021. "A Timeline of COVID-19 Developments in 2020." *American Journal of Managed Care*, January 1. https://www.ajmc.com/view/a-timeline-of-COVID19-developments-in-2020.

Anderson, Stephen. 2020. "COVID-19 and Leisure in the United States." *World Leisure Journal* 62 (4): 352–56. https://doi.org/10.1080/16078055.2020.1825259.

Asp, David. 2021. "Hatch Act of 1939 (1939)." In *The First Amendment Encyclopedia*. https://www.mtsu.edu/first-amendment/article/1046/hatch-act-of-1939.

Baldwin, Edward R. 1932. "Saranac Lake and the Saranac Laboratory for the Study of Tuberculosis." *Milbank Memorial Fund Quarterly Bulletin* 10 (1): 1–16.

Beiner, Guy. 2006. "Out in the Cold and Back: New-found Interest in the Great Flu." *Cultural and Social History* 3 (4): 496–505.

Beiner, Guy, ed. 2021. *Pandemic Re-awakenings: The Forgotten and Unforgotten "Spanish" Flu of 1918–1919*. Oxford: Oxford University Press.

Bennett, Gillian. 2005. *Bodies: Sex, Violence, Disease, and Death in Contemporary Legends*. Jackson: University of Mississippi Press.

Bodner, John, Wendy Welch, Ian Brodie, Anna Muldoon, Donald Leech, and Ashley Marshall. 2021. *COVID-19 Conspiracy Theories: QAnon, 5G, the New World Order and Other Viral Ideas*. Jefferson, NC: McFarland.

Bonotti, Mateo, and Steven T. Zech. 2021. "The Human, Economic, Social, and Political Costs of COVID-19." *Recovering Civility during COVID-19* 3:1–36.

Briggs, Charles L. 2004. "Theorizing Modernity Conspiratorially: Science, Scale, and the Political Economy of Public Discourse in Explanations of a Cholera Epidemic." *American Ethnologist* 31 (2): 164–87.

Briggs, Charles L., with Clara Mantini-Briggs. 2003. *Stories in the Time of Cholera: Racial Profiling during a Medical Nightmare.* Berkeley: University of California Press.

Brunvand, Jan Harold. 1989. *Curses! Broiled Again! The Hottest Urban Legends Going!* New York: Norton.

Buchanan, Larry, Quoctrug Bui, and Jugal K. Patel. 2020. "Black Lives Matter May Be the Largest Movement in U.S. History." *New York Times,* July 3. https://www.nytimes.com/interactive/2020/07/03/us/george-floyd-protests-crowd-size.html.

Centers for Disease Control and Prevention. 2020. "First Travel-Related Case of 2019 Novel Coronavirus Detected in the United States," January 21. https://www.cdc.gov/media/releases/2020/p0121-novel-coronavirus-travel-case.html.

Cohut, Maria. 2020. "The Flu Pandemic of 1918 and Early Conspiracy Theories." *Medical News Today,* September 29. https://www.medicalnewstoday.com/articles/the-flu-pandemic-of-1918-and-early-conspiracy-theories.

Davies, Pete. 1999. *Catching Cold: 1918's Forgotten Tragedy and the Scientific Hunt for the Virus That Caused It.* London: Michael Joseph.

Davis, Ryan A. 2013. *The Spanish Flu: Narrative and Cultural Identity in Spain, 1918.* New York: Palgrave Macmillan.

Devenyns, Jessi. 2021. "Survey: 7 in 10 Consumers Say they Will Keep Cooking at Home After the Pandemic." *Food Dive,* January 19. https://www.fooddive.com/news/survey-7-in-10-consumers-say-they-will-keep-cooking-at-home-after-the-pand/593532/.

Doheny, Kathleen. 2020. "Toxic Methanol in Hand Sanitizers: Poisonings Continue." *WEBMD Health News,* August 17. https://www.webmd.com/lung/news/20200817/toxic-methanol-in-hand-sanitizers-poisonings-continue.

Emekci, Şeyda. 2021. "Balcony: A Remembered Architectural Element amid the Pandemic—Evidence from Digital Media." *Journal of Urban Studies* 12:609–30.

Erll, Astrid. 2020. "Afterword: Memory Worlds in Times of Corona." *Memory Studies* 13 (5): 861–74. https://doi.org/10.1177/1750698020943014.

Freeman, D., F. Waite, L. Rosebrock, A. Petit, C. Causier, A. East, L. Jenner, A. L. Teale, L. Carr, S. Mulhall, E. Bold, and S. Lambe, S. 2022. "Coronavirus Conspiracy Beliefs, Mistrust, and Compliance with Government Guidelines in England." *Psychological Medicine* 52 (2): 251–63. https://doi.org/10.1017/S0033291720001890.

Goldstein, Diane E. 2004. *Once upon a Virus: AIDS Legends and Vernacular Risk Perception.* Logan: Utah State University Press.

Gutman, Rachel. 2020. "Sorry to Burst Your Quarantine Bubble." *Atlantic,* November 30. https://www.theatlantic.com/health/archive/2020/11/pandemic-pod-bubble-concept-creep/617207/.

Henley, Jon, and Niamh McIntyre. 2020. "Survey Uncovers Widespread Belief in 'Dangerous' COVID Conspiracy Theories." *Guardian,* October 26. https://www.theguardian.com/world/2020/oct/26/survey-uncovers-widespread-belief-dangerous-COVID-conspiracy-theories.

Hiiemäe, Reet, Mare Kalda, Mare Kõiva, and Piret Voolaid. 2021. "Vernacular Reactions to COVID-19 in Estonia: Crisis Folklore and Coping." *Folklore* 82:1–32.

Kasulis, Kelly. 2020. "'Patient 31' and South Korea's Sudden Spike in Coronavirus Cases." *Aljazeera,* March 3. https://www.aljazeera.com/news/2020/03/31-south-korea-sudden-spike-coronavirus-cases-200303065953841.html.

Kelley, Greg. 2020. "Doctor Beaky, the Four Thieves, and *De Fabulis Pestis.*" *Contemporary Legend* 3 (10): 48–72.

King, Ellie M., Paul Smith, Paul F. Wilson, and Mark A. Williams. 2021. "Digital Responses of UK Museum Exhibitions to the COVID-19 Crisis, March–June 2020." *Curator: The Museum Journal* 64 (3): 487–504.

Kitta, Andrea. 2012. *Vaccinations and Public Concern in History: Legend, Rumor, and Risk Perception.* New York: Routledge.

Kitta, Andrea. 2019. *The Kiss of Death: Contagion, Contamination, and Folklore.* Logan: Utah State University Press.

Lantis, Margaret. 1960. "Vernacular Culture." *American Anthropologist* 62 (2): 202–16.

Lee, Jon D. 2014. *An Epidemic of Rumors: How Stories Shape Our Perception of Disease.* Logan: Utah State University Press.

Leng, Trystan, Connor White, Joe Hilton, Adam Kucharski, Lorenzo Pellis, Helena Stage, Nicholas G. Davies, Centre for Mathematical Modelling of Infectious Disease 2019 nCoV Working Group, Matt J. Keeling, and Stefan Flasche. 2020. "The Effectiveness of Social Bubbles as Part of a COVID-19 Lockdown Exit Strategy: A Modelling Study." *Wellcome Open Research* 5:213. https://doi.org/10.12688/wellcomeopenres.16164.2.

Lévi-Strauss, Claude. 1966. *The Savage Mind.* Chicago: University of Chicago Press.

McNeill, Lynne. 2007. "Portable Places: Serial Collaboration and the Creation of a New Sense of Place." *Western Folklore* 66 (3–4): 281–99.

Mould, Tom, ed. 2018. "Fake News: Definitions and Approaches." Special Issue of *Journal of American Folklore* 131 (522).

Newall, Mallory. 2020. "More Than 1 in 3 Americans Believe a 'Deep State' Is Working to Undermine Trump." *Ipsos,* December 30. https://www.ipsos.com/en-us/news-polls/npr-misinformation-123020.

O'Kane, Caitlin. 2021. "Texas Man Sentenced to 15 Months in Prison for Spreading COVID-19 Hoax on Facebook." *CBS News,* October 6. https://www.cbsnews.com/news/COVID-19-hoax-facebook-texas-christopher-charles-perez-15-months-prison/.

Oliver, J. Eric, and Thomas J. Wood. 2014. "Conspiracy Theories and the Paranoid Style(s) of Mass Opinion." *American Journal of Political Science* 58 (4): 952–66.

Primiano, Leonard Norman. 1995. "Vernacular Religion and the Search for Method in Religious Folklife." *Western Folklore* 54 (1): 37–56.

Richter, Felix. 2020. "Etsy Thrives amid Pandemic—and It's Not Just Masks." *Statista,* December 9. https://www.statista.com/chart/23729/etsy-gross-merchandise-sales/.

Ritchie, Hannah, Edouard Mathieu, Lucas Rodés-Guirao, Cameron Appel, Charlie Giattino, Esteban Ortiz-Ospina, Joe Hasell, Bobbie Macdonald, Diana Beltekian, and Max Roser. 2022. "Coronavirus Pandemic (COVID-19)." *OurWorldInData.org,* accessed on March 1. https://ourworldindata.org/coronavirus.

Rouhier-Willoughby, Jeanmarie. 2020. "Editors' Introduction to the *Folklorica* Special Issue 'Vernacular Responses to the COVID-19 Pandemic.'" *FOLKLORICA—Journal of the Slavic, East European, and Eurasian Folklore Association* 24: ii–xix.

Sanders, Linley. 2020. "The Difference between What Republicans and Democrats Believe to Be True about COVID-19." *YouGovAmerica,* May 26. https://today.yougov.com/topics/politics/articles-reports/2020/05/26/republicans-democrats-misinformation.

Schaeffer, Katherine, 2020. "A Look at the Americans Who Believe There Is Some Truth to the Conspiracy Theory That COVID-19 Was Planned." *Pew Research Center,* July 25. https://www.pewresearch.org/fact-tank/2020/07/24/a-look-at-the

-americans-who-believe-there-is-some-truth-to-the-conspiracy-theory-that-COVID
-19-was-planned/.

Sepe, Marichela. 2021. "COVID-19 Pandemic and Public Spaces: Improving Quality and Flexibility for Healthier Places." *Urban Design International* 26:159–73.

Shahsavari, Shadi, Pavan Holur, Tianyi Wang, Timothy R. Tangherlini, and Vwani Roychowdhury. 2020. "Conspiracy in the Time of Corona: Automatic Detection of Emerging COVID-19 Conspiracy Theories in Social Media and the News." *Journal of Computational Social Science* 3 (2): 279–317.

Smith, Paul. 1990. "'AIDS—Don't Die of Ignorance': Exploring the Cultural Complex." In *A Nest of Vipers: Perspectives on Contemporary Legend*, vol. 5, edited by Gillian Bennett and Paul Smith, 113–41. Sheffield, UK: Sheffield Academic Press.

Spinney, Laura. 2018. *Pale Rider: The Spanish Flu of 1918 and How It Changed the World.* London: Vintage.

Taylor, Derrick Bryson. 2021. "A Timeline of the Coronavirus Pandemic." *New York Times*, March 17. https://www.nytimes.com/article/coronavirus-timeline.html.

Terry, Mark. 2021. "Updated: Comparing COVID-19 Vaccines: Timelines, Types and Prices." *BioSpace*, July 28. https://www.biospace.com/article/comparing-covid-19-vaccines-pfizer-biontech-moderna-astrazeneca-oxford-j-and-j-russia-s-sputnik-v/.

Turner, Patricia A. 1993. *I Heard It through the Grapevine: Rumor in African-American Culture.* Berkeley: University of California Press.

Turner, Victor. 1974. "Liminal to Liminoid, in Play, Flow, and Ritual: An Essay in Comparative Symbology." *Rice Institute Pamphlet* 60 (3).

Vallee, Mickey. 2020. "Doing Nothing Does Something: Embodiment and Data in the COVID-19 Pandemic." *Big Data and Society* 7 (1): 1–12.

Wannigamage Dulakshi, Michael Barlow, Erandi Lakshika, and Kathryn Kasmarik. 2020. "Analysis and Prediction of Player Population Changes in Digital Games during the COVID-19 Pandemic." In: *AI 2020: Advances in Artificial Intelligence*, edited by Marcus Gallagher, Nour Moustafa, and Erandi Lakshika, 458–69. https://doi.org/10.1007/978-3-030-64984-5_36.

Wilson, Anika. 2013. *Folklore, Gender, and AIDS in Malawi: No Secret under the Sun.* New York: Palgrave MacMillan.

Woodward, Theodore E. 1994. "Edward L. Trudeau: Pioneer Climatologist." *Transactions of the American Clinical and Climatological Association* 105:19–35.

World Health Organization. 2015. "World Health Organization Best Practices for the Naming of New Human Infectious Diseases." *World Health Organization*, May. https://apps.who.int/iris/bitstream/handle/10665/163636/WHO_HSE_FOS_15.1_eng.pdf.

World Health Organization. 2020. "Weekly Epidemiological Update." *World Health Organization*, December 29. https://www.who.int/publications/m/item/weekly-epidemiological-update---29-december-2020.

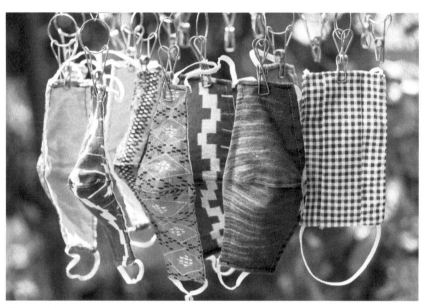
Figure 1.0. Homemade face masks

Section I
The Vernacular to the Rescue
Community, Creativity, and Coping with COVID-19

THE EARLY STAGES OF COVID-19 THRUST THE WORLD into a liminal state, spurring both anxieties about the unfamiliar virus and eager attempts to creatively adjust to "the new normal." The daily rhythms, work schedules, and expected routines many people were accustomed to had been thrown out the window, prompting individuals and groups to turn to artistic expressions and outlets as means of coping or establishing community with others. Holiday vacations were replaced with Zoom hangouts, nightly movies were paused to cheer on essential healthcare workers outside, and additional hours of free time were filled with long neighborhood walks, newly planted "victory gardens," and perfected sourdough recipes.

While the pandemic first and foremost is associated with hardships and tragedies, the communal responses to the public health crisis remain culturally significant and, at their best, heartwarming and empowering. The three chapters that open this book examine case studies of people turning to artistic expressions to navigate the uncertainties wrought by COVID-19. From neighborhood street art in the UK through traditional folk art in the midwestern US to the widely popular trend of baking, each chapter considers how humans exercised their creative muscles in response to uneasy and isolating times. Although all three expositions concentrate on the early stages of COVID, they offer insight into the types, processes, and impacts of artistic vernacular expressions that emerged in later stages of the pandemic as well.

https://doi.org/10.7330/9781646424818.p001

1

Rainbows, Snakes, and Scarecrows
Creative Vernacular Interventions in Response to COVID-19—A View from the United Kingdom

Andrew Robinson

INTRODUCTION

Utilizing this author's extensive photographic documentation and material available online, this chapter will review and consider the wide range of COVID-related transitory and ephemeral material artifacts produced in both physical and virtual contexts to reveal the nature and context of individual and communal responses to the COVID crisis across the UK. What was the meaning and importance of these displays, customs, and rituals, and the material artifacts they produced? How did they develop and what did they mean for both those who created them and for their audience? What factors prompted their production during the thirteen weeks of the first UK lockdown in the spring of 2020? What do they reveal about the British experience of, and response to, the COVID crisis and the resulting restrictions on freedom?

The aim is not to exhaustively capture all forms of creative response, but rather to identify, document, and study a range of key responses as case studies of the manner in which the population of the nation with the highest infection and death rate in Europe outside Russia sought and found personal and communal expression at this challenging time.

METHODOLOGY

The primary visual research upon which this chapter is based was largely collected during the first UK COVID-19 lockdown, which lasted from March 23 until June 23, 2020. During the early part of lockdown, people's

https://doi.org/10.7330/9781646424818.c001

movements were severely restricted, limiting the scope of collection to the author's local neighborhood of Mapperley, Nottingham along with further material from Buxton, Derbyshire and Baildon, West Yorkshire when travel to these locations was permitted to care for vulnerable elders. Material collected by colleagues from the Centre for Contemporary Legend at Sheffield University, Dr. David Clarke, Diane Rogers, and Sophie Parkes-Nield, along with photographs kindly provided by Andrew Rodgers, further extended the reach of the research. Throughout the first UK lockdown, creative visual displays of vernacular art produced in response to the COVID crisis were widely shared across social media, usually by the makers themselves, and received extensive coverage in local and national news media, allowing the author to further extend the scope of the research across the whole UK.

The material collected and discussed, while not in any way exhaustive, is nevertheless representative of the types of display that became common on almost every street around the country during the UK's first lockdown, although these responses were not repeated in subsequent stages of the crisis. Other organizations, including the Elphinstone Institute at the University of Aberdeen and the Museum of Childhood at the Victoria and Albert Museum in London, recognized the value of this ephemeral material culture and were also engaged in documenting and collecting similar items.

THE VIRUS ARRIVES

The first outbreak of the virus within Europe was confirmed in France on January 24, and the first confirmed case recorded in the UK was on January 29 (Aspinall 2020). However, the virus spread most quickly across northern Italy and Spain, with Italy entering a national lockdown on March 9 and Spain and France following a week later, on March 16 and 17, respectively (*Reuters* 2020). In the early weeks of the COVID crisis, the UK government moved slowly, seeming hesitant and reluctant to make any firm decisions. Although a public information campaign focusing on handwashing was introduced in early February (Department of Health and Social Care 2020), the country's borders remained open, people traveled to the Alps and Spain during February half-term holidays, and there were no restrictions on gatherings despite growing concern that the UK government should be closing borders and taking action. People in the UK were thus able to watch as restrictions and then lockdowns were imposed in other countries before their own government took similar action in late March 2020.

The UK government finally closed all schools, pubs, restaurants, and other venues on Friday, March 20, and the prime minister notified the public of a national lockdown in an 8:00 p.m. broadcast on Monday, March 23 (Johnson 2020c). It should be noted that while the devolved governments of England, Scotland, Wales, and Northern Ireland introduced slightly different measures, much of the experience was nevertheless shared across the UK, especially during the period of the first lockdown covered by this chapter. Under lockdown, everyone was confined to their homes, allowed outside only to buy food and essentials, take daily exercise, care for vulnerable people, and work (but only if they couldn't work from home). In addition, all vulnerable people were instructed to shield for twelve weeks (Johnson 2020a). As in many countries, overnight parents faced the challenge of childcare and homeschooling while trying to work from home and deal with the stress and worry of the spreading virus and rising death toll. Families were encouraged to take daily walks for exercise, and it is these walks and the interested audiences they attracted—along with the challenge of coping with the isolation resulting from lockdown—that prompted many of the individual and communal responses in the form of vernacular displays and interventions that this chapter will explore.

THE MYSTIC AND THE RAINBOW

The most noticeable visible response during the initial stage of the first UK lockdown was that many households used their front windows and gardens as vehicles for individualistic expression in response to their isolation in their homes. This is particularly surprising given the typical national reserve toward such expressions of individuality and identity. For instance, during the recent Euro 2020 football championship (held in May and June 2021), in which England's national team had its greatest success since winning the World Cup in 1966, this author had to pass between fifty and a hundred residences before finding one proudly showing support by displaying posters or flying flags. Aside from occasionally extravagant displays of Christmas lights during the festive season and increasingly popular window and garden displays at Halloween, there is a certain reluctance to use one's home for the display of political posters, national flags, or other expressions of individual identity, beliefs, or political opinion. This reserve may be related to the importance of privacy in English culture which, as Kate Fox observes, is "impossible to overstate" (Fox 2004, 43). Bhatti et al. (2014) explain that although gardens are semi-public outdoor spaces, "privacy in a garden is highly prized" and the British make gardens for themselves, their families, and their friends. Nevertheless, during the first COVID lockdown in the spring of 2020, in response to lockdown isolation, front windows and gardens across the nation quickly came to be used as canvases for a multitude of creative vernacular displays and interventions—often borrowed from other nations that had entered lockdown earlier—displayed to be viewed by others.

One of the first and most persistent vernacular responses was the appearance of rainbows in a multitude of forms, from drawings and paintings to collages of tissue paper, woven ribbons, garlands, stickers, balloons, chalk drawings, and even decorative icing (see figure 1.1). These, often accompanied by messages of hope and positivity, were usually displayed in street-facing windows or pinned to gates and hedges (see figure 1.2). The image of the rainbow—a spectral visual phenomenon, an optical illusion produced by sunlight refracting through raindrops in the sky to produce a multicolored arc, a vision that seems to move away as we approach, with its proverbial pot of gold always just out of reach at the distant end—itself went viral as the virus spread. According to Christian and Jewish scriptures, the first rainbow appeared following Noah's release from self-isolation in the ark after the retreat of the great flood, a sign of God's covenant with all creatures of the Earth never again to destroy all life by the waters of a flood (Genesis 9:13–16). As such, the rainbow is a positive, life-affirming sign symbolizing the survival of life on Earth after a storm, deluge, or other worldwide disaster thanks to the faith of the people in the protection of God.

The rainbows seen in the UK were inspired by news and social media coverage from Italy, where displays of rainbows and positive messages of hope began appearing in a number of regions in late February and early March as Italy moved toward lockdown. On March 5, Italian newspapers carried stories of the appearance of small, anonymous post-it notes with the phrase "Tutto andrà bene" ("Everything will be fine!") accompanied by the image a heart on front doors, letterboxes, and bus stops across Lombardy (Vinci 2020). These notes, credited with sparking the widespread use of this phrase during the lockdown in Italy, have been claimed as a "collective poetic act" by Francesca Boifava and Patrizia Catterin, two commenters on an Italian blog. At a birthday party they attended on February 20, 2020, all twenty-six guests—inspired by the Bresciana poet Luciana Landolfi—filled a hundred-sheet block of post-it notes with the phrase and distributed them around their communities in the following days to create a "poetic wave" and "cultivate hope and love" (MoVimento 5 Stelle 2020). Similar notes had appeared in China during the early weeks of lockdown with the Cantonese phrase *jiāyóu*, an expression of encouragement and support meaning "Don't give up" or "Keep up the fight," which was also chanted from apartment windows in Wuhan during its lockdown in early January (*Guardian* 2020).

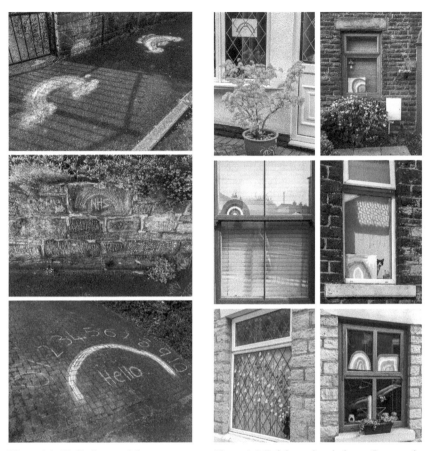

Figure 1.1. Chalk-drawn rainbows: Sherwood and Mapperley, Nottingham (*top and bottom*); and Baildon, West Yorkshire (*middle*).

Figure 1.2. Rainbows in windows: Crosspool, Sheffield (*top left*; photograph © Diane Rodgers); Greenfield, Saddleworth (*top right*); and Mossley, Greater Manchester (photographs © Sophie Parkes-Nield).

The phrase "Tutto andrà bene" (or "Andrà tutto bene") has been linked to the teachings of the medieval English mystic Julian of Norwich (Maccioni 2020), an anchoress who had chosen a life of isolation in a cell attached to St. Julian's Church in King Street, Norwich. On the evening of May 8, 1373, when she was approximately thirty years old and gravely ill, Mother Julian experienced a series of fifteen divine visions or "shewings" conveying God's love for humankind followed by a sixteenth vison the subsequent evening. Julian recovered and recounted her visions in the first known book written in English by a woman, *The Revelations of Divine Love* (Crampton 1994). In her text, Julian placed greatest emphasis on her last four revelations (chapters

27–86), especially the topic of the thirteenth revelation, which largely dealt with her struggle to understand and accept evil and the presence of sin in the world. She experienced a loss of faith that was only restored during her final revelation the following night. Julian's doubts are directly addressed by God, who explains, "I may make all things well, I can make all things well, I will make all things well, and I shall make all things well; and thou shalt see thyself that all manner of things shall be well" (33).

Historian and TV presenter Janina Ramirez (2016), author of *Julian of Norwich: A Very Brief History*, suggests that St. Julian may have lost her family during the Black Death, which struck Norwich in 1349, when she was approximately six years old. Ramirez posits that living in the wake of the Black Death, Julian practiced a form of self-isolating not just to preserve her life but also as a way of "finding calm and quiet and focus in a chaotic world" (quoted in Rigby 2020).

Clearly, Julian of Norwich's self-imposed isolation and her life-affirming positive interpretation of her mystical visions had resonance for those facing the lockdown in the early weeks of March 2020 in Italy, where, thanks to recent General Audiences by Pope Benedict XVI (2010) and Pope Francis (2016), her teachings remain fairly well known. The phrase "Everything will be fine" quickly gained traction and people across Italy were soon displaying signs and banners with the phrase from windows and balconies and sharing related videos and photographs online. Many of these banners and signs accompanied the text with hearts and rainbows. In addition to their Christian connotation, rainbows are a well-established symbol of peace and happiness in Italy. The Italian rainbow flag of peace, often displaying the word PACE across its center, was created in the early 1960s by Italian pacifist philosopher Aldo Capitini and has been carried at peace marches and demonstrations ever since (Associazione Amici di Aldo Capitini 2003). (The flag has gained increasing popularity since the 1980s and was widely displayed as part of the "peace from all balconies" campaign during the buildup to the Iraq War in the autumn of 2002.)

In this context, the rainbow, symbolizing God's promise never to destroy the creatures of the Earth, becomes a visual expression of the phrase "Tutto andrà bene," a promise that humankind will ultimately survive and prosper thanks to God's love, as revealed in a vision to a fourteenth-century mystic. Text and image, operating in both virtual and physical worlds, expressed the hope and belief that individuals, communities, and humankind would survive the growing pandemic.

Inspired by news reports and social media coverage of lockdown in Italy, COVID rainbows accompanied by positive messages began to be appear in domestic settings across the UK in the days immediately preceding the closure of schools on Friday, March 20, and were widely reported in the press over the weekend that followed. Prior to its more recent adoption by the Gay Pride Movement and LGBT+ community, the rainbow's cultural significance within the UK has been most closely associated with children and childhood. Rainbow designs are commonly used as decoration in preschool and primary school settings and prove a popular subject for children's drawings. Images of rainbows are also often found on children's bedding, clothing, and nursery equipment. *Rainbow* was also the name of a popular and fondly remembered UK children's series, originally inspired by *Sesame Street*, which aired on the ITV network from 1972 to 1992 (Sheridan 2004, 211). The rainbow also has associations with the UK counterculture movement dating back to the late 1960s, when rainbow designs were commonly found on badges, shoelaces, T-shirts, and other items as well as incense sticks, oversize cigarette papers, and hubble-bubble pipes found in hippie shops and at festivals. Although the display of rainbows during the early days of the UK lockdown was clearly influenced by the use of the rainbow as a symbol of unity and hope in other countries, in the UK, their production by children can be seen to fall largely within cultural norms. However, the manner in which rainbows were displayed in front windows and gardens across the country, and their heartfelt messages of hope and goodwill, breaks with traditional British reserve and the normal privacy of home and garden.

A number of different individuals have been credited with introducing the practice to the UK by the media. Crystal Stanley of Ipswich, inspired by social media posts from Italy, set up a "Rainbow Trail" Facebook page on Thursday, March 19, 2020, encouraging people to display rainbows as a sign of positivity, hope, and togetherness and to create a trail for children to follow on their daily walks. Over 4,000 people joined in the first two days, and within three weeks, the group had more than 182,000 members worldwide (*BBC News: Suffolk* 2020). On the same day, Alice Aske from Somerset launched a Facebook page and Twitter hashtag called "Chase the Rainbow" to provide an activity for children that avoided "touching for fear of passing on the virus," attracting close to 65,000 followers in the first twenty-four hours (Scarlett and Wallis 2020). Kezia Roberts from Horsforth near Leeds, in self-isolation herself, also set up a Facebook group called "Chase the Rainbow" on March 20 (Roberts 2020) to foster unity and to "cheer people up in these tough times" (*BBC News: Leeds* 2020). Once again, inspiration came from media reports of mothers in the city of Bari in the Italian region of Puglia using Facebook to encourage others to leave positive messages around their communities (Moss 2020).

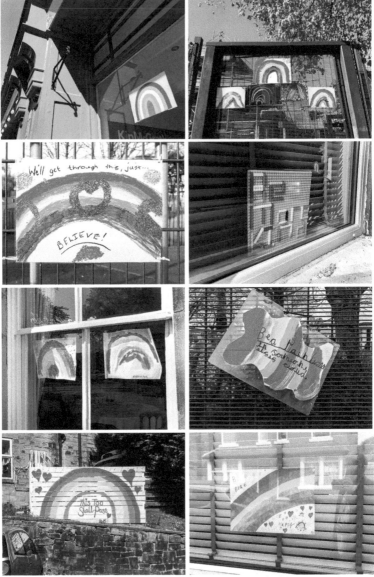

Figure 1.3. Rainbows with positive messages: Buxton, Derbyshire; Mapperley, Nottingham (*second row left and bottom right*); and Mossley, Greater Manchester (*bottom left*; photograph © Sophie Parkes-Nield).

Media reports from the northeast of England on Saturday, March 21, recounted that rainbows had been seen in windows around Newcastle and North Tyneside as part of a "Cheerful Windows" campaign promoted by local schools (Sharma 2020). Angela Ruthven explains that the initiative "has offered a positive approach. It's bringing families together at home to create a rainbow, making people smile if they are spotted in windows. It's bringing our wonderful school and even the world together . . . showing that we are all in this together" (quoted in Sharma 2020).

While not overtly adopting the phrase "Everything will be fine," the rainbows displayed in the UK during the early days of lockdown were accompanied by other life-affirming symbols such as hearts, smiley faces, and shining suns along with positive messages like "Hope," "Be kind" (Sharma 2020), and "Be confident and brave" (*BBC News: England* 2020). Moreover, both parents and children stated in interviews that their motivation was to challenge the fear and negativity of the lockdown, to "brighten someone's day" and to "keep children and friends connected during an uncertain time" (Wallis 2020). Shona Richardson, a head teacher from Rosewell, Midlothian, told the BBC: "We did not want it all to be doom and gloom for the children. We thought this would be a really visual way of bringing hope at a time when there is not much out there. It also sends a message to the elderly people to say we are thinking of you and hopefully it will give them some joy too. These children won't be able to see their friends so much so it's a way they can communicate together" (*BBC News: England* 2020).

Most rainbow drawings adopted the traditional simple semicircular arch design, with red on the outside and blue on the lower inner side of the arc, although examples employing a wide range of creative and at times seemingly random color combinations were to be found (see figure 1.3). Others adopted the more contemporary design starting and ending in clouds and often contained short positive messages such as "Stay safe" or "Keep on smiling." Although some used printable sources online, most rainbows were hand-drawn and colored using crayons, felt tips, or sharpies, while other rainbows were collaged from paper and cloth, sculpted from clay or papier-mâché, or created on the computer (see figure 1.4). Knitted rainbows and Hama Bead creations were found hanging from trees in Avebury, Wiltshire, and Stone Middleton in Derbyshire; rainbow-colored hearts were strung from a street sign in Lambley, Nottingham; and rainbow paper chains appeared in a window overlooking the Pavilion Gardens in Buxton (see figure 1.5). The vast majority documented, however, were in the form of fairly simple hand-drawn depictions.

Rainbow displays spread ever more rapidly following the full lockdown announced on Monday, March 23, and continued to be reported by the press and widely shared on social media for many weeks. Images of rainbows were included in the queen's television address broadcast on April 5 when she suggested that such new traditions and customs were a symbol

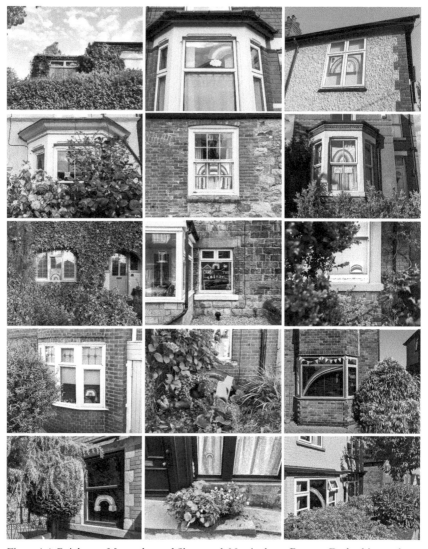

Figure 1.4. Rainbows: Mapperley and Sherwood, Nottingham; Buxton, Derbyshire; and Warminster, Wiltshire.

of "our national spirit" that would "help to define our future" (Elizabeth II 2020).

The displays of the rainbow and its symbolic reminder that the sun will follow a storm and all will be well thanks to God's covenant, while having the prosaic function of occupying children and the social function of providing a positive message for those on walks to view, could also be seen as an

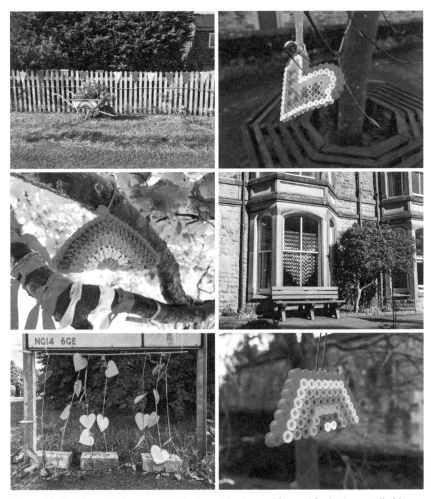

Figure 1.5. Rainbows: Calverton, Nottinghamshire (*top and bottom left*); Avebury, Wiltshire (*middle left*); Stoney Middleton, Derbyshire (*top and bottom right*); and Buxton, Derbyshire (*middle right*).

apotropaic sign, a ritual symbol to ward off evil and to keep the virus at bay. There is similarity here with the Amabie craze that swept Japan during early March 2020. The legendary Japanese *yokai* (or spirit) Amabie—a whimsical and mischievous mermaid-like creature with a bird's head, human hair, and the body of a fish—which according to popular folklore originally rose from the ocean in 1846 advising people that "should an epidemic come, draw me and show to the people, so that you can be free from disease" (Kuhn 2020). The activity of drawing Amabie is seen as a cathartic process by which fears and hopes are transferred from the subconscious to the paper. Amabie first resurfaced in a tweet on January 30, and tweets grew to as many as forty-six thousand a day by March 14 (Furukawa and Kansaku 2020) as paintings, drawings, and personalized depictions appeared on social media. People displayed drawings of the spirit in their windows and sushi boxes, fabric, and other items were adorned with depictions of the creature (Saunders 2020). The creature also appeared accompanied with the slogan "Stop the Spread of the Virus" in Ministry of Health posters to promote COVID safety (Furukawa and Kansaku 2020). It's hard to judge the extent to which people believed in the protection provided by Amabie; nevertheless, drawing and sharing the character has similar benefits to those associated with the drawing and display of rainbows in the UK: providing a positive activity and bringing a sense of togetherness and community in difficult times, motivations referenced frequently by parents of the children who engaged in this uncharacteristic mass outpouring of unity and hope.

STAY AT HOME, PROTECT THE NHS, SAVE LIVES

Very quickly in the UK, the meaning of the rainbows shifted from a message of positivity and peace to a display of support for and solidarity with the National Health Service and care workers (see figure 1.6). Indeed, the vast majority of communal and individual responses to the COVID crisis and the isolation resulting from the lockdown from this point onward focused on the NHS as much as, or in place of, positive expressions of hope or support for those at most risk from the virus, sending messages of goodwill and encouragement to key workers and raising funds to support them. There was also a shift away from children as the main producers of rainbows as their use, display, and function broadened. There are a number of possible reasons for this shift in the symbolism of UK rainbow displays during the early stages of lockdown.

The Conservative government's messaging as the country entered lockdown placed increasing emphasis on the UK population observing the restrictions not to protect themselves, their families, or their communities, but rather to "flatten the curve" and protect the NHS (Johnson 2020b). The lockdown was a part of the government's "delay" strategy following an unsuccessful "contain" strategy, with the aim of delaying the spread of the virus to ensure that the NHS could cope with the increasing numbers of COVID cases. The three-part slogan, "Stay at Home, Protect the NHS, Save Lives," was used throughout the early period of the lockdown and seen on the podiums at daily press conferences, online, and on billboards

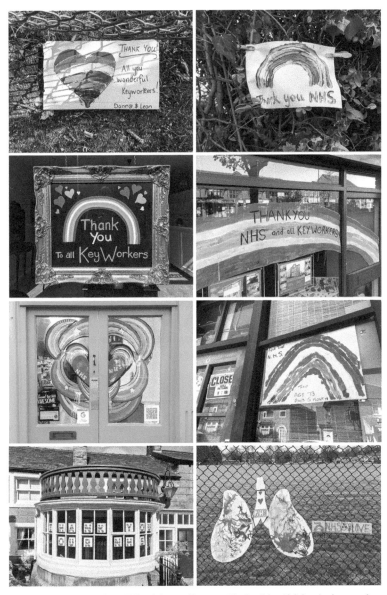

Figure 1.6. Support the NHS rainbows: Buxton, Derbyshire (*left-hand column and bottom right*); and Mapperley, Nottingham (*right-hand column*).

across the country (*ITV News* 2020b). In using the NHS as a motivating factor for compliance, the government was playing on the British public's special (some might say sentimental) relationship with the publicly funded, universal, and free at the point of delivery National Health Service. This treasured gem of the British welfare state, founded in 1948 by Aneurin Bevan, minister for health in the postwar Labour government, was memorably celebrated (despite Tory attempts to prevent it) as part of Danny Boyle's opening ceremony for the 2012 London Olympics (Osborne 2016). For many, there is some irony in the Conservative Party's sudden enthusiasm for the NHS, given their long-standing reputation for underfunding and privatizing the service, along with a series of recent funding cuts described by *Guardian* columnist Polly Toynbee (2019) in the October before the virus arrived as "brutal."

As can be seen, the British public was well primed for response should the NHS be invoked as part of a call to arms, and the message "Support the NHS" soon became ubiquitous across all government briefings, media coverage of the crisis, and the leaflets, posters, and online graphics offering advice and guidance relating to COVID-19. Calls for the return to work of health practitioners, the rapid building of extra capacity in the form of the temporary NHS "Nightingale" hospitals, and concerns over health workers' safety and the supply of PPE kept the NHS at the top of the news agenda and at the forefront of people's experience of the crisis throughout the lockdown. The NHS was the front line in the battle against the virus, healthcare workers were the army, and the public would become casualties unless they stayed at home, supported the NHS, and thus saved lives (war metaphors will emerge again later in this chapter).

It seems likely that the linkage of the rainbow to the widespread concern and public support for the NHS was influenced by a campaign introduced by the NHS in 2018 to support the LGBT+ community in healthcare settings by the wearing of a rainbow. The NHS Rainbow Badge, a special rainbow version of the standard NHS "lozenge" badge, originated at Evelina London Children's Hospital (Guy's and St. Thomas' NHS Foundation Trust 2018) as part of a campaign to encourage NHS workers to signify their understanding and willingness to support LGBT+ patients and workers. Lenny Byrne, chief nurse and director of Integrated Clinical Professions at Plymouth NHS Trust, explains, "The NHS Rainbow Badge is a simple visible symbol to let people know that you can talk to us about who you are, your identity, and how you are feeling—without being judged" (Byrne 2019).

Thus, in the year leading up to the first wave of the virus, the NHS logo was increasingly seen accompanied by the rainbow design on the uniforms of NHS workers, within hospitals and health settings, and on websites. Matt Hancock, the UK health secretary, appeared at the daily government COVID briefing the day after lockdown was imposed wearing an NHS rainbow badge, prefiguring the association between rainbow and support for the NHS that would soon follow.

The rainbow design used in these settings was the six-banded rainbow that has been a symbol of gay pride since Gilbert Baker hand-dyed silk in rainbow colors to create flags for a gay pride parade in San Francisco in June 1978 (Haag 2017). For the original gay pride flag, Baker added a pink band to the top of the standard seven-banded rainbow, with each color being ascribed its own meaning. The pink band, however, was removed soon after (pink silk apparently proving too expensive), and the flag's indigo and blue bands were combined as royal blue to leave the six bands used today.

As the British public searched for rainbows on flags and badges to show solidarity with both their community and the NHS, they often used the six-banded gay pride version of the rainbow, readily available online as a symbol of gay pride. Indeed, some eBay sellers who had been marketing the NHS rainbow badges as "LGBT+ badges" renamed them as "Support the NHS" badges. Many other NHS-related rainbow products quickly became available (see figure 1.7).

All of this, however, was not without controversy. Members of the LGBT+ community felt that a symbol representing their hard-fought struggle for acceptance, used to symbolize safe spaces and understanding, had been co-opted and stolen from them for another purpose. This criticism created fierce debate in both the media and on online forums. Writing in the *Huffington Post*, Rachel Charlton-Dailey explains the problem: "To LGBT people like me, it symbolises hard-fought representation, and refusing to live in the shadows. Unfortunately, it now feels like it's been taken from us, and that our message is being shouted over by, for the most part, cisgender straight people who don't really care about queer issues . . . I wish the public had chosen another symbol. What would have been wrong with a love heart, a dove for peace, or even some flowers? . . . I applaud the vital key workers in the pandemic, but this was never their flag to wave" (2021).

Others, such as Green Party candidate James Taylor (2020), have critiqued the use of the rainbow as a symbol of support for the NHS as a diversionary tactic that helped to essentially depoliticize the public view of the emergency services through its association with a children's symbol, suggesting that "the innocence of the child's hand remained unsullied by the real and fierce debates that featured in adult conversation about how underfunding and unpreparedness had left NHS staff in danger." Nevertheless, the rainbow became a potent symbol of the British public's support for the NHS and healthcare workers, which was shared in a range of different contexts and settings and continues to be displayed in windows across the country.

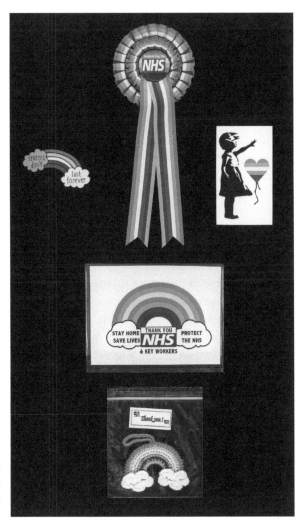

Figure 1.7. COVID
rainbow products
purchased on eBay, May
2020 (originals in color).

Another expression of support for the NHS during the early weeks of the lockdown was the weekly clapping that took place across the country at 8:00 p.m. every Thursday night. The ritual was started by London-based Dutch yoga teacher Annemarie Plas via posts on Instagram and Twitter using the hashtag #ClapForOurCarers. Her original Facebook post explains, "During these unprecedented times, they need to know that we are grateful. Please join us on 26th of March at 8pm for a big applause (from front doors, garden, balcony, windows etc) to show all nurses, doctors, GPs and carers our appreciation for their ongoing hard work and fight against this virus" (MacLellan 2020).

Plas had been inspired by the communal clapping and singing reported from other countries that had entered lockdown earlier, which had been widely reported in the media. However, unlike the often daily and impromptu expressions of solidarity and community seen across Europe and beyond, the UK's Clap for Carers was specifically organized in support of the NHS and limited to a single evening a week, with the streets and avenues of the nation largely silent on other nights. Clap for Carers was picked up by the media, circulated widely, and—following intensive coverage of the first week's clapping—the ritual was observed nationally and repeated on successive Thursday nights for the following nine weeks (Howard 2020). Prime Minister Boris Johnson, who was suffering from COVID-19 and in self-isolation, praised the "inspirational" NHS and stepped out of his apartment on Downing Street to give his support (Clifton 2020), and a video shared by the NHS included messages from Sir Elton John, Sir Paul McCartney, and David Beckham, among others (*Telegraph* 2020).

The Thursday night ritual was designed to allow people to show appreciation for the NHS and other key workers but it also provided an important opportunity for people to engage in a communal custom and meet and talk with neighbors. On the author's normally quiet street, where neighbors value their privacy and largely keep to themselves, residents took part in the clapping each week, staying outside for up to thirty minutes afterward talking and sharing stories as car horns and fireworks echoed around the valley. After a neighbor played a few wartime tunes to celebrate V-E Day, the weekly event developed into a music celebration with the addition of a French horn, a violin, and a guitar (see figure 1.8).

After an initial positive response, as the weeks progressed, the ritual received increasingly negative coverage from political commentators and medical workers as issues with the supply of ventilators and PPE for health workers were reported. Plas decided to bring it to an end after ten weeks, saying that she thought it would be "good to stop it at its peak" amid increasing concerns that the event was becoming politicized: "I think the narrative is starting to change and I don't want the clap to be negative" (Coffey 2020). After the official clapping ended, people on the author's street decided to continue to socialize on Thursday evenings and, the following week, gathered on a neighbor's drive for a socially distanced get-together (heavy rain on the following two Thursdays ultimately ended the ritual).

Shortly after Clap for Carers ended, YouGov research reported that as many as 69 percent of the population had taken part, with 29 percent doing so every week. However, it also revealed that a third of those surveyed felt

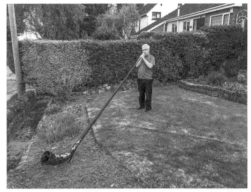

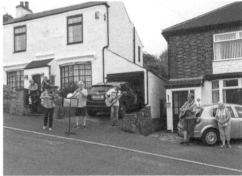

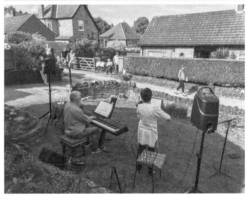

Figure 1.8. Clap for Our Carers (*top and middle*) and V-E Day (*bottom*): Mapperley, Nottingham (originals in color).

the practice had been hijacked for politic gain and the majority (63 percent) felt it was right to end it after the tenth week (Abraham 2020).

Clapping wasn't the only performative expression of communal resilience to be heard echoing around Britain's streets during lockdown. For more than twelve weeks, the town of Belper in Derbyshire held a daily "Moo" at 6:30 every evening, during which people stepped outside their houses to moo like a cow as loudly as they could for two minutes (*BBC*

News: East Midlands 2020). The event was first performed the same week that Clap for Carers began and wasn't expected to last., However, social media allowed the Moo to grow as people posted videos on the event's Facebook page. It became a fun affair attracting large numbers of parents and children every evening and was performed as far afield as Japan, India, and the United States. A competitive element evolved whereby people used smart phone decibel meters to measure the loudness of their moo, with some reaching levels as high as 123.8 decibels.

The bizarreness of the Moo attracted local and national media attention, and a range of souvenirs were sold to raise funds for local charities. The last Moo of the first lockdown took place on Saturday, June 13, but the Moo has been subsequently revived on a number of occasions. A book has been published about the practice and a Moo festival took place in Belper in early June 2021 to raise money for local charities (The Belper Moo 2021).

TEDDY BEARS, SCARECROWS, AND CURBSIDE GIFTS

While rainbows quickly became a national symbol of resilience, community spirit, and support for the NHS, as lockdown continued, many other creative vernacular displays were to be found uncharacteristically displayed in windows, attached to gates and hedges, and installed on driveways and sidewalks across the country. Such displays served multiple functions as people strove to motivate and entertain children while homeschooling; provide interventions to brighten up neighbors' daily walks for exercise; and attempt to break the increasing monotony and stress of the ongoing lockdown. The examples included here, collected by the author from his local neighborhood during lockdown, are representative of many similar others shared and reported from across the country.

On one leafy suburban street in Nottingham, fairy doors appeared at the base of every tree, providing interest for eagle-eyed children on daily walks (see figure 1.9). These survived for over three months, and some are still to be found untouched over a year later. On a nearby street, small inspirational quotes written on rainbow-colored scratch-off cards were pinned at eye level to every tree by an anonymous resident, offering a wealth of philosophical advice to passersby and those visiting the nearby shops (see figure 1.10). The cards contained positive messages such as "A smile is the best make up a girl can wear" and "A day without laughter is a day wasted," along with motivational statements ("It's not whether you get knocked down, it's whether you get up"), advice for dealing with the fear and anxiety of lockdown ("Never let your fear decide your future"),

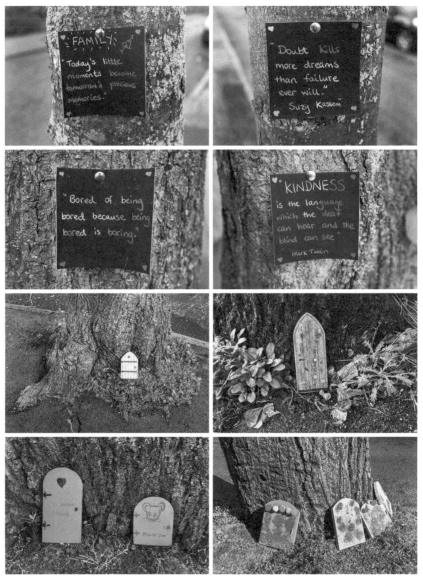

Figure 1.9. Positive quotes on Bennett Road and fairy doors on Kenrick Road, Mapperley, Nottingham.

and professions of communal responsibility ("Act as if what you do today makes a difference—it does!").

Alongside rainbows, teddy bears were also often to be found displayed in people's front windows and gardens as part of a scavenger bear hunt,

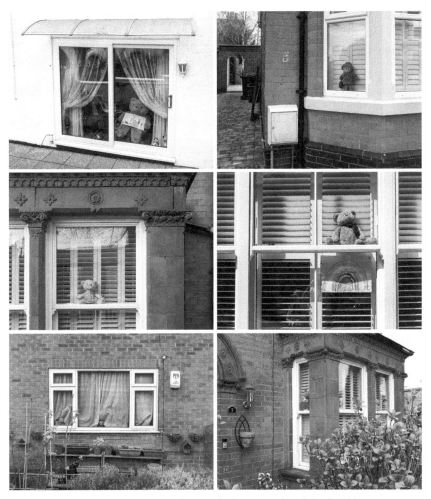

Figure 1.10. Teddy bear hunt, Mapperley, Nottingham, March and April 2020.

an idea again borrowed from elsewhere via social media and news reports (see figure 1.10). The idea was based on existing activities linked to the popular children's book by Michael Rosen, *We're Going on a Bear Hunt*, whose motto is "We're not scared" (Rosen 1993). Lockdown bear hunts may have started in Japan (Linton-Hatfield 2020), but their wider circulation seems to have been prompted by a Facebook post by the public group Project Quarantine (later renamed Project Village), which was started on March 13, 2020 by Lauren Schmidt Ross in Denver, Colorado as a "community space for sharing resources, support, and inspiration to help us all stay strong through the pandemic" (2020). The idea spread quickly via Facebook and

WhatsApp groups, and soon people across the world were organizing bear hunts that were documented and promoted on social media. News reports soon picked up on the trend, ensuring even greater participation. By the end of March, bear hunts were reported in London, Japan, Australia, Germany, Scotland, Reykjavík, Australia, New Zealand, Belgium, the Netherlands, and all fifty states of the US (Fortin 2020). As with many lockdown displays, the activity was designed to keep children entertained and encourage families to go out for walks during isolation, but it also helped preserve a sense of community during lockdown.

The hunt took on added poignancy when it was learned that seventy-four-year-old Michael Rosen, to whom many bear hunters were sending images, was unwell with what he thought was a bad case of the flu. It wasn't revealed until much later that he had actually been suffering from COVID-19, spending seven weeks in intensive care before he slowly recovered (Hattenstone 2020). Although many in the UK participated, bear hunts never gained the same popularity as the displays of rainbows drawings and messages of support for the NHS.

Another common sight during early lockdown and especially the Easter holidays were scarecrows, which began to pop up on suburban streets around the country. Scarecrow festivals and trails are common in the spring and summer in rural villages across the UK as a means of attracting and entertaining visitors and raising funds for local organizations and charities. Festivals are typically themed, often around a topical subject, and villages may provide simple maps and invite visitors to vote for the best display. Kettlewell in the Yorkshire Dales, for example, has been holding an annual scarecrow festival since 1994. The first festival, with displays depicting villagers' professions, was organized to raise funds for the local primary school (Kettlewell Scarecrow Festival 2022). As lockdown continued, many communities in both urban and rural settings organized COVID-19-themed scarecrow trails, providing further displays of unity and resilience, an additional creative activity for parents and children, and further motivation for daily walks.

A sign in Calow near Chesterfield where numerous scarecrows appeared explains: "During the lockdown, why not brighten up the streets of Carlow by making a scarecrow. This will help brighten up Everyone's daily walk" (see figure 1.11). Many scarecrows explored COVID-related themes, showing support for healthcare and other key workers but also providing humorous commentary on subjects such as COVID-related panic buying, government incompetence, and the monotony of lockdown (see figure 1.12).

An NHS superhero wearing a Zorro mask and rainbow wig made by children from a nursery on the site of the royal hospital appeared in Calow,

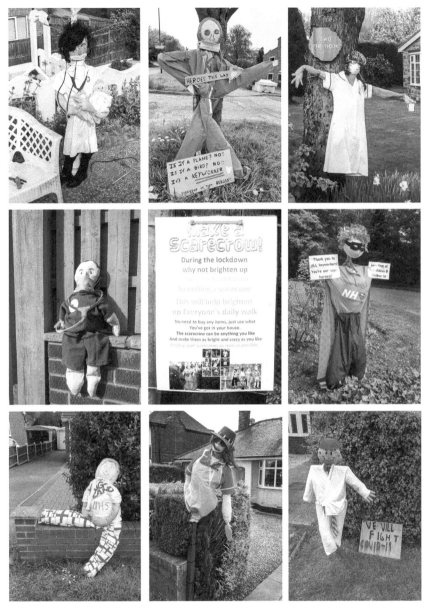

Figure 1.11. COVID-19 scarecrows: Stannington, Derbyshire (*top left;* photograph ©
David Clarke); Greenfield, Saddleworth (*top right;* photograph © Sophie Parkes-Nield); and
Mapperley, Nottingham (*top center*). Scarecrow trail, Calow, Chesterfield (*lower two rows;* pho-
tographs © Andrew Rodgers).

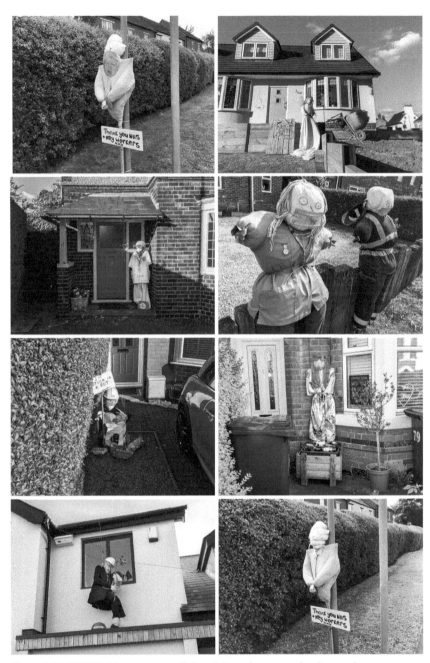

Figure 1.12. COVID-19 scarecrows: all from Mapperley except for the one from Papplewick (*second row right*), Nottinghamshire.

Chesterfield, where another scarecrow in a judo outfit promises to fight COVID-19. Stannington in Sheffield has its own superhero key worker, while a doctor with a stethoscope, wearing a white gown and blue protective gloves, is seen holding a newborn in an Italianate garden in Mapperley, Nottingham. Nearby, a scarecrow seated on a toilet reading a book is down to its last roll of toilet paper (a reminder of panic buying in the early weeks of lockdown). On another street, a woman is floating above a recycling bin overflowing with wine bottles; the accompanying chalkboard reads, "When your bin goes out more than you do" (see figure 1.14). A workman is buried to his knees holding a sign explaining "I'm stuck in a rut" counting off seven weeks of lockdown, while other displays depict health workers as superheroes and angels. One display recounts the embarrassing moment when, as mayor of London, Boris Johnson, with Union flags in hand, got stuck "Like a Damp Towel on the Line" (Addley 2019) above the onlooking crowds while on a zip wire during a photo op for the London 2012 Olympics (Sich 2012).

Crocheted and knitted items also appeared in many places during lockdown, displayed in windows, gardens, and other public places (see figure 1.13). Easter- and summer-themed postbox covers appeared in the village of Burton Joyce near Nottingham, and a tree outside the local store was decorated with crocheted flowers. The gates to the Moravian church in the author's home village of Baildon, West Yorkshire, were adorned with more than a hundred brightly colored crocheted flowers, pom-poms, and knitted dolls made by elderly women members of a church craft group who could no longer meet in person. Crocheted postbox toppers, rarely if ever seen before COVID, have since become a common sight. Knitting groups, Women's Institutes, and Townswomen's Guilds share patterns and coordinate installations online without, it appears, assistance from the Royal Mail. The UK Post Box Toppers and More Facebook group was formed in March 2021 as "a place to share ideas and ask questions about yarn bombing pillar boxes and bollards and anything you can put a hat on in the UK!" and currently has 23,700 members (UK Post Box Toppers and More Group 2022). The resulting crocheted creations often mark the passing of the seasons, with Christmas-, Easter-, and Halloween-themed designs proving popular, or celebrate national events such as the queen's Platinum Jubilee in June 2022 or her passing in September 2022.

As lockdown continued, people used free time to clear out closets, attics, and garages. Because local tips and charity shops were closed, items were left on suburban driveways and pavements for people to take. Fascinating collections of offerings were presented to those on their daily walks (see figure 1.14). One neighbor, slowly clearing out a host of items from both

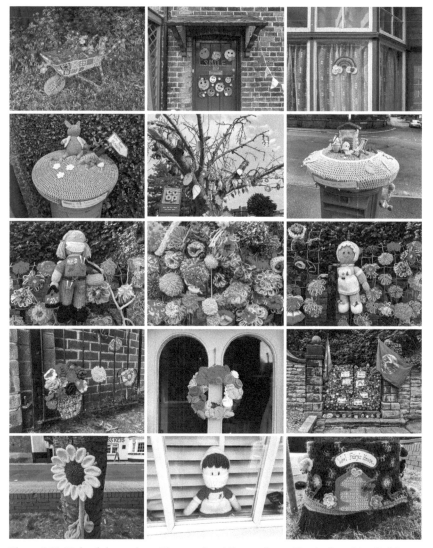

Figure 1.13. Knitted decorations: Sherwood and Burton Joyce, Nottinghamshire; Baildon, West Yorkshire; Castleton, Derbyshire; and Warminster, Wiltshire.

attic and garage, presented weekly offerings on their driveway. While it has become fairly common in recent years for people to leave scrap metal at the edge of their property for collection by metal recyclers, who tour the streets on a regular basis, leaving such a wide range of items outside gates and driveways for neighbors to take for free is a new practice that has continued, albeit on a much smaller scale, post lockdown.

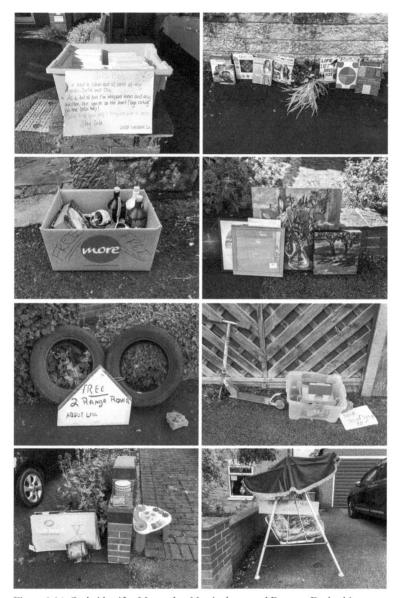

Figure 1.14. Curbside gifts: Mapperley, Nottingham; and Buxton, Derbyshire.

THE BLITZ SPIRIT AND THE CULT OF CAPTAIN TOM

On the Thursday following Easter, after three weeks of lockdown, the UK government announced that restrictions would continue for at least another three weeks, and while there was general support for this, the public was becoming increasingly frustrated with isolation, homeschooling, remote working, and the increasing death toll. Having exhausted the potential of rainbows, teddy bears, and scarecrows, a new distraction was perhaps needed; one arrived in the form of Captain Tom Moore.

On April 6, the ninety-nine-year-old war veteran began to take daily walks, aiming to walk one hundred lengths of his garden before his birth-day twenty-four days later. In doing so, he hoped to raise £1,000 for NHS Charities Together to say thank you for the care he received during recent treatment for a fractured hip and a cancer scare, and as an expression of support for the NHS during the COVID crisis. He reached his initial target in just four days, and media interest increased dramatically following a short interview with singer Michael Ball on BBC Radio 2 on Sunday, April 12. Donations reached £1 million just two days later (Huddleston 2020).

Captain Tom's positive, optimistic outlook, summed up in his oft-repeated phrase "Tomorrow will be a good day" (reminiscent of "Tutto andrà bene"), along with his down-to-earth manner, humor, and strength of personality, led to him becoming a media celebrity overnight. The ritual-istic daily performance of his walk—slowly pushing his walking frame back and forth outside his house—and the rapidly increasing donations led an almost rolling news coverage of the story, with Tom giving more than 150 media interviews and participating in a number of documentaries about his life (*ITV* 2020). He reached his target of one hundred lengths by April 16 and recorded "You'll Never Walk Alone" with Michael Ball, becoming the oldest person ever to have had a UK number one record (*ITV News* 2020a). Captain Tom kept walking, and by the time his JustGiving page closed on the evening of his birthday, he had raised more than £32,796,475 from 1.5 million supporters.

April saw an outpouring of creative vernacular tributes inspired by Captain Tom's achievement and encouraged by the media frenzy surrounding coverage of the story, mainly in the form of portraits in every imaginable style and media, which were displayed in windows, installed in gardens, painted on walls and houses, and widely shared on social media, both while in production and as finished artifacts. Pencil drawings were popular, as were paintings, col-lages, window installations, and sculptures. Many people sent their portraits to Captain Tom; others sold or raffled artwork online to raise funds; and murals celebrating his efforts were painted on walls across the country, including in Pontefract, Abergavenny, Cambourne, Tamworth, and Thetford.

Most representations of Captain Tom were taken from press photo-graphs of his walk, where he was commonly pictured dressed in his blazer adorned with service medals, pushing his walking frame, and giving the thumbs-up gesture. Others portrayed Tom as a dashing mustachioed soldier, based on archive photographs of him taken during World War II, and other potent symbols of the lockdown, including the NHS logo, rainbows, and other wartime references were almost always present.

Sonya and Ian Kinnie of Yarm commissioned graffiti artist Drew Allen to create a painting for the front window of their home including Captain Tom, and Carl Fredricksen (from the Pixar film *Up*) in front of a large rainbow, with Fredricksen's house held aloft by a collection of rainbow-colored balloons. Fredricksen was chosen as "another member of the older generation" who exhibited "true grit and determination, courage in the face of adversity" (Nolan 2020). Other creations were more lighthearted or eccentric; the Welsh artist and social media celebrity Nathan Wyburn creating a "foot painting" of Moore in uniform (Owen 2020), and balloonist Craig Cash sculpted a life-size balloon replica to mark his hundredth lap, sending a version to the captain on his birthday (Fieldhouse 2020).

Time and again, references to Captain Tom's military past and World War II were made. Glen Folan painted Tom pushing his walking frame, wearing his service medals, and casting a shadow of a younger soldier on the wall behind. Jacqueline Hurley's *Tomorrow Will Be a Good Day* pictured Tom leading a line of young soldiers across a black-and-white battlefield with a series of brightly colored sculpted poppies in the foreground, all framed by barbed wire (Winspear 2020). Rosie McLoughlin from Newtownabbey in County Antrim created a window painting with a portrait of Tom alongside a saluting solider instructing viewers to "Salute Our Heroes," accompanied by a Spitfire, a Lancaster bomber, the NHS logo, and a kneeling solider praying beside a wartime grave in a field of poppies (Keenan 2020).

Captain Tom thus provided a focal point for a number of intersecting themes relating to the British experience of the lockdown and isolation, including an expression of national resolve; an attitude of resilience and camaraderie, often mythologized as the "Blitz spirit"; a show of support for the NHS and other key workers; and a life-affirming positive message during COVID. By producing depictions of Captain Tom and displaying them outside their homes, sharing them online, or sending them to Tom himself, the British public celebrated both Tom and his fundraising efforts along with those to whom he was paying tribute. At the same time, the public increasingly mythologized him as a hero supporting other COVID heroes. This hero worship resulted in a wealth of symbolic material artifacts that functioned as expressions of national resolve. Historian Charlie Hall suggests that when under threat or facing crisis or hardship, Britain often looks back to the "moment in history when it overcome its greatest challenge: the second world

war" (quoted in Wood 2020), and Captain Tom, himself a World War II veteran, provided the perfect vehicle for such retrospective expressions, which
chimed with the narrative and messaging promoted by the government.

Early in their response to the spread of the virus, Boris Johnson and
the British government utilized metaphors describing the fight against the
pandemic as a war. In the daily briefing broadcast on March 17, 2020, two
days before all schools were closed and five days before the full lockdown
was imposed, Johnson explained that the government had been forced to
take "steps that are unprecedented since World War II" and that in respond-
ing to the threat of the virus it "must act like any wartime government."
In closing his speech, he consolidated his use of wartime metaphors to
emphasize the need to follow the scientific advice underpinning the government guidelines: "Yes, this enemy can be deadly, but it is also beatable—and
we know how to beat it and we know that if as a country we follow the
scientific advice that is now being given, we know that we will beat it. And
however tough the months ahead, we have the resolve and the resources to
win the fight" (Johnson 2020b).

As Elena Semino (2021) has pointed out, war metaphors have multiple
applications for the pandemic, including the virus as enemy, health professionals as an army, the sick or the dead as casualties, and the elimination of
the virus as a victory. Writing in the *Guardian* on March 21, 2020, Simon
Tisdall suggests that the use of war metaphors "do nothing but breed fear,"
while Henry Irving feels that evoking the Blitz spirt may be actively dangerous, as it could breed a complacency that could make the difference
between life and death, proposing that we need to define a coronavirus
spirit of our own (2020). Dr. Charley Hall (quoted in Wood 2020), while
rejecting the passive response suggested by the omnipresent "Keep Calm
and Carry On" slogan (popularized since the discovery of an unused and
forgotten World War II poster in a bookshop in Alnwick, Northumberland,
in 2000; see Hughes 2009), suggests two active elements of the Blitz spirit
that would be beneficial in a response to COVID-19: first, the importance
of people grasping the seriousness of the situation and adjusting their lifestyles accordingly, and second, adhering to government restrictions and
supporting one another as people did in the Blitz. Semino (2021) suggests
that conflict metaphors, while in many ways problematic, may be relevant
and useful in the early weeks of a pandemic or crisis when "an urgent threat
requires an immediate collective effort"; such metaphors have the power to
help frame complex issues and convey their dangers, promote a sense of
collective responsibility, and justify the imposition of limits on individual
freedom in the service of a common purpose.

The British public got to know Thomas Moore as "Captain Tom," and his exploits were often viewed through a rose-tinted wartime lens, his military service forming an essential part of his narrative. Wartime photographs illustrated his JustGiving page and accompanied numerous media reports, in which he was usually pictured proudly wearing his regimental blazer and the medals received for service in India and Burma during World War II. He'd kept in touch with his regiment, organizing the yearly reunion for sixty-four years, and the Yorkshire Regiment provided a guard of honor on the day he completed his walk. He was made an honorary colonel of the Army Foundation Collage and his birthday was celebrated with two military flypasts over his home. Captain Tom himself used war metaphors to describe his motivation, explaining, "We're a little bit like having a war at the moment. But the doctors and the nurses, they're all on the front line, and all of us behind, we've got to supply them and keep them going with everything that they need, so that they can do their jobs even better than they're doing now" (*BBC News: Beds Herts and Bucks* 2020).

Wartime references were further consolidated by the fact that Captain Tom's fundraising coincided with the buildup to the seventy-fifth celebration of V-E (Victory over Europe) Day on May 5, 2020, an event focusing on national unity and perseverance in times of national crisis. The public was encouraged to create displays, organize street parties, and hang bunting to celebrate the event, which was widely covered in both local and national media (Chamberlain 2020; Lindsay 2020).

Reports on Captain Tom's progress were often broadcasted alongside media coverage of preparations for the V-E Day celebrations and historical retrospectives of the war. He was also immortalized in numerous V-E Day displays, including a bus shelter installation in the rural village of Lambley in Nottinghamshire that also featured Union flags, other V-E Day imagery, and signs showing support for the NHS (see figure 1.15).

As such, Captain Tom provided an ongoing expression of Boris Johnson's metaphoric battle against the virus, with the ninety-nine-year-old war veteran's daily walk and the large amounts of money he raised for the NHS illustrating a hard-fought, single-handed campaign against the viral enemy then invading the country, helping to maintain the "We're all in this together" mentality and further unifying public support for their health heroes. In recognition of his service, he was knighted in person by the queen on July 17, 2020, at Windsor Castle and has since received numerous other awards and accolades, including being featured as Man of the Year on the cover of *GQ Magazine* shortly before his unfortunate death from COVID on February 2, 2021.

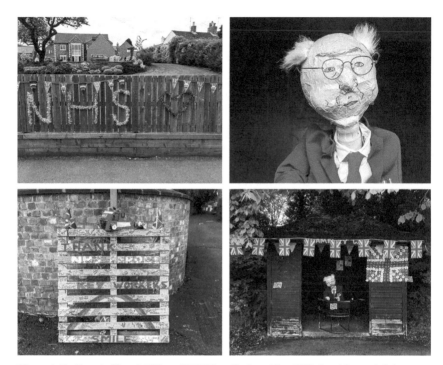

Figure 1.15. Captain Tom, NHS, and V-E Day displays, May 2020, Lambley and Calverton (*bottom left*), Nottinghamshire.

SNAKES AND VILLAINS

On May 10, after seven weeks of lockdown, the UK government announced that restrictions would continue until at least the middle of June before a slow and progressive lifting could take place (Johnson 2020d). As May progressed and people took advantage of the increased freedom to meet outdoors, a new COVID custom began to be reported in the press: the creation of "COVID-19 snakes"—links of brightly painted pebbles in public parks and gardens across the country. In Buxton, Derbyshire, a COVID snake gradually grew along the side of the Pavilion Gardens, amassing more than two thousand pebbles and remaining until autumn. Similar snakes have appeared in other towns.

As with other COVID displays, many stones represented three key COVID themes: rainbows, messages of support for the NHS, and further tributes to Captain Tom. The Buxton stone snake, for instance, included a wide range of creatively painted stones, the majority depicting positive symbols such as suns, brightly colored flowers, bumblebees, and numerous rainbows accompanied by related phrases such as "Bring me sunshine,"

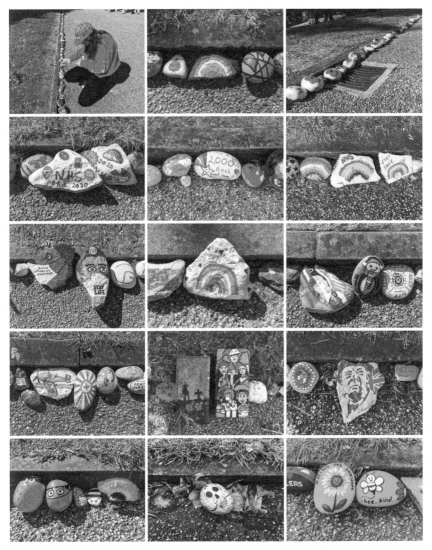

Figure 1.16. COVID stone snake, Pavilion Gardens, Buxton, Derbyshire, May 2020.

"Bee kind," and "Stay safe" (see figure 1.16). There were many representations of masked NHS practitioners and key workers. A number of stones referenced the war and V-E Day, including numerous poppy stones, a painting of a Spitfire, a portrait of Churchill, and another of a soldier before a grave in a field of poppies alongside the phrase "Lest we forget, 75 years." Only one with a more negative message was to be seen: a stone painted with a skull's face staring up ominously from the path.

As the first UK lockdown of 2020 began to draw to a close in late May and early June, the positive "Keep Calm and Carry On" attitude of the early weeks had already began to fade, fueled in part by boredom and frustration but also by increasing accounts of government mismanagement, incompetence, and cronyism along with the widespread sharing of conspiracy theories. The murder of George Floyd on May 25 in the Powderhorn Park neighborhood of Minneapolis, Minnesota, and the resulting lockdown-breaking demonstrations and statue toppling further added to the general unrest; posters supporting Black Lives Matter appeared alongside rainbows in some windows. This all added to a growing sense of frustration, anger, and despair at both the situation in general and the UK government in particular. The weather may also have had an influence; in 2020, Britain experienced the warmest spring and April on record before the weather finally broke in the first week of June (Madge 2020).

If Captain Tom Moore had arrived as a hero to act as a focus for positive feelings of resolve during the first half of lockdown, the second half had a villain in the form of the prime minister's special advisor Dominic Cummings, who became a focus for the growing anger and disillusionment at the government and wider establishment. The full glare of the media spotlight was shone on Cummings when it was revealed that in late March, just after the UK lockdown had begun, he had traveled the length of the country in breach of the government's own lockdown rules to visit his family in Durham at a point when he believed both he and his wife had just contracted the virus (Weaver 2020). This was followed by a further breach of the rules when he took his family for a drive to enjoy the river views at Barnard Castle—allegedly to test his eyesight following his illness—leading to numerous public displays of dissent. Further creative interventions utilizing effigies of Cummings became popular, such as Jason Hall's cutout figures of Cummings, which appeared in and around Nottingham (Locker 2020). The story dragged on, especially in the tabloid press, and for many people the "Cummings Effect" undermined both their trust in the government and their willingness to continue to follow the lockdown guidelines. The UK government experienced a dramatic nine-point drop in the polls in a single week, and one in three of those who broke lockdown rules at this time cited Cummings as justification (Curtis 2020).

A phased reopening of schools began on June 1, with nonessential shops reopening on the June 15 before most restrictions were lifted on June 23, 2020. By this time, the COVID customs and creative interventions so characteristic of the first stage of the lockdown had largely ceased, and they failed to return in the subsequent lockdowns that followed in the autumn of 2020 and the spring of 2021.

SUMMARY

The production of lockdown artifacts along with the performative aspects of their display in both physical and virtual worlds and the ritual performance of clapping (and mooing) provided both individuals and groups with membership of a wider community through replication and repetition of established tropes. At the same time, such activities provided opportunity for participants to assert their individuality through the form, materials, and expressions chosen. These physical, tangible, real-world activities occupied legitimate space and time in the lives of those who took part in both making and viewing them, while at the same time being inspired by and shared via online forums and social media. The rainbows, bear hunts, and clapping were no sooner begun in one small neighborhood in one particular country than they were being adopted in communities around the world, often within less than twenty-four hours, with local adaptions and modifications of both meaning and expression.

While the vernacular British response to the first lockdown had many similarities with that of other countries—and indeed activities were often inspired by reports from those that had entered lockdown earlier—activities across the UK and the resulting material culture they produced nevertheless acquired a distinctive British flavor. Central to this were the numerous demonstrations of support for and solidarity with the NHS and other key workers along with the numerous references to a sense of national resolve embodied in the notion of the "Blitz spirit." This was evoked by the use of wartime metaphors and further consolidated thanks to the efforts of Captain Tom and the celebration of V-E Day in early May. Captain Tom himself became mythologized as a hero representing both the nation's sense of resolve and the belief that "tomorrow will be a good day." Conversely, the prime minister's special advisor Dominic Cummings become mythologized as an anti-hero representing the hypocrisy, entitlement, and incompetence that many accused the government of in its mismanagement of the crisis.

The vast majority of the artifacts produced during lockdown were ordinary and utilitarian in their artistry and production. Drawings, paintings, and other creations were shared on social media and reported in the press not on the basis of their artistic merit, craftsmanship, or aesthetic value, but rather on their symbolic meaning and their contribution to an ongoing narrative of resilience, support for the NHS, and celebration of Captain Tom. Time and again, when interviewed about their motivation for engaging in these lockdown customs and rituals and the benefits this brought, people provided very similar explanations: to occupy both parent and child, to provide an outlet for feelings about the pandemic and lockdown, to give a purpose to daily walks for exercise, to structure and maintain a sense of local community during lockdown and isolation, and to provide a sense of belonging to a wider worldwide online community.

The sense of community, belonging, and escape these activities offered was an important part of many people's experiences of lockdown, providing key benefits during an unprecedented time of worldwide anxiety and concern. Writing in the *Guardian*, Rafael Behr (2020) suggests that the changes wrought by our response to the virus, including the customs and rituals observed during the lockdown, are "cultural rather than political" and that "societies are shaped by custom and ritual as much as they are held together by legislation." Concerning the impact of the lockdown on the individual mind, he warns that we should not "underestimate the aggregate effect of curtailing millions upon millions of micro-niceties," such as a handshake, a slap on the back, or sharing food, which "exercised muscles of empathy and diplomacy." Public engagement in the COVID-related customs and activities discussed here perhaps provided opportunities for new forms of "micro-niceties" in which residents could show solidarity with their neighbors and maintain contact with their wider community at a time when they were unable to mix with friends, colleagues, and others in normal ways.

If, as Grassby (2005) has suggested, material objects can provide a defense against a "fleeting memory and a precarious identity in a mutable world," then the physical artifacts created during lockdown and their online sharing might well have functioned to provide people with a reminder of pre-COVID times, acting as a means of solidifying individual and communal identity and hope when we were threatened by lockdown restrictions and facing an uncertain future.

ACKNOWLEDGMENTS

I would like to extend my thanks to my colleagues at the Centre for Contemporary Legend at Sheffield Hallam University for their help and advice while I was writing this chapter, in particular to Dr. David Clarke, Diane Rodgers, Sophie Parkes-Nield, and Andrew Rodgers for permission to use their photographs, and to Sophie for proofreading the draft. A special thank-you to my daughter Beatrice for accompanying me on our daily "COVID walks," during which most of these photographs were taken and the ideas originated. This research was supported by the Department of Media and Communication at Sheffield Hallam University. All photographs © Andrew Robinson unless otherwise noted.

REFERENCES

Abraham, Tanya. 2020. "Third of Britons Think Clap for Carers Has Been Politicised." *YouGov*, June 4. https://yougov.co.uk/topics/politics/articles-reports/2020/06/04/third-britons-think-clap-carers-has-been-politicis.

Addley, Esther. 2019. "'Like a Damp Towel on a Line': The Day Boris Johnson Got Stuck on a Zip Wire." *Guardian*, July 16. https://www.theguardian.com/politics/2019/jul/16/stuck-zip-wire-boris-johnson-london-2012-olympics.

Aspinall, Evie. 2020. "COVID-19 Timeline." *British Foreign Policy Group*, April 8. https://bfpg.co.uk/2020/04/COVID-19-timeline.

Associazione Amici di Aldo Capitini. 2003. "La bandiera della Pace." https://web.archive.org/web/20030618184553/http://www.comitatopace.it/materiali/bandieradella pace.htm.

BBC News: Beds Herts and Bucks. 2020. "Coronavirus: Captain Tom Moore Raises More Than £9m for NHS." April 15. https://www.bbc.co.uk/news/uk-england-beds-bucks-herts-52290076.

BBC News: East Midlands. 2020. "Coronavirus: Belper Moo Relieves Lockdown Misery." April 11. https://www.bbc.co.uk/news/uk-england-derbyshire-52252003.

BBC News: England. 2020. "Coronavirus: Rainbow Pictures Springing Up across the Country." March 21. https://www.bbc.co.uk/news/uk-england-51988671.

BBC News: Leeds. 2020. "Families Decorate Windows with Rainbows to Cheer People." March 23. https://www.bbc.co.uk/news/av/uk-england-leeds-52008155.

BBC News: Suffolk. 2020. "Coronavirus: Rainbow Trail Success Surprises Ipswich Mum." April 11. https://www.bbc.co.uk/news/uk-england-suffolk-52214965.

Behr, Rafael. 2020. "The Lockdown in Our Minds Will Be the Last Restriction to Be Lifted." *Guardian*, April 28. https://www.theguardian.com/commentisfree/2020/apr/28/lockdown-restrictions-solidarity-coronavirus-social-distancing.

The Belper Moo. 2021. Facebook. https://www.facebook.com/thebelpermoo.

Benedict XVI. 2010. "Julian of Norwich—General Audience." *The Vatican*, December 1. https://www.vatican.va/content/benedict-xvi/en/audiences/2010/documents/hf_ben-xvi_aud_20101201.html.

Bhatti, Mark, Andrew Church, and Amanda Claremont. 2014. "Peaceful, Pleasant and Private: The British Domestic Garden as an Ordinary Landscape." *Landscape Research* 39 (1): 40–52. https://doi.org/10.1080/01426397.2012.759918.

Byrne. Lenny. 2019. "The NHS Rainbow Badge—What Does It Mean?" *University Hospitals Plymouth NHS Trust.* https://www.plymouthhospitals.nhs.uk/nhs-rainbow-badge.

Chamberlain, Zoe. 2020. "15 VE Day Party Ideas You Can Enjoy in Your Home and Garden." *Birmingham Live*, May 7. https://www.birminghammail.co.uk/whats-on/family-kids-news/15-ve-day-party-ideas-18211531.

Charlton-Dailey, Rachel. 2021. "The Pandemic Is Easing. Give the 'NHS Rainbow' Back to the LGBT Community." *HuffPost*, April 23. https://www.huffingtonpost.co.uk/entry/nhs-rainbow-flag_uk_60828b2de4b0e7cb020dcee1.

Clifton, Katy. 2020. "Boris Johnson Hails 'Inspirational' NHS as He Claps for Key Workers on Downing Street Doorstep during Self-Isolation." *Evening Standard*, April 2. https://www.standard.co.uk/news/uk/boris-johnson-self-isolation-clap-for-nhs-a4405676.html.

Coffey, Helen, 2020. "Clap for Our Carers Event Should Stop After Next Thursday, Says Founder." *Independent*, May 23. https://www.independent.co.uk/life-style/clap-our-carers-thursday-event-stop-nhs-coronavirus-annemarie-plas-a9528596.html.

Crampton, Georgia Ronan, ed. 1994. *The Shewings of Julian of Norwich.* Kalamazoo, MI: Medieval Institute Publications.

Curtis, Chris. 2020. "How Dominic Cummings' Lockdown Travels Changed Public Opinion." *iNews*, May 28. https://inews.co.uk/opinion/dominic-cummings -lockdown-durham-public-opinion-431599.

Department of Health and Social Care. 2020. "Coronavirus Public Information Campaign Launched across the UK." February 3. https://www.gov.uk/government/news /coronavirus-public-information-campaign-launched-across-the-uk.

Elizabeth II. 2020. "The Queen's Broadcast to the UK and Commonwealth." *Royal.UK*, April 5. https://www.royal.uk/queens-broadcast-uk-and-commonwealth.

Fieldhouse, John. 2020. "Father and Daughter Salute Captain Tom Moore with Their Balloon Skills!" *Lincolnshire World*, April 20. https://www.lincolnshireworld.com /news/people/father-and-daughter-salute-captain-tom-moore-with-their-balloon -skills-2543953.

Fortin, Jacey. 2020. "Children Are Hunting Teddy Bears during the Coronavirus Outbreak." *New York Times*, April 3. https://www.nytimes.com/2020/04/03/style /teddy-bear-scavenger-hunt.html.

Fox, Kate. 2004. *Watching the English: The Hidden Rules of English Behaviour.* London: Hodder & Stoughton.

Francis. 2016. "The Easter Triduum during the Jubilee of Mercy—General Audience." *The Vatican*, March 23. https://www.vatican.va/content/francesco/en/audiences/2016 /documents/papa-francesco_20160323_udienza-generale.html.

Furukawa, Yuki, and Rei Kansaku. 2020. "Amabié—A Japanese Symbol of the COVID-19 Pandemic." *JAMA* 324 (6): 531–33. https://jamanetwork.com/journals/jama/full article/2768645#247314471.

Grassby, Richard. 2005. "Material Culture and Cultural History." *Journal of Interdisciplinary History* 35 (4): 591–603.

Guardian. 2020. "'Wuhan Jiāyóu': Chants of Solidarity Spread across City at Epicentre of Coronavirus." January 28. https://www.theguardian.com/science/video/2020/jan /28/wuhan-jiayou-chants-of-solidarity-spread-across-city-at-epicentre-of-corona virus-video.

Guy's and St Thomas' NHS Foundation Trust. 2018. "Have You Spotted Our NHS Rainbow Badges?" *Guy's and St Thomas' NHS Foundation Trust.* https://www.guys andstthomas.nhs.uk/about-us/equality/nhs-rainbow-badges.aspx.

Haag, Matthew. 2017. "Gilbert Baker, Gay Activist Who Created the Rainbow Flag, Dies at 65." *New York Times*, March 31. https://www.nytimes.com/2017/03/31/us/obituary -gilbert-baker-rainbow-flag.html.

Hattenstone, Simon. 2020. "Michael Rosen on His COVID-19 Coma: It Felt Like a Pre-Death, a Nothingness." *Guardian*, September 30. https://www.theguardian.com /books/2020/sep/30/michael-rosen-on-his-COVID-19-coma-it-felt-like-a-pre -death-a-nothingness.

Howard, Harry. 2020. "Let's Clap for the NHS EVERY Week." *Mail Online*, March 27. https://www.dailymail.co.uk/news/article-8159617/Dutch-yoga-teacher-started -Clap-Carers-movement-wants-repeat-Thursday.html.

Huddleston, Gemma. 2020. "Captain Tom Moore's 100th Birthday Walk for the NHS." *Just Giving*, March. https://www.justgiving.com/fundraising/tomswalk.

Hughes, Stuart. 2009. "The Greatest Motivational Poster Ever?" *BBC News Magazine*, February 4. http://news.bbc.co.uk/1/hi/magazine/7869458.stm.

Irving, Henry. 2020. "Blitz Spirit Won't Help 'Win the Fight' against COVID-19." *History and Policy, Opinion Articles*, March 20. https://www.historyandpolicy.org/opinion -articles/articles/blitz-spirit-wont-help-win-the-fight-against-COVID-19.

ITV. 2020. "Captain Tom's War." May 8. https://web.archive.org/web/20200513113250 /https://www.itv.com/hub/captain-toms-war/10a0141a0001.

ITV News. 2020a. "Captain Tom Moore and Michael Ball Land UK Number One with Charity Single." April 19. https://www.itv.com/news/anglia/2020-04-19/captain -tom-moore-and-michael-ball-land-uk-number-one-with-charity-single.

ITV News. 2020b. "Government Launches New Coronavirus Advert with Stay at Home or 'People Will Die' Message." April 2. https://www.itv.com/news/2020-04-02/stay-at -home-or-people-will-die-government-launches-new-coronavirus-ad-blitz.

Johnson, Boris. 2020a. "Prime Minister's Statement on Coronavirus (COVID-19): 16 March 2020." *Prime Minister's Office, 10 Downing Street,* March 16. https://www.gov .uk/government/speeches/pm-statement-on-coronavirus-16-march-2020.

Johnson, Boris. 2020b. "Prime Minister's Statement on Coronavirus (COVID-19): 17 March 2020." *Prime Minister's Office, 10 Downing Street,* March 17. https://www.gov .uk/government/speeches/pm-statement-on-coronavirus-17-march-2020.

Johnson, Boris. 2020c. "Prime Minister's Statement on Coronavirus (COVID-19): 23 March 2020." *Prime Minister's Office, 10 Downing Street,* March 23. https://www.gov .uk/government/speeches/pm-address-to-the-nation-on-coronavirus-23-march -2020.

Johnson, Boris. 2020d. "Prime Minister's Statement on Coronavirus (COVID-19): 10 May 2020." *Prime Minister's Office, 10 Downing Street,* May 10. https://www.gov.uk/govern- ment/speeches/pm-address-to-the-nation-on-coronavirus-10-may-2020.

Keenan, Shaun. 2020. "Captain Tom Moore Tribute Appears on Co. Antrim Window." *Belfast Live,* April 24. https://www.belfastlive.co.uk/news/captain-tom-moore -tribute-appears-18140756.

Kettlewell Scarecrow Festival. 2022. https://www.kettlewellscarecrowfestival.co.uk/history .php.

Kuhn, Anthony. 2020. "In Japan, Mythical 'Amabie' Emerges from Nineteenth-Century Folklore to Fight COVID-19." *National Public Radio,* April 22. https://www.npr.org /sections/coronavirus-live-updates/2020/04/22/838323775/in-japan-mythical-am abie-emerges-from-19th-century-folklore-to-fight-COVID-19?t=1625246847208.

Lindsay, Kali. 2020. "VE Day 2020: How You Can Celebrate the 75th Anniversary of VE Day during Lockdown." *Chronicle Live,* May 3. https://www.chroniclelive.co.uk /whats-on/ve-day-2020-how-you-18189414.

Linton-Hatfield, Danielle. 2020. "Project 2020 Quarantine—Bear Hunt." *Marshall Democrat-News* [Missouri], March 27. https://www.marshallnews.com/gallery/36878.

Locker, Joseph. 2020. "You're Disposable, I'm Essential—Dominic Cummings Cutout Tied to Left Lion." *Nottingham Post,* May 31. https://www.nottinghampost.com /news/nottingham-news/frustrated-artist-who-feels-hes-4178451.

Maccioni, Riccardo. 2020. "Coronavirus. 'Andrà tutto bene': dalla visione della beata Giuliana lo slogan antivirus." *Avvenire,* March 17. https://www.avvenire.it/chiesa /pagine/andra-tutto-bene-ecco-com-e-nata-la-frase.

MacLellan, Kylie. 2020. "Britons to Laud Healthcare Workers with Nationwide Applause." *Reuters,* March 26. https://www.reuters.com/article/health-coronavirus-britain -applause-idINKBN21D1Q0.

Madge, Grahame. 2020. "May 2020 Becomes the Sunniest Calendar Month on Record." *Met Office,* June 1. https://www.metoffice.gov.uk/about-us/press-office/news /weather-and-climate/2020/2020-spring-and-may-stats.

Moss, Rachel. 2020. "Rainbow Trails Are Popping Up Everywhere." *HuffPost,* March 31. https://www.huffingtonpost.co.uk/entry/rainbow-trails-artwork-the-story_uk _5e8202e5c5b6256a7a2e8db2.

MoVimento 5 Stelle. 2020. "Andrà tutto bene, ecco dove è nata la frase della speranza!" *Il blog delle stelle,* March 23. https://www.ilblogdellestelle.it/2020/03/andra-tutto-bene -ecco-dove-e-nata-la-frase-della-speranza.html.

Nolan, Laura. 2020. "Yarm Couple Have Artwork Made for Captain Tom Moore." *Northern Echo*, April 23. https://www.thenorthernecho.co.uk/news/18400747.yarm -couple-artwork-made-captain-tom-moore/.

Osborne, Samuel. 2016. "Danny Boyle Claims Tories Tried to Axe NHS Celebration in London 2012 Olympics Opening Ceremony." *Independent*, July 10. https://www.inde-pendent.co.uk/news/uk/politics/danny-boyle-nhs-celebration-tories-london-2012 -olympics-opening-ceremony-a7129186.html.

Owen, Cathy. 2020. "Watch the Amazing Painting of Captain Tom Britain's Got Talent Artist Makes Using Only His Feet." *Wales Online*, April 19. https://www.walesonline .co.uk/news/wales-news/captain-tom-nhs-amazing-painting-18113980.

Ramirez, Janina. 2016. *Julian of Norwich: A Very Brief History*. London: SPCK.

Reuters. 2020. "Timeline—How the Global Coronavirus Pandemic Unfolded." September 9. https://www.reuters.com/article/health-coronavirus-timeline -idUSL1N2GN04J.

Rigby, Nic. 2020. "Coronavirus: Mystic's 'Relevance' to Self-Isolating World." *BBC News, East*, March 30. https://www.bbc.co.uk/news/uk-england-norfolk-52020227.

Roberts, Kezia. 2020. "About—Chase the Rainbow Horsforth." *Facebook*. https://www .facebook.com/groups/823432101484731/about.

Rosen, Michael. 1993. *We're Going on a Bear Hunt*. London: Walker Books.

Ross, Lauren. 2020. "Project Village." *Facebook*. https://www.facebook.com/groups /projectvillage/about.

Saunders, Rebecca. 2020. "Amabie: The Japanese Monster Going Viral." *BBC Travel*, April 23. https://www.bbc.com/travel/article/20200422-amabie-the-japanese-mon-ster-going-viral.

Scarlett, Sara, and Tiffany Wallis. 2020. "Mother's Plea to Cheer Up the Community Leads to Thousands of Households across the UK Putting Children's Rainbow Paintings in Their Windows." *Mail Online*, March 20. https://www.dailymail.co.uk/news/article -8135805/Mothers-plea-cheer-leads-Chase-Rainbow-campaign.html.

Semino, Elena. 2021. "Not Soldiers but Fire-fighters—Metaphors and COVID-19." *Health Communication* 36 (1): 50–58. https://doi.org/10.1080/10410236.2020.1844989.

Sharma, Sonia. 2020. "Why Rainbow Paintings Are Popping Up in North East Windows during Coronavirus Crisis." *Chronicle Live*, March 23. https://www.chroniclelive.co .uk/whats-on/family-kids-news/why-rainbow-trail-windows-coronavirus-17965407.

Sheridan, Simon. 2004. *The A-Z of Classic Children's Television: From Alberto Frog to Zebedee*. Richmond, UK: Reynolds & Hearn.

Sich, Adam. 2012. "Mayor of London Boris Johnson Gets Stuck on a London 2012 Olympic Games Zip Line in Victoria Park." *On Demand News*. YouTube, August 2. https://www.youtube.com/watch?v=3hRwnXmdRCo.

Taylor, James Piers. 2020. "Rally round the Flag." *WordPress*, May 8. https://jamespierstay-lor.wordpress.com/2020/05/08/rally-round-the-flag/.

Telegraph. 2020. "Clap for Our Carers: Celebrities Thank NHS Staff in Heartwarming Video." YouTube, April 9. https://www.youtube.com/watch?v=q7WBssQ8Nps.

Tisdall, Simon. 2020. "Lay Off Those War Metaphors, World Leaders. You Could Be the Next Casualty." *Guardian*, March 21. https://www.theguardian.com/commentisfree /2020/mar/21/donald-trump-boris-johnson-coronavirus.

Toynbee, Polly. 2019. "These Brutal Cuts to the NHS Will Haunt the Conservatives." *Guardian*, October 25. https://www.theguardian.com/commentisfree/2019/oct/25 /boris-johnson-conservatives-nhs-funding.

UK Post Box Toppers and More Group. 2022. "About." *Facebook*. https://en-gb.facebook .com/groups/876920579707070/about.

Vinci, Alessandro. 2020. "Coronavirus, spuntano in Lombardia decine di biglietti solidali anonimi: 'Tutto andrà bene!'" *Corriere della sera*, March 5. https://www.corriere.it /tecnologia/20_marzo_05/coronavirus-spuntano-lombardia-decine-biglietti-solidali -anonimi-tutto-andra-bene-a29b7edc-5ed0-11ea-bf24-0daffe9dc780.shtml.

Wallis, Tiffany. 2020. "Chase the Rainbow—Kids' Drawings of Rainbows Placed in Thousands of Windows across UK to Lift Spirits in Coronavirus Crisis." *Sun*, March 20. https://www.thesun.co.uk/news/11218992/children-rainbow-drawings -windows-coronavirus/.

Weaver, Matthew. 2020. "Pressure on Dominic Cummings to Quit over Lockdown Breach." *Guardian*, May 22. https://www.theguardian.com/politics/2020/may/22 /dominic-cummings-durham-trip-coronavirus-lockdown.

Winspear, Paul. 2020. "Captain Sir Tom Moore's 100th Birthday Portraits to Be Auctioned by Sworders to Raise Money for His Own Charity." *Bishop's Stortford Independent*, October 30. https://www.bishopsstortfordindependent.co.uk/whats-on/sworders -to-auction-off-captain-sir-tom-100th-birthday-portraits-for-charity-9128459/.

Wood, Sam. 2020. "The Reality of Blitz Spirit during COVID-19." *University of Kent News Centre*, May 5. https://www.kent.ac.uk/news/society/25315/expert-comment-the -reality-of-blitz-spirit-during-COVID-19.

2

Silver Linings
Chronicling Cultural Sustainability at the Geographic
Center of North America

Troyd Geist, Pieper Bloomquist, and James I. Deutsch

THE GEOGRAPHIC CENTER OF NORTH AMERICA LIES somewhere in North Dakota—though residents may dispute whether its exact location is closer to Rugby, as calculated by the US Geological Survey in 1928, the aptly named Center, some 150 miles southwest, or even the tiny community of Orrin, 30 miles south, where a resident built a large stone shrine commemorating an apparition he had of the Virgin Mary declaring that his farmstead was the actual center (Daley 2017). Accordingly, when the state recorded its first positive test for COVID-19 on March 11, 2020, it was clear that the disease had penetrated from elsewhere to the heart and soul of North America (North Dakota Department of Health 2020).

North Dakota is a large, rural, sparsely populated state with an abundance of open spaces, which the state's residents cherish. North Dakota is also known for its rich cultural heritage, where one's ethnic background, identity, and traditions are steadfastly and proudly held. After all, this is a state whose Ukrainian American *pysanka* (Easter egg) artists visited Ukraine after the dissolution of the former Soviet Union, which had suppressed religious and ethnic identity, to reteach the millennia-old art form to their long-separated family members.

The separation of family members, friends, and colleagues during the coronavirus pandemic of 2020 and beyond brought significant challenges to the lives of North Dakotans—as it did to life throughout the United States. Not surprisingly, many North Dakotans relied on their cultural and artistic heritage to connect with each other—both culturally and socially—to adapt, better understand, and cope with the worst viral pandemic in more than one hundred years.

https://doi.org/10.7330/9781646424818.c002

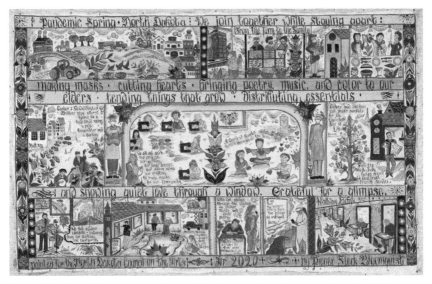

Figure 2.1. Pieper Bloomquist's painting *Silver Linings* chronicles cultural sustainability during the pandemic. (Photo courtesy of NDCA.)

This chapter explores the artistic practices, traditions, and cultural heritage of both individuals and communities during the first months of the pandemic in North Dakota. As elsewhere, the interactions of artists and musicians within community and individual traditions were reimagined to sustain culture and to meet the emotional, physical, and spiritual needs of the state's citizens. These interactions and connections were particularly important to elders in care facilities, who were especially vulnerable to the illness.

The essay highlights several examples of cultural sustainability and healing—primarily through the support of the Folk Arts and Art for Life programs of the North Dakota Council on the Arts (NDCA). One theme that unites these examples is how traditional artistic expressions have helped North Dakotans not only to better understand the pandemic, but also to ameliorate their isolation. As a result, Art for Life became "art for health and wellness" in many communities throughout North Dakota. In a state where empty spaces abound, the NDCA's programs brought people together at a time when those connections were most needed.

Medical practitioners and therapists have thoroughly documented some of the most important connections between art and wellness, especially among aging populations. For instance, Dr. Gene Cohen, a pioneer in the field of geriatric psychiatry at the George Washington University

Center on Health, Aging, and Humanities, reported that "professionally conducted, community-based, cultural programs resulted in higher overall ratings for physical health, fewer doctor visits, less medication use, fewer instances of falls, fewer miscellaneous health problems, better morale, less loneliness, and increased activity for the participants" (Geist 2017, 27). One explanation, according to Cohen, is that "the arts provide some of the best opportunities to experience a new sense of control or mastery. In the arts, the opportunities to create something new and beautiful are endless and offer an enormous sense of satisfaction and empowerment"—and this has positive effects on the immune system (Cohen 2006, 9).

Similarly, Dr. Charles B. Hall of Albert Einstein College of Medicine in New York studied individuals in their seventies and eighties who were engaged in "leisure activities . . . defined as activities that individuals engage in for enjoyment or well-being, independent of work or activities of daily living," such as playing music or games that were mentally challenging (Hall et al. 2009, 357). The results demonstrated that although "participating in these activities did not prevent the onset of Alzheimer's disease, it may have delayed the rapid memory loss, thinking problems, and other symptoms that occur with the disease" (Geist 2017, 29).

Further support for the importance of social engagement comes from a research team at Brigham Young University (BYU) that observed, "Being socially connected is not only influential for psychological and emotional well-being but it also has a significant and positive influence on physical well-being and overall longevity" (Holt-Lunstad et al. 2015, 227). The researchers concluded that "the increased likelihood of death was 26% for reported loneliness, 29% for social isolation, and 32% for living alone" (233).

At a time when the coronavirus pandemic was forcing elderly individuals to isolate and quarantine in care facilities—which is exactly what the BYU team advised against—the NDCA's Art for Life program safely brought people together in ways that helped to relieve their loneliness and isolation.

Moreover, the NDCA commissioned folk artist Pieper Bloomquist of Grand Forks, North Dakota, in 2020 to commemorate individual and community responses to the historic pandemic through the exquisite technique of Swedish *bonadsmålning*. Some of the scenes documented by Bloomquist are specific to the state and represented with images of real people, while others are shared across the country and globally. Using her own gesso substrate and egg tempera paints, Bloomquist created a forty-two-by-sixty-three-inch bonadsmålning painting on linen titled *Silver Linings* (see figure 2.2). The images or stories are divided into three broad panels that encapsulate the emotions and interactions: (1) Pandemic Spring North Dakota—We

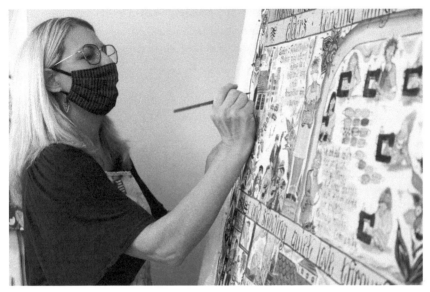

Figure 2.2. Wearing a mask, Pieper Bloomquist paints *Silver Linings*. (Photo courtesy of NDCA.)

join together while staying apart; (2) making masks, cutting hearts, bringing poetry, music, and color to our elders, tending things that grow, distributing essentials; (3) showing quiet love through a window, grateful for a glimpse.

By way of background, bonadsmålning is a traditional style of painting whereby important biblical, allegorical, community, family, and historical events are commemorated in a series of colorful framed images. In Sweden, especially from the mid-eighteenth to the mid-nineteenth century, the paintings, typically made of paper or linen, "were hung in peasants' homes at various times of the year, or . . . were permanently fastened to the walls, in imitation of aristocratic tapestries and wall paintings" (MacBrayne 1972, 85). Their distinctive stylistic features include the use of multiple narrow panels or borders featuring various events happening simultaneously; panels divided by horizontal script in Fraktur-type font with calligraphic designs; floral, circle clouds, and drapery motifs used as fillers throughout; and compact design displaying the *horror vacui* (fear of empty spaces) common in medieval tapestry designs, especially in northern Europe.

In contrast to some of the broader spatial effects common in Italian Renaissance art, artists in northern Europe "maintained a more medieval and decorative horror vacui coupled with multiple, static narratives climbing flattened compositions" (Adelson 2002, 522). The result is what one scholar termed "the collective conception of medieval art as a paragon of crowded spaces, which strives . . . to plug and veneer every possible gap by whatever means necessary, generating meanings through sheer profusion." (Gertsman 2018, 801). Some of the best-known manifestations include "book margins teeming with grotesques, the profusion of sculpture on church portals, [and] images colonizing road interstices on maps" (801).

Needless to say, medieval artists had to contend not only with a metaphorical horror vacui but also, and more precariously, with the literal horror of widespread plagues and pandemics that dwarf today's coronavirus pandemic in both scope and scale. For instance, the bubonic plague (known as the Black Death) that ravaged Europe in the fourteenth century caused "Europe's population [to fall] from 94 million in 1300 to 68 million in 1400, a drop of more than a quarter," according to one estimate (Scheidel 2017, 296). One much higher estimate is that perhaps between "75 and 200 million people died in a few years' time, starting in 1348 when the plague reached London" (Shipman 2014, 410).

Whatever the numbers, one response to the Black Death from the artistic community was to venerate "those saints deemed to be most willing to intercede on behalf of suffering humankind" (Snowden 2019, 65). Particularly meaningful was Saint Sebastian, who was "tied to a stake for his faith, while archers pierced his body with arrows, which were a conventional symbol for plague" (66). While millions were dying of the plague, and as the "bonds of community broke down during the pestilence, the example of a heroic martyr who had confronted death without flinching was comforting" (66).

The reference to a degree of comfort provided by artists amid this horror also brings to mind the observation about the plague made by the *National Enquirer*, one of the highest-circulation newspapers of the late twentieth century. Its headline of May 6, 1986, proclaimed, "Even though 55 million died, Black Death That Wiped out Europe Had a Good Side!" (quoted in Getz 1991, 265). As medical historian Faye Marie Getz observes, the *Enquirer* article "ends with the comforting observation that this awesome slaughter indeed had 'a silver lining.'" According to Getz, the thesis that the article presents, wedged though it may be between advertisements for secret good-luck charms and miracle diet pills, is that the Black Death "put an end to those dismal Middle Ages" and "nurtured geniuses like Michelangelo and Leonardo da Vinci" (265).

Whether the coronavirus pandemic may yield a similar "silver lining" remains to be seen, but Bloomquist's bonadsmålning titled *Silver Linings* documents some of the ways in which North Dakotans connected with each other during the first year of the pandemic. Moreover, the contrast between North Dakota's empty spaces and the horror vacui design of

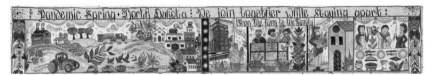

Figure 2.3. The USDA Farmers to Families Food Box program supported many of those impacted by the pandemic. (Photo courtesy of NDCA.)

bonadsmålning, which employs a "fear of empty spaces," may seem contradictory. Yet consider the state's history and geography. The state's first inhabitants, Native Americans, gathered to hold ceremonies such as the Sun Dance to seek visions and spiritual aid under the ever-present sun in a vast sky and landscape that can make one feel inconsequential, like a speck on the land. Moreover, from the state's early European settlers grew stories of people driven mad by loneliness while trying to establish homesteads. North Dakotans appreciate the benefits of empty spaces but also acknowledge the physical and psychological challenges of isolation, highlighting the essential need to be connected for human well-being. Taking a closer look at some of the specific elements in Bloomquist's painting suggests more harmony than contradiction. Now, just as years ago, North Dakotans used art, music, and other forms of cultural expression to join together and interact across the state's empty spaces.

One example appears in the top panel of Bloomquist's painting (see figure 2.3), which documents the USDA Farmers to Families Food Box program, a national effort in which many individuals and communities took part. This program was designed to support those impacted by the closure of hotels, restaurants, and other food-source businesses. Due to disruptions in the food-supply line, farmers' products—meat, dairy, and produce—were at risk of spoiling. So these products were purchased at the source, boxed, and transported to distribution centers such as food banks and faith-based organizations to feed those in need. On the left of the panel we see the farms of North Dakota and a truck carrying food to towns and cities. The center of this panel shows workers wearing masks unloading a truck and redistributing the food into boxes that can then be brought home and enjoyed at the table. The table scene is stylized in a way typical of bonadsmålning, with altered perspective and depictions of food and serving ware. The pandemic seemed to bring people closer to an understanding of where their food comes from. Many people started their own gardens.

Bonadsmålning is modeled after medieval woven tapestries, and like those tapestries, the most important scenes may be centered in the painting

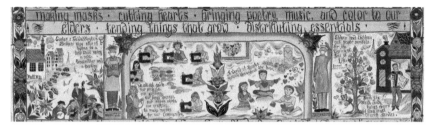

Figure 2.4. The middle panel of *Silver Linings* depicts essential activities under an archway and floral spray. (Photo courtesy of NDCA.)

under an arch (see figure 2.4). In the center of *Silver Linings'* middle panel are two scenes divided by a large vertical floral spray. One illustrates an activity that quickly spread throughout our nation and globally—the making of protective facemasks. With the pandemic spreading and the lack of sufficient numbers of masks, those who could sew immediately put aside their own projects to make facemasks for others, often distributing them for free to healthcare workers and eldercare facilities. Quilters and quilting guilds especially contributed.

The panel also illustrates the World of Hearts Facebook campaign. #aworldofhearts was started by Mandy Gill of Bismarck, North Dakota, and within forty-eight hours, more than one hundred thousand people were following and posting. Soon thereafter hundreds of thousands more from around the world were participating. The movement involved people creating paper cutouts of hearts and putting them on the windows and walls of homes, businesses, hospitals, and other buildings to share love, support, and solidarity at a time when so many felt alone and isolated. In March 2020, inspired by this campaign, the state Capitol building's lights were lit to create a beacon in the shape of a giant heart.

The center arch is flanked by our ever-present essential workers (see figure 2.5), the food service employee and the healthcare worker, both wearing full PPE (personal protective equipment).

Flanking the center arch on either side, Bloomquist continues the theme of community fellowship, highlighting two examples of North Dakota musicians adapting to support their spiritual communities. In early spring 2020, religious services and institutions throughout the country were shuttered in response to the coronavirus pandemic, resulting in many protests and defiance. This led to some of the earliest efforts at cultural sustainability since religious services play an integral role in maintaining community values and a sense of identity throughout North Dakota. Some services moved to an online format and added radio broadcasts for those who do

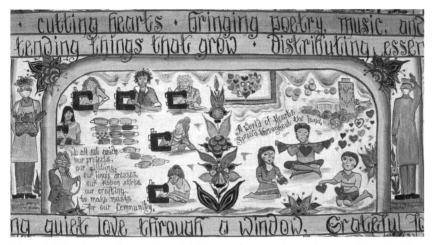

Figure 2.5. People sew face masks and children make paper hearts for essential workers in food service and healthcare. (Photo courtesy of NDCA.)

not use social media. For instance, Judy Larson, who lives just north of the South Dakota border, was able to keep the music alive even though her local Reformed Presbyterian Church had canceled in-person services.

To re-create the hymns and songs that are so vital to the services, Larson and her family first repurposed an outbuilding on their farm and turned it into a recording studio, complete with sound equipment and what she called "ratty blankets or quilts" hung up to dampen the sound. Then she and her family—husband Todd and five children ranging in age from ten to nineteen—recorded the hymns selected by their pastor, Spencer Allen. Todd played the bass, as well as both electric and acoustic guitars, and all provided vocals.

The only thing missing was a piano, so Larson substituted her accordion (see figure 2.6). It's an instrument she had started playing only five years previously, but she had also recently studied in depth with master North Dakota musician Chuck Suchy through the NDCA's Folk and Traditional Arts Apprenticeship program. Learning from Suchy about the traditional music played by North Dakotan settlers originally from Germany, Bohemia, and Norway, Larson understood how "people worked with what they had," even if they may not have been "the best players in the world."

Larson and her family provided music for the church services—both online and on the radio—from mid-March through mid-May 2020. Much like the traditional music played for entertainment in small North Dakota communities on a Saturday night, the Sunday morning "church services

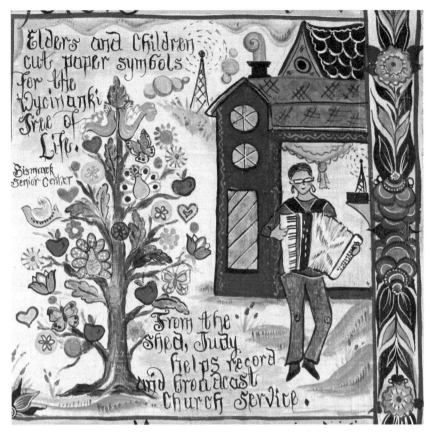

Figure 2.6. Judy Larson plays traditional music on her accordion. (Photo courtesy of NDCA.)

brought people together in a way that they can participate together even though they had to stay separated," Larson observed.

Similar ingenuity amid coronavirus restrictions throughout the state brought a "drive-in" Easter Sunday concert of church music and hymns at the Hettinger County Fairgrounds in Mott on April 12, 2020. Understanding the importance of music in traditional Easter services, pastor Corey Warner had approached a group of local musicians, the Waddington Brothers, with the idea of playing for congregants in their cars. Originally from Montana, the Waddington Brothers have performed both at bluegrass festivals and in churches throughout the United States and Canada. True to their name, they are indeed a band of brothers, consisting of Seth on guitar, twins Ethan and Jacob on banjo and mandolin, and Job on bass (see figure 2.7).

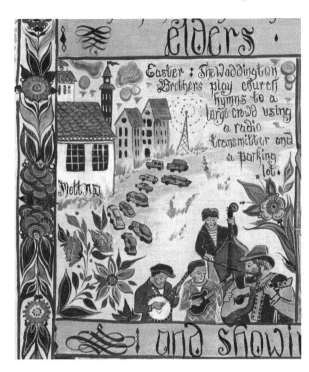

Figure 2.7. The four Waddington Brothers play bluegrass music for Easter Sunday services. (Photo courtesy of NDCA.)

Realizing that the band would need massive sound equipment to play music loud enough for congregants to hear through their car windows, Seth and his wife Rachel came up with the idea of using an FM transmitter instead. By tuning in on their car radios, the passengers in some sixty automobiles heard a traditional Easter service—complete with pastoral readings, a sermon, and music and hymns. Instead of applause, the passengers honked their car horns, even before this type of honking became a feature at campaign rallies during the presidential campaign of 2020. "It was an honor to be able to play for people even though they couldn't come sit in a chair and I couldn't see them right in the face and speak to them," Seth reflected. "It was a blessing to be able to have an Easter service and fellowship with the community."

That sort of fellowship and community cohesion is one of the goals behind the NDCA's Art for Life program. It seeks to improve the emotional and physical wellness of elders—both those in care facilities and those living independently—through ongoing art and artist interaction. Program partners are community artists, arts agencies, eldercare facilities, and schools. The strict quarantines initiated in response to the pandemic isolated many elders, who suddenly lacked the interpersonal connections so vital to their quality of life and life itself. In fact, eldercare activity directors have reported that they believe the stress, isolation, and loneliness associated with the quarantine resulted in rapid deterioration in health, mental acuity, and even in the loss of life.

Chuck Suchy, the master musician and folk singer from Mandan with whom Judy Larson apprenticed, conducted a special effort within the Art for Life program during the height of the quarantine in 2020. Safely distanced on the phone, he visited with elders from Bismarck, Enderlin, and Jamestown, asking about their lives, thoughts, and experiences to help alleviate their stress and loneliness. Then, using words of inspiration generated from those conversations, Suchy wrote, recorded, and shared songs that revealed the elders' strength, humor, and wisdom during these difficult times of isolation. Those songs then were shared with elders in care facilities and their families to spark new conversations with loved ones.

Suchy's music for elders in three places of North Dakota perfectly illustrates one observation by Dr. Oliver Sacks, a physician and professor of neurology: "Music can lift us out of depression or move us to tears—it is a remedy, a tonic, orange juice for the ear. But for many of my neurological patients, music is even more—it can provide access, even when no medication can, to movement, to speech, to life. For them, music is not a luxury, but a necessity." Although often mistakenly attributed to Sacks's *Musicophilia: Tales of Music and the Brain* (2007), this quotation first appeared on a series of Starbucks coffee cups, according to an email to Pieper Bloomquist on October 18, 2021, from Kate Edgar, executive director of the Oliver Sacks Foundation.

By poignantly conveying the need for and strength of human connection in a time of quarantine, Suchy's lyrics about sharing and togetherness strongly reinforce Sacks's observation. One of Suchy's songs is titled "How Will I Know Your Heart?"

> Clover bows, gentle wind
> Earth revolves
> with life we're in
> Winter's brown, to green of spring
> Listen now, the robins sing
>
> How will I know your heart
> if I can't hold your hand?
> How can we touch apart
> each other understand?

Did we know who we were
before the world came here?
How can we love impart?
How will I know your heart?

What is it we can trust
if all we've known is lost?
We must become an us
sharing a common cost

If I know your heart
I believe it's true
I (we) have a place to start
I believe in you

Everything, everywhere
Every good, each smile we share
Weary eyes, wrought with fear
Healing love, healing tears

Now that you know my heart
bound'ries and borderlines
No longer keep apart
love in your heart from mine

Now that I know your heart
we'll build a world anew
Love is the place we'll start
I believe in you

Now that you know my heart
Now that I know your heart

The bottom panel comprises four sections divided by decorative vertical borders (see figure 2.8). Each section features other positive efforts from the NDCA's Art for Life program to help elders cope while isolated in healthcare and eldercare facilities. Windows are a consistent visual in many of these scenes. Windows have become a bittersweet symbol associated with new ways of safely connecting during the pandemic. Suchy's song lyrics express that sentiment, as does Bloomquist's painted text: "We join together while staying apart [and] showing quiet love through a window, grateful for a glimpse." Windows served as portals to both joyful reunion and the heart-wrenching sadness experienced by too many.

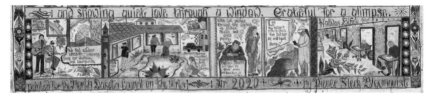

Figure 2.8. Windows and doorways are symbols of ways of interacting and connecting during the pandemic. (Photo courtesy of NDCA.)

In many examples of folklore, windows and doorways serve as portals or points of transition between opposing forces: life versus death, natural versus supernatural, opportunity versus uncertainty, and fortune versus danger. Folktales are particularly rich in these metaphors. For instance, the story known as "Beauty and the Beast" has taken many forms, not only as oral literature but as feature-length films. The story first appeared in print in 1740, as a novel written in French by Gabrielle-Suzanne Barbot de Villeneuve, in which Beauty (known as Belle in French) must live in the palace of the Beast in exchange for her father having plucked a rose from the Beast's property. Much about the Beast's palace is magical, but especially striking are the windows. As described by scholar Virginia Swain, the "magical windows of the grand salon," on one hand, are able to place Belle "in touch with the upper-class social life of Paris," but at the same time they "serve to reinforce Belle's isolation" because the Parisian scene is only an optical illusion: "What she had believed to be real was only an artifice" (2005, 206). Another example is "The Sea-Hare," also known as "Hiding from the Devil (Princess)," in which a princess possesses "magic windows which give her the power of seeing everything. She assigns her suitors the task of hiding themselves from her. Those who fail have their heads placed on stakes before the palace" (Thompson 1946, 106). The lines between fortune versus danger and life versus death could not be clearer.

In similar fashion, doorways and thresholds often act as portals between the natural and supernatural worlds. According to the *Standard Dictionary of Folklore, Mythology and Legend*, in the British Isles, "All the doors in the house were opened when someone was dying to ease the passage of the soul, and it was wrong to stand or kneel between the dying one and any door" (Leach 1949, 321). At the opposite end of life, "The opening of all doors to ease and quicken childbirth is a common practice among Indonesian peoples" (321). In many cultures, the door serves "as a protection from everything that threatens from the outside. Not only the door itself . . . but all the parts of the doorway: lintel, doorposts, and threshold" (321).

In eldercare facilities, windows and doorways became focal points in many manifestations of being together while staying apart. During the pandemic, healthcare workers were stretched thin and worked valiantly not only to protect against the virus but to fight off the negative health effects of boredom, depression, stress, and isolation for our elders in facilities. They did so partly through stoking, through art and human connection, such psychoneurological effects as increase in immune cell messengers, dopamine production, and general stress release beneficial to the immune system.

In one segment of the lower panel, Bloomquist has depicted Art for Life program artist Melissa Gordon creating colorful chalk drawings on sidewalks outside Prince of Peace Care Center/Evergreen Place Assisted Living in Ellendale and Good Shepherd Home in Watford City. Both facilities worked in collaboration with their local arts agencies to book Gordon for this project. As Gordon drew, some residents watched from their windows while others, sporting protective masks, monitored her progress from a safe distance. The images that emerged from the chalk drawings—such as a pastoral scene featuring a big red barn, or delicate pink and purple blossoms—resonated deeply with the viewers. Because many residents had spent most of their lives on North Dakota farms and ranches, the drawings sparked strong memories and feelings of nostalgia. "Everybody was talking about it, how excited they were," observed Cyndal Glynn, a registered nurse at Evergreen Place. "They kept checking in. It gave them a lot of joy to go out and see something that's outside the norm, especially given the quarantine."

At Good Shepherd, Gordon created personalized chalk marker drawings directly on residents' windows in response to the requests of the residents. "Socialization is such a big part of their day, so to maintain those guidelines of distance but to keep them engaged with their families and each other has been a challenge," explains Alicia Glynn, Evergreen Place housing manager. "It was something to talk to their families about. It was neat for them to share that connection with each other, too." Kristin Rhone, activity director at Good Shepherd Home, agrees: "Art helps us take care of the resident as a whole, and helps us honor them—mind, body, and soul."

It is typical of bonadsmålning to include images from varying times and places together in the same scene. In the same painted segment depicting Melissa, one sees a truck with a scissor lift. It features the Fargo/Moorhead area family that rented a lift to raise them to the upper-story window to help the family's grandmother celebrate turning ninety years old during the quarantine. Again, the window in this depiction is a portal for joyful togetherness.

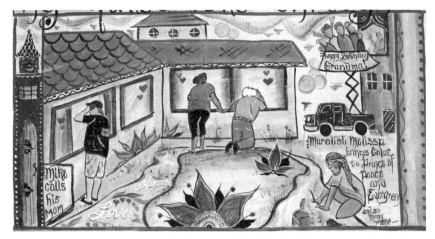

Figure 2.9. Melissa Gordon creates chalk art on a sidewalk while Pieper Bloomquist's husband, Mike, talks on a phone with his mother through her window. (Photo courtesy of NDCA.)

Yet for many others, windows carry the dual symbolism of both reunion and separation. Also in this segment, Bloomquist included images of family members standing at the windows of their loved ones at a healthcare facility. Such scenes became all too common during the spring of 2020 for many families, including Bloomquist's. During the weeks she was creating this painting, her husband's mother entered a healthcare facility and was in isolation for the entirety of her brief illness before her death. Bloomquist painted her experience of the day her mother-in-law was moved to a ground-floor room where Mike, her husband, could finally see his mom—through a window. This scene fit with the theme of *Silver Linings* because of the love that shone—and was being shown—through the windows on that day. The joy and relief that came when Mike could see his mom's face and hear her voice on the phone were immeasurable. Eventually, it was many of these same windows that witnessed a painful separation, bringing sadness when family could only watch helplessly through them as they said their last farewell to a dying loved one.

Melissa Gordon created artistic chalk murals of encouragement on the sidewalks and windows at the eldercare facilities she visited (see figure 2.9), using words like *joy*, *hope*, *love*. Those words were meant for all of us: those ill and under quarantine, those separated, and those hoping to catch a glimpse.

In eldercare facilities, not only were elders quarantined from people outside their facility, they also were often quarantined from people within the same building—confined to their rooms for days, weeks, and months at a time. During these times, eldercare activity directors and staff worked

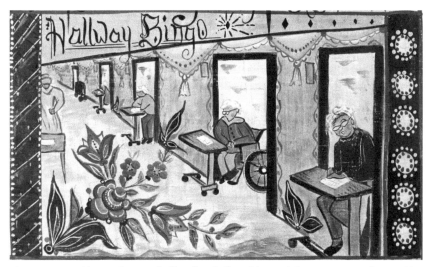

Figure 2.10. Residents of a care facility play "hallway bingo." (Photo courtesy of NDCA.)

tirelessly to create joyful interactions and connect elders with each other safely. For example, Maple Manor Care Center in Langdon, North Dakota, like many other places, reimagined a staple of eldercare activity, bingo, by conducting "hallway bingo" (see figure 2.10). Residents were wheeled to or seated at the threshold of their rooms facing the hallway—daubers and bingo cards placed on the wheeled tables in front of them—as someone down the hall called out the numbers. In this example, the doorway is indeed a transition point between loneliness and companionship, danger and safety.

Social contact opportunities outside the eldercare facility were creatively reimagined in several ways. Through the Art for Life program, Maple Manor worked with artists like Mindi Lill, the local art teacher, who spoke with residents via phone and then painted pictures inspired by those conversations on the windows of elder residents' rooms. When the weather warmed, musicians David Gorder and Shawn Carrier provided an outdoor concert in the courtyard. The musicians moved from window to window playing sets of songs so that every elder had their own personal concert to lift their spirits.

Bloomquist especially wanted to capture what a healthcare worker would be experiencing from inside a hospital room or eldercare facility. She struggled with that. As a nurse, she is aware of what the actual environment looks like and what healthcare workers were experiencing in the wake of the pandemic, but at the time she was creating her bonadsmålning, her husband's mother was facing isolation and eventual death in one of those healthcare facilities. So in her painting, the perspective of the family's emotion took precedence. She represented healthcare workers as she saw and experienced them: accurately dressed head to toe in full PPE, aiding not only with medications and basic needs, but also with social media and communication opportunities for a population of elders not accustomed to the technology. Healthcare workers brought elders to their windows and doorways and expressed upbeat emotions of positivity with smiles and laughter.

Bloomquist was inspired by a photograph of a friend in full PPE outside her workplace. Her friend's wave and smiling eyes expressed the optimism better than anything Bloomquist could have imagined. She captured her friend's cheerful energy by including her likeness in this painting.

All these projects—from music at religious services to art for elders—are designed in part to create positive memories in spite of the great anxiety and often tragic consequences of the coronavirus pandemic. North Dakotans have indeed used art and cultural heritage to cope with the coronavirus pandemic.

Even though artists have not been able to facilitate in-person activities with residents of eldercare facilities, they have continued to find ways to connect and create despite visiting restrictions. Bloomquist is currently working on a bonadsmålning with elders residing at Maryhill Manor in Enderlin, North Dakota. Instead of hosting daily painting activities in the facility, Bloomquist interviews residents via Zoom on an iPad. She is compiling their stories into a large storyboard and will create an outline on canvas, which will then be brought to the facility and painted by residents working with the activity directors. The project will then be returned to Bloomquist so she can embellish and add the elements that will make the finished piece typical of the bonadsmålning folk art.

Another recent NDCA project uses the memories of elders to create poems that evoke both the quiet moments and major milestones of their lives. Thanks to a grant from the Art for Life program, fourteen elders served by the Burleigh County Senior Center in Bismarck held telephone conversations to share some of their memories with writers Matthew Musacchia and Maureen McDonald-Hins (see figure 2.11). After the conversations, the writers shaped those memories using the "I'm From" poetic template developed by George Ella Lyons to create poems, which were compiled into book form. The poems—and the memories and experiences expressed in them—served as vehicles for social connection between the elders and the friends and family members with whom the poems were shared.

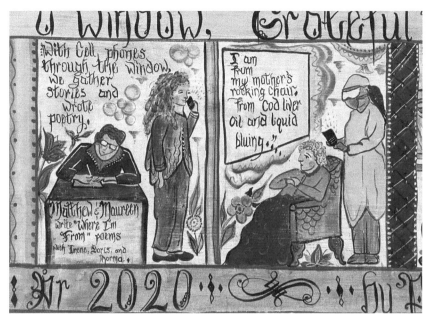

Figure 2.11. Matthew Musacchia and Maureen McDonald-Hins interview elders to develop poems about their lives. (Photo courtesy of NDCA.)

I'm from My Mother's Rocking Chair

I am from my mother's rocking chair,
    From cod liver oil and liquid bluing.
I am from many houses, including one that was haunted,
    The fragrance of lilacs and fresh-baked bread.
I am from Dad's big garden, us kids collecting potato bugs in a coffee can of kerosene,
    The big gnarled oak tree and its swing.
    We would climb as high as we could and hang upside down on the branches.

I'm from singing together and Mom's beautiful voice,
    From Babe, Sonnie, Rene, and Crooked Neck.
I'm from Dad playing the Jew harp and Sunday drives in a borrowed car,
    And from rolling down the hill on the old museum lawn.
I'm from "If you cry in the cold, your face will freeze that way."
    And "Two Little Children" and "Letter Edged in Black."
I'm from listening to the radio show *Fibber McGee and Molly*.

I'm from a little log cabin along River Road in Bismarck and English royalty,
    Pasta dishes and simple foods.

From a brother smoking a "dead" firecracker on the Fourth of July,
    Blowing up and tearing his mouth open—wide open.
Grandma's one-hundred-year-old buffet,
    Letters from the war safely tucked away in my cedar chest.
News reels at movie theaters informing us of the war front.

Irene Walter, April 13, 2020

Initially some of the elders were skeptical: "I thought, 'Oh, dear, my life is not exciting,'" said Nanc Skaret with a laugh. "But I found a lot of things to write about. I hadn't thought about some of this stuff for years."

Lisa Bennett, site manager at the senior center, felt that the poetry project was both a responsible and a timely way to process the complicated feelings stirred up by a global health crisis. Reading the memories of elders who lived through the 1930s Depression and World War II, Bennett gained a new appreciation for the people she serves. "It taught me that they all lived really full lives," she explained. "It just proved to me that the human race is very resilient. It was a very good reminder at a perfect time."

Bennett's observations confirm some of the ways in which the artistic practices and cultural traditions of NDCA's Art for Life program enhanced the lives of many North Dakotans across the state during the first year of the coronavirus pandemic. Anecdotal evidence seems to support the findings of medical researchers, such as Dr. Gene Cohen, Dr. Charles Hall, Dr. Julianne Holt-Lunstad, and others that art, music, and similar activities may improve both mental and physical well-being by helping to sustain an individual's emotional and spiritual needs.

Those activities are the sparks. Equally important is the structure that allows that artistic energy to travel and help ignite well-being. Dr. Cohen ascribes, partially, the arts' positive impact on health and wellness to brain plasticity, the ability of the brain to adapt by forming and strengthening new brain cells. This happens "when branchlike extensions (known as dendrites) from one brain cell (neuron) achieve contact with extensions of other neurons [and] new synapses [contact points] are formed" (2006, 10). Analogously, consider neurons as individuals, dendrites as social structures and traditions, and synapses as art (see figure 2.12). We connect and come together with other people through our social structures, relationships, and traditions which, too, have their own power in health and wellness, and they set in motion that point of contact, that spark, which oftentimes is art.

All the scenes depicted in Bloomquist's bonadsmålning *Silver Linings* beautifully illustrate community connections and togetherness, and their positive effects on health and wellness. There may be plenty of empty spaces

Pathways and Points of Interaction

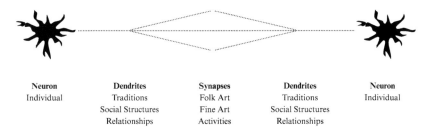

Neuron	Dendrites	Synapses	Dendrites	Neuron
Individual	Traditions	Folk Art	Traditions	Individual
	Social Structures	Fine Art	Social Structures	
	Relationships	Activities	Relationships	

Figure 2.12. Pathways and Points of Interaction. (Graphic courtesy of NDCA.)

throughout North Dakota, but the lack of empty space in Bloomquist's painting confirms the closeness of human culture. North Dakota is not only at the geographical center of North America; its Art for Life program places it also at the center of social engagement and cultural sustainability.

ACKNOWLEDGMENTS

Reporting for parts of this narrative comes from Matthew Musacchia, a country/folk musician who has been working with the North Dakota Council on the Arts since 2014; Alicia Underlee Nelson, an author and freelance writer/photographer who covers history, travel, art, and culture for numerous publications; and Nita Ritzke, a poet and writer who is an associate professor of communication at the University of Mary. The Smithsonian Institution provided support for the contributions of James I. Deutsch.

REFERENCES

Adelson, Candace J. 2002. "New York Renaissance Tapestries." *Burlington Magazine* 144 (August): 521–23.

Cohen, Gene D. 2006. "Research on Creativity and Aging: The Positive Impact of the Arts on Health and Illness." *Generations: Journal of the American Society on Aging* 30 (1): 7–15.

Daley, Jason. 2017. "New Calculations Reposition the Geographical Center of North America." *Smithsonian Magazine*, January 30. https://www.smithsonianmag.com /smart-news/new-calculations-reposition-geographical-center-north-america-1 -180961932/.

Geist, Troyd A. 2017. *Sundogs and Sunflowers: An Art for Life Program Guide for Creative Aging, Health, and Wellness.* Bismarck: North Dakota Council on the Arts.

Gertsman, Elina. 2018. "Phantoms of Emptiness: The Space of the Imaginary in Late Medieval Art." *Art History* 41 (5): 800–37.

Getz, Faye Marie. 1991. "Black Death and the Silver Lining: Meaning, Continuity, and Revolutionary Change in Histories of Medieval Plague." *Journal of the History of Biology* 24 (2): 265–89.

Hall, Charles B., Richard B. Lipton, Martin J. Sliwinski, Mindy Joy Katz, Carol A. Derby, and Joe Verghese. 2009. "Cognitive Activities Delay Onset of Memory Decline in Persons Who Develop Dementia." *Neurology* 73 (5): 356–61.

Holt-Lunstad, Julianne, Timothy B. Smith, Mark Baker, Tyler Harris, and David Stephenson. 2015. "Loneliness and Social Isolation as Risk Factors for Mortality: A Meta-analytic Review." *Perspectives on Psychological Science* 10 (2): 227–37.

Leach, Maria, ed. 1949. *Funk and Wagnalls Standard Dictionary of Folklore, Mythology and Legend.* New York: Funk & Wagnalls.

MacBrayne, Lillian D. 1972. "Southern Swedish Painted Bonader." *Art Institute of Chicago Museum Studies* 7:85–122.

North Dakota Department of Health. 2020. "First Case of Novel Coronavirus Confirmed in North Dakota as Work Continues to Prevent Spread." *North Dakota Health News*, March 11. https://www.health.nd.gov/news/first-case-novel-coronavirus-confirmed -north-dakota-work-continues-prevent-spread.

Sacks, Oliver. 2007. *Musicophilia: Tales of Music and the Brain.* New York: Knopf.

Scheidel, Walter. 2017. *The Great Leveler: Violence and the History of Inequality from the Stone Age to the Twenty-First Century.* Princeton: Princeton University Press.

Shipman, Pat. 2014. "The Bright Side of the Black Death." *American Scientist* 102 (6): 410–13.

Snowden, Frank M. 2019. *Epidemics and Society: From the Black Death to the Present.* New Haven: Yale University Press.

Swain, Virginia E. 2005. "Beauty's Chambers: Mixed Styles and Mixed Messages in Villeneuve's *Beauty and the Beast.*" *Marvels and Tales: Journal of Fairy-Tale Studies* 19 (2): 197–223.

Thompson, Stith. 1946. *The Folktale.* New York: Dryden.

3

Kneading Comfort, Community, Craftsmanship
Home Baking in the Coroniverse

Lucy M. Long and Theresa A. Vaughan

INTRODUCTION

An unexpected response to the COVID-19 pandemic in the US was a rise in home baking, particularly of bread (Marvar 2020; Mull 2020).[1] We say unexpected because recent trends had been moving away from the reliance on bread as a staple of the foodways practices that had historically defined mainstream, British-based American food culture (Levenstein 1988; Wallach 2013). Prior to the pandemic, concerns over the impact of carbohydrates from grains on body weight and a rise of awareness of gluten sensitivities had limited the consumption of bread. Those concerns seemed to be dismissed with the arrival of the pandemic, and there appeared to be a return to bread as the staff of life—or at least the staple for meals—for many Americans. Baking itself emerged as an activity frequently discussed on social media, and the necessary ingredients went into high demand. A wide variety of types and forms of bakery items were shared and celebrated, both virtually and in real life. These include what are considered "artisanal" breads, but also other baked goods, both sweet and savory—pies, cakes, cookies, muffins, biscuits, turnovers, and a host of other pastries. While concerns over the safety of grocery shopping and the availability of supplies motivated some of this activity,[2] baking's popularity seemed to go far beyond nutritional needs. Drawing from social media, news accounts, ethnographic data, and personal experiences,[3] we examine this popularity, exploring the functions baking served. Recognizing that all foodways activities can have multiple meanings, we identify three themes around baking that offer insights into why and how individuals participated in baking: comfort, community,

https://doi.org/10.7330/9781646424818.c003

and craftsmanship. These themes demonstrate ways in which home baking offered creative ways to cope with the pandemic. In many cases they overlap and support each other, reflecting the interconnected nature of motivations as well as of social networks. These themes also illustrate the rise of vernacular strategies and expertise, with "vernacular" referring to everyday cultural practices and expressions of specific groups.

In his influential 1995 article on religion, Leonard Primiano joined scholars such as Henry Glassie and Margaret Lantis (1988) in calling for the use of *vernacular* rather than *folk* as the qualifier for the subject of folklorists' study.[4] This word represented a shift away from some of the simplistic and inaccurate dichotomies between official and unofficial cultures and between folk and elite cultures made by earlier scholars. It also, in Primiano's formulation, asserted a methodology and perspective that addressed lived experience and personal interpretation as the bases for artistry and practice (Primiano 1995, 43). He recognized that the vernacular exists within a dynamic and dialogic relationship with the institutions and groupings within a society that represent hierarchies of power and authority. Primiano's theorizing challenged the ways in which scholars were approaching the study of belief, but more relevant to home baking, it emphasized the potential for individuals to assert their own meanings and identities.

Vernacular culture from this perspective can be understood as challenging the larger, more dominant structures—the official policies and teachings, mass-mediated culture, and individuals that are held up as the official authorities of culture. We suggest that this is what happened with home baking during the pandemic—although, somewhat ironically, often through social media—a type of mass-mediated culture in which the individual is the producer rather than the consumer. We also recognize that many of the participants in this vernacular response were most likely from social classes and identities that, in "normal" times, would be part of those dominant structures. While we were not able to determine the socioeconomic standing of individuals, we can assume in most cases a certain amount of privilege. The ability to work from home as well as to have access to ingredients, cooking facilities, and the skills and knowledge needed for baking implies a certain social standing that reflects the disparities of race, class, and gender in American society. As one observer concluded about the sourdough trend, it "upheld white privilege, racism, and classism by widening gaps in food access and marginalizing Black bakers" (Dadalt 2021). We agree, however, also to recognize the complexity of individuals working within whatever constraints face them and to admit the possibility for change. Sociologists studying "foodie" trends before and during the pandemic came to a similar conclusion: "These experiences involve privilege, but they are not straight-forwardly restricted to self-described foodies or upper-middle class white eaters. In a world of tremendous uncertainty and risk, preparing and enjoying food can feel deeply comforting, providing a soothing balm against the hardships of the outside world" (Oleschuk et al. 2021).[5]

Shortages of flour and yeast followed the sudden demand for those ingredients, but instead of dampening enthusiasm, they inspired creativity, innovation, and sharing. Concerns over gluten sensitivities led to experimentation with flour varieties as well as virtual interactions with other people to find solutions. Previous admonitions by the weight loss industry to cut back on carbohydrates were ignored, and individuals focused on the emotional and social qualities of baked goods rather than their caloric or nutritional ones. The offerings by professional chefs of recipes for gourmet "comfort foods" and the food industries' definitions of that category were taken as inspiration for individuals to create what was personally meaningful to them rather than as prescriptions that had to be followed. Furthermore, such baking asserted identities and values, and established and confirmed membership in social groups and relationships.

Home baking, then, represents vernacular culture finding ways to cope with the pandemic that went beyond the biological need for food. It offered a way in which individuals could address the isolation and fears accompanying the pandemic, providing an avenue for creativity, for distraction from the tedium of lockdowns, and for a sense of control during a time of uncertainty. It also brought attention to individuals who might have previously been overlooked, allowing them to emerge as knowledge-holders and authorities. In some cases, it was the basis for the development of groups that then challenged the values and structures of contemporary society and the industrial food complex. These emergent communities and practices around home baking are asserting the value of vernacular culture during this pandemic.

COMFORT

One of the most obvious and oft-cited reasons for baking was comfort (Easterbrook-Smith 2021; Ocklenburg 2020; Güler and Haseki 2021; O'Connell 2021). Food media as well as social media posts, oral history interviews, and our own experiences all attested to the comforting effects of both preparing and consuming baked goods. This is particularly interesting because before the pandemic in the US, bread, pastries, and the like tended to fall into the category of fattening, carb-laden foods of which people watching their weight and cholesterol levels should be wary. The concept of comfort food in the context of the pandemic has been explored elsewhere (Long 2020; Long et al. 2021), but categorizing these items as "comfort food" gave "permission" for people to eat those foods when under stress, relieving them of the moral associations with such eating as indicating a lack of self-discipline or an unhealthy interest in "things of the flesh" (Jones 2017; Jones and Long 2017; Long 2022).[6]

The pandemic was a period of stress filled with uncertainty about the future, fears of sickness and death, social isolation, and worries about meeting the challenges of daily life as well as the tedium of lockdowns. Baking was presented in food media as a way to deal with this stress, and social media quickly became filled with postings of photographs and accounts of making bread, pastries, cakes, pies, cookies, and other baked "goodies" (Giorgis 2020; Goldberg 2020). A closer look at the needs fulfilled by comfort food offers explanations for the popularity of baked products as a comfort food as well as of baking itself as a "comfort foodway." Those needs have been identified by medical sociologists and psychologists as physical comfort, nostalgia, indulgence, convenience, and belonging (Locher 2002; Locher et al. 2005; Troisi and Gabriel 2011).[7] Each of these needs is addressed through baking as a vernacular practice, especially when we shift the emphasis to the processes and practices involved and not just the product. The needs also are not mutually exclusive but can be fulfilled simultaneously or highlighted at different points in the processes surrounding baking.[8] Looked at from the psychological point of view, baking as pandemic activity fulfills not just the lowest level of Maslow's hierarchy of needs (physiological) but also the higher-level needs for belonging, love, and esteem (Ocklenburg 2020).

Of the five needs, one of the most obvious ones initially was physical comfort. The pandemic was recognized at different times across the world, but it struck throughout the winter of 2020. In the US, the colder weather made it sensible to warm the house by using the oven, something less likely to be attractive in seasons and places with higher temperatures. The aroma of breads and other products baking added to the physical comfort offered, and the heat they exuded when done physically warmed eaters who were too impatient to wait for them to cool off.

Beyond the warmth of the breads themselves was the physical comfort gained from the exertions involved in sifting flours, kneading dough, and lifting loaves from the oven. For the many individuals involved in remote work, even the movements involved in reaching for ingredients or simply walking from other parts of the house to the kitchen offered a respite from sitting in front of the computer screen. The kneading of bread further seemed to offer physical comfort to many. Its very repetitiveness can have a meditative quality, and it seemed to force an attentiveness to the process that individuals found calming (Siragusa 2021). The taste of the bread can also be seen as a physical comfort that engaged all the senses, giving an embodied sense of pleasure as well as a focusing of attention.[9] According to one study, baking not only served as a "hedonic" activity—one that gave fleeting pleasure and sensory stimulation—but also offered eudaimonic, or self-actualized, experiences (Güler and Haseki 2021).

Indulgence, another of the needs identified, was also openly recognized. The uncertainties during the pandemic around food shortages and the future made concerns about calories seem irrelevant. A frequently expressed attitude on social media was encapsulated in the familiar proverb "Eat, drink, and be merry, for tomorrow we may die." In any case, the stress accompanying the pandemic and the lack of other familiar outlets for comfort seemed to give public permission to indulge in what we could—and that was formerly forbidden baked goods. Indulgence was also closely tied to physical comfort in that baking offered sensory pleasure and aesthetic engagement, two qualities frequently pushed aside in the usual higher valuing of productivity and achieving tangible goals.[10]

A third need potentially met by comfort food is that of nostalgia, a longing or sentimental affection for the past. It assumes that our memories of the past are positive and warm and will evoke feelings of affirmation. Such memories oftentimes are romanticizations of childhood and earlier times, while negative memories are ignored or dismissed.[11] The idea that bread is automatically a fond part of each American's past speaks to the assumption that "proper"[12] mainstream American food culture is based on British and other western European culinary traditions.[13] Bread in a variety of forms was historically as well as today a basic staple in western European food cultures. Yeast breads made from wheat tended to be the provenance of the wealthy and privileged in those cultures, but they became normative for what was considered mainstream healthy eating in the US.

The reality in the US, though, is that homemade bread was not necessarily the stuff of American childhoods. Not all residents grew up on a bread-centric diet. For those who did, commercially produced soft white breads made from highly processed wheat was the staple of many American homes and was pushed by home economists as early as the 1890s as being healthier and more acceptable than the coarser, denser, and darker breads of many of the European immigrants with peasant or laborer backgrounds (Levenstein 1988; Wallach 2013). In terms of gendered labor in the United States, this move from baking bread in the home effectively removed baking from being largely the domain of women to being produced commercially by men. Although women seemed to welcome the convenience of store-bought bread and baked goods, this change follows a familiar pattern of women's work becoming monetized when it is taken up by men (Easterbrook-Smith 2021).

Homemade breads in the much of the twentieth-century US represented either pioneer lifestyles that persisted in rural farmhouses or poor mountain homes or the "hippie" ethos of the 1960s counterculture (Belasco [1993] 2014; Deutsch 2019; Dutch 2018). Baking bread at home was seen in mainstream culture as odd and unnecessary. Lucy can attest from personal experience growing up in both urban and rural areas of the South that children who brought to school sandwiches made of such bread were looked upon with pity or disdain and were oftentimes teased, while Theresa, who grew up in a multicultural university town, saw less of this. Home-baked desserts, however, were appreciated, and now that commercial products are so easily available, tend to carry high social value. Home-baked bread also regained status in the 2000s, seen as reflecting skill, cosmopolitan and sophisticated tastes, and possession of leisure time (Dutch 2018). The "foodie" trend in the US, with its obsession on the origins and preparation of dishes, has contributed to this perception, but part of that value may be derived from the association of home-baked breads with cultures in which artisanal breads are perceived as a daily staple and life seems to feature a successful balance of work and pleasure. The food cultures of France, Italy, and Spain have long been held up as models of refined cuisines, and all feature wheat-flour yeast breads. Similarly, there is currently a trend toward appreciating the heartier breads of eastern and central Europe as well as of Ireland. The nostalgia fulfilled through eating these breads, then, may be more a matter of imagined, romanticized pasts than the realities of individual histories.

The fourth need identified by scholars as fulfilling needs for comfort is convenience. At first glance, this need does not seem to be especially relevant during the pandemic. After all, home baking usually involves time and effort and results in numerous dishes and surfaces to clean afterwards. The final product, however, can be seen as a convenient meal or snack. A slice of bread can easily be made a meal by adding toppings, and it can conveniently be served on a napkin or plate and held in the hand. A piece of pie or cake might require utensils and dishes, but homemade cookies can be picked up by hand. Any of these can be eaten whenever and wherever is convenient for the consumer.

Another aspect of convenience is that lockdown orders and remote work meant that many people were now at home for long hours (Faludi and

Crosby 2021). This made it convenient to find the time for kneading dough, waiting for it to rise, and then baking it. While these processes would not normally be seen as convenient, since they tend to take extensive stretches of time as well as effort and equipment, they could now be fit in between other chores or work and provided much-needed breaks from computer screens and virtual meetings. This suggests class and gender issues around the question of who was working at home and under what circumstances.[14] Furthermore, the living situations and specific circumstances of individuals and groups would shape whether or not taking the space and time to bake would be convenient.[15]

Belonging was also identified by researchers as a need fulfilled by comfort food (Troisi and Gabriel 2011). In studies of people with "secure attachment" (those with positive relationships with others), researchers found that those individuals enjoyed comfort food more when they felt isolated or their relationships were threatened. The corollary was that comfort food fulfilled the natural need social beings have to belong, for a sense that they have a place in society and matter to other people (Troisi et al. 2015). Home baking fulfilled this need in several ways, both physically and virtually. Family and friend relationships were built and affirmed through exchanges of knowledge, ingredients, and final products, even if necessarily done at a distance by phone, email, or social media. Baking cakes from a recipe passed down over generations can reinforce a sense of belonging to a particular place and people, as does baking items from one's cultural heritage.[16] Sharing sourdough starters, equipment, or cookbooks established networks that could then develop into social relationships, creating what can be seen as folk groups built around a common experience. Knowing that there were people sharing that experience made individuals feel less isolated and alone.

The need to belong was heightened during the pandemic by the closing of public spaces and the need to social distance as a way of curtailing the virus. In response, a number of individuals intentionally started virtual groups to meet their own social needs. There also emerged awareness of the isolation others might be experiencing and mindfulness of the need to reach out to them. Out of these shared experiences and recognitions there then emerged a number of communities, some probably short-lived, but others perhaps lasting beyond the pandemic (see figure 3.1).

Judging from social media accounts, ethnographic research, and personal experiences, home-baked goods and practices offered comfort to many people on a number of levels. The vernacular practices of finding comfort through food and foodways, however, challenge the food industry's appropriation of the concept (Long 2022). Rather than focusing on specific

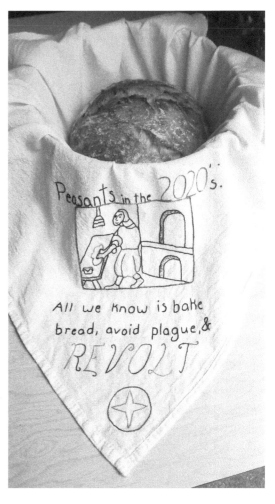

Figure 3.1. Theresa Vaughan, a member of the Facebook group Modern Hand Embroidery, learned to bake bread during the pandemic, and in March 2021 embroidered a kitchen towel she used to keep her bread warm. (Photo by Sarah Romes Walker, used with permission.)

products that reflected a definition of "proper" American eating as being of British heritage and pioneer-based, the new vernacular conceptions of comfort food recognized the diversity of backgrounds and identities that make up the nation. Chefs offered comfort foods from their own childhoods outside the US mainstream, and some social media sites encouraged individuals to look beyond the mainstream for potential comfort.[17] Posts on social media of baked goods such as bagels, South American empanadas, steamed Chinese rice-flour buns, and pastries with "exotic" ingredients illustrated this expansion. According to the Human Relations Area Files at Yale, comfort food, which could be ramen noodles, curries, Spam, soup dumplings, congee, and other foods of different cultural origins, saw an explosion of interest during the pandemic. For families who were scattered across borders, sharing pictures of or exchanging recipes for familiar home food brought a sense of personal connection and comfort to isolated individuals and communities.[18]

Vernacular responses also are challenging the morality implied in the use of the phrase "comfort food," presenting food and foodways as comforting without the associated guilt or shame (Long 2022). The initial impetus for preparing and consuming home-baked goods may partially have been to relieve stress—and thereby "justified"—but their consumption emphasized the aesthetic experience and delight that came from them. Individuals did at times bemoan weight gained from these foods (Koenig 2020), but nevertheless there seemed to be a shift in values recognizing the importance of such experiences.

Responses also seem to emphasize the potential sociability of sharing baked goods and of consuming them together—whether virtually or physically. That commensality is now recognized by the general public as well as some scholars[19] as being just as important, and perhaps even more so, as the nutritional qualities of a dish. In this way, the individual uses of comfort food challenged medical-nutritional mainstream approaches to healthful eating, asserting that food is more than just the calories and nutrients it contains.

COMMUNITY

The need to belong pushed some people into affirming previously established relationships as well as creating new ones. Family, neighborhood, religion, work, and personal interests had oftentimes brought people together in the past, and those networks continued to form the basis for social interactions during the pandemic, whether virtual or physical. Numerous other social groups emerged, and a number of these focused on some aspects of foodways—gardening; shopping for groceries; eating together; sharing cooking knowledge, recipes, ingredients, or equipment; and, of course, baking, particularly of bread. Groups focused on bread and baking, like other groups, varied in purpose, structure, and medium for interacting. Some emerged in response to fears of shortages of foodstuffs (flour and yeast, notably); some grew out of the search for specific ingredients, recipes, or know-how; and others were established or affirmed by sharing the final products of baking. Some were intentionally developed around baking, but others were brought together by factors such as shared hobbies, having children in the same school, or simply living in the same neighborhood or apartment building. Lucy, for example, met regularly with a small number of people to play old-time music, and the group oftentimes shared baking stories and successes. Many of the groups were virtual, while others included physical proximity or face-to-face interaction (hopefully with masks and social distancing). Whether these numerous groupings will last beyond the pandemic remains to be seen, but they were commonly referred to as "communities."

The word *community* is used colloquially to refer to a group that has a welcoming and friendly attitude. The group can exist in physical space or can be virtual, but the essential criterion for being a member of a community tends to be an emotional perception that one belongs. There is also an implication of mutual concern, respect, and consideration between members, so that there is an expectation that people within a community will come to each other's assistance if needed (Long 2015, 52–53). If they do not, the group fails as a community.

This sense of mutual obligation to and responsibility for each other was highlighted during the pandemic, so that people frequently invoked those references in talking about groups they were in, as well as larger geographic and political regions surrounding them. A strong sense of community developed around food: not just sharing food, but also in sharing the labor in producing, harvesting, preparing, and preserving it. To understand how and why these communities developed, it is helpful to step back and analyze them first as folk groups.

A folk group is any group of people who share a commonality and develop expressive traditions out of that commonality (Bauman 1972). Those traditions reflect not only the commonality but also the individual interests, identities, circumstances, and abilities of specific members of that group. Because the members of groups differ, no two folk groups will be the same even though they may share a great deal in common. ideally, this also makes them dynamic, adaptable to new needs and individuals, although the need to adapt oftentimes calls into question the identity of the group and of power hierarchies within it. Two conditions are needed for folk groups to develop: proximity or contact and regular interaction (Noyes 2003; Sims and Stephens 2005). That interaction allows for traditions to emerge and for the nature of the group to be negotiated. This dynamic quality also means that there are primary commonalities that bring people together and then secondary ones that can affirm the group—or act as the impetus for the emergence of a smaller group.

The pandemic offered a commonality—COVID-19—that was shared globally. Not everyone had the same experiences or the same interpretations, however, so the initial sense of a worldwide community joined in a common fight seemed to fracture, in the US at least, into numerous subgroups. Similarly, food as a culturally constructed category and the biological need to eat are also shared commonalities that tend to define humanity across the world. Those topics were frequent subjects of discussion in news and social media as well as in virtual and face-to-face social interactions. Also, the shortages of certain items as well as concerns about entering public spaces to shop for groceries acted as a commonality for some. Bread, yeast, and flour were all difficult to acquire at different times and places due to breaks in the supply chain, shortages of supermarket staff, and a need for more production time to meet demand (Castrodale 2020). This inspired groups to share either those materials or the knowledge of how to make or find substitutions for the commercial products. Theresa recounts that a social network developed among her friends and neighbors around the getting and sharing of ingredients for baking:

> I began scouring Amazon, King Arthur, and several other websites for flour and yeast, as well as other items I couldn't find locally. Some things weren't available there, and flour and yeast could be had but only in fifty-pound bags or huge commercial blocks intended for commercial baking . . . This is when it occurred to me that others were experiencing the same issues finding staples. I connected with friends and colleagues on Facebook to ask if there were any sightings of flour or yeast. Lots of friends reported being astonished that it had all disappeared. We bemoaned the fact that people were hoarding as we put our heads together to try to figure out how to get supplies. Some of us would go to grocery stores early in the morning looking for flour, yeast, baking supplies, and other staples and would send out an alert to others saying what store and what time had what supplies so we could hopefully get there before everything was gone. Some people bought the overpriced fifty-pound bags of flour and shared them with friends. Some of us kept our eyes on online sites and reported where we found items. I eventually checked the online site of a flour mill in Arkansas that I had visited on vacation. As soon as they began to restock, I ordered flour and, as a bonus, they were giving away yeast with the flour.
>
> Socializing in person gave way to making stronger connections through social media and Zoom meetings—and baking gave us something to talk about besides how overworked we were or our grief over not seeing friends, or worse, having those close to us become ill and sometimes die. While the pandemic kept us physically apart, a shared experience, need for comfort and diversion, and strategizing about getting the supplies we needed brought us together in a different way.

The yeast shortage in particular seemed to inspire the emergence of social networks.[20] The scarcity of yeast was caused by a number of factors: demand for it spiked during a period when suppliers expect lower demand (after the winter holidays), yeast can only be grown and processed so fast, and pandemic lockdowns and closures caused issues with packaging supplies and packaging businesses (Mak 2020). Sourdough starters, a mixture of dough that has been allowed to "capture" and carefully nurture wild yeasts floating in the air, were shared and passed along among people in physical proximity (Delap 2020). These starters were then used in place of yeast to make bread (and other foods such as pancakes), giving a slightly tangy taste to the final product. Some extolled the virtues of sourdough for its healthful properties, noting also that the acidic nature of the bread that comes from the fermented yeast results in a longer shelf life (Sofo et al. 2021). Posts on social media disseminated knowledge of how to capture wild yeasts and create a starter. It seemed popular also for people to name their starters and to recount their provenance, creating something like a lineage that connected the lucky recipient of the starter to other people or places. Theresa's first starter, for example, was named Audrey after the friend who had given it to her. In some cases, sharing starters created groups whose members then shared the final products, coming full circle and reinforcing the sense of community.

These sourdough starter "communities" also illustrate the complexity of these types of groups. Many had other commonalities that had brought them together prior to the pandemic—physical proximity in a neighborhood, hobbies, work, family ties—providing a preestablished network. Not everyone in those groups was interested in sourdough, but sharing the starter both reinforced those existing ties and offered a basis for a new group.

One sourdough group Lucy participated in as a consumer illustrates this layering of commonalities. All the members played old-time and contradance music and oftentimes got together to jam. Some also participated in other activities—dancing, kayaking, camping, hiking. Lucy met at a campground with a subset of the total group to share loaves of bread made with a sourdough starter that had been passed around among them several weeks earlier. As a musician and camper, she was invited into the group even though she had not participated in the sharing of the starter—primarily because she lived too far away. Also, one individual had used the starter for gluten-free bread, made specifically for his spouse. This bread reflected the ways in which an item can represent both a group as a whole and an individual member.

The need to acquire the skills for making bread was also a commonality for a number of groups. Prior to the pandemic, these groups would have included physical gatherings, but the need to social distance forced them to interact virtually. A Facebook group to which Lucy belonged was started by a well-known old-time musician, Bruce Molsky, specifically to share information, knowledge, and experiences around baking. Fiddle and Dough was a "closed group"—people had to be allowed to join by the administrator. Molsky established the group in February 2020, very early in the pandemic, but he lived in New York, one of the first "epicenters" of COVID-19 in the US. In Molsky's words, "This group is for players and lovers of all kinds of traditional and roots music who love to bake bread! Let's share recipes, photos of our baking successes and failures, tips, stories, links and advice. Let's let our love of one of the most simple and important foods bring us together in a satisfying, yeasty and fermented way. The biga the story, the better. Ok, sorry. Let's have some fun with this!" (quoted with permission).

The invitation delineates the commonalities of the group—a love of traditional music and of baking bread—and there is an expectation that any new members will appreciate those commonalities. There is also an in-joke that would signal to readers that the group is serious about baking and suggests a certain amount of previous knowledge and experience. Spelling "bigger" as "biga" refers to a form of single-use "yeasted pre-ferment" oftentimes used in Italian bread baking. One member of the group responded with a similar pun: "Can't believe I missed your penny wise & pound 'poolish' 'biga' joke." *Poolish* is another baking term, originally the Polish word for the pre-ferment. Whether or not the individual posting it has a connection to Poland is unclear—and unnecessary, since the joke references additional knowledge about baking practices, speaking to the group based on its common interest in baking rather than ethnic identity.

Other groups focused on baking as their primary commonality, some even specifying types of breads or grains.[21] Some groups formed around baking were less formal in their structure and intent, using baking simply as a focus for virtual gatherings. For example, a friend of Lucy's began a monthly cooking/eating Zoom event, inviting a small number of individuals who had all worked together previously. Each month, one person would select a dish and send out recipes. Everyone would collect the ingredients and then, while on Zoom, prepare the food, consume it simultaneously, and critique the end result. These conversations inevitably turned into discussions of a personal nature, an indication that the group was a community in which members felt welcomed and accepted.

This group focused on baking twice. In the run-up to Christmas 2020, they held a cookie-decorating party, trying to re-create virtually the ritual cookie decorating and exchanges that are frequently a part of that holiday's

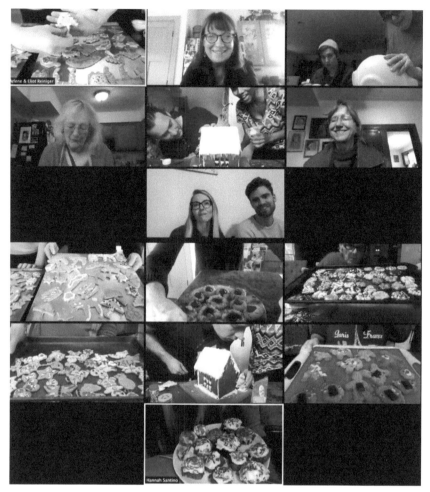

Figure 3.2. Virtual Christmas cookie decorating, December 2020. (Photos by Susan Eleuterio, used with permission.)

celebration. One member sent a number of recipes from which individuals selected the cookies they wanted to make and prepared them ahead of time. The time together on Zoom was spent decorating the cookies, discussing the process, and recounting past attempts at such endeavors. There was also a great deal of aesthetic satisfaction—and envy—as everyone shared their final products on the screen (see figure 3.2).

Similarly, for St. Patrick's Day, Lucy shared a recipe for Irish soda bread and led an online cooking demonstration of how to make it the Northern Irish style, on a stovetop griddle instead of in the oven. In both cases, the baking was an affirmation of friendships that already existed, but the activity also added a layer of commonality that turned the group into what feels now like a community.

Family groups that baked together seemed to have an additional purpose of passing along traditions. Baking was an excuse to connect virtually, but it also involved familial identity and history through the recipes and knowledge that were being celebrated—and preserved. One participant in the comfort food project recounted how she began teaching a niece to make family recipes via Zoom:

> I gave her a cooking lesson. I gave her the recipe ahead of time and then she and I made blintzes together, it was so much fun. So she loved that, and next on our list is cinnamon rolls, which [my] grandmother, my bubbeh, . . . used to make these amazing yeast cinnamon rolls. She would make them for everybody . . .—she had four kids and all these grandchildren, she would make a big pot of them for everybody and either my cousin and she find somebody to deliver them on Friday morning, so we would have them for Saturday morning breakfast. (H.G.S., Comfort Foodways Oral History interview, Summer 2020)

This sampling of the variety of groups that developed around bread and baking raises the question of whether or not they could be considered communities in the scholarly sense. Not everyone was welcome in them; each set parameters for membership, and some, especially the ones focusing more on artisanal breads and pastries, seemed to require a certain amount of technical baking knowledge and skill to fully participate.[22] As these were voluntary groups, however, individuals, particularly in the virtual networks, could easily disengage or fade into the background. Also, in a number of cases, administrators and organizers of the groups emphasized that learning and sharing knowledge were purposes of the group and that interactions needed to be respectful and helpful. Such rules encouraged the sense of those groups being communities in that they would accept members' individual abilities, identities, and interests as long as they agreed on the commonality. In this way, the groups are perhaps more typical of face-to-face interactions.

The significance of these groups being perceived as communities is obvious given the circumstances of the pandemic. COVID-19 crossed national borders and ignored the usual lines drawn in societies around race, class, gender, religion, and even abilities.[23] It had the potential of affecting the health of every individual across the globe. It also affected some communities, nations, and regions more than others. In the United States, for example, the high mortality and morbidity rates in some Indigenous nations were tragic, and the loss of elders keenly felt (McLernon 2021). For those who recognized that threat or felt the economic, social, or psychological repercussions of it, the idea of community was both a comfort and a solution. As a global pandemic, COVID-19 was a commonality reflecting and emphasizing the connectedness of all people. Closing down borders ironically affirmed those connections, although a number of individuals then interpreted the closings as threats to their own well-being. It is no surprise, however, that communities would emerge around the commonality of food. The specific focus on bread and baking in the US reflects the symbolism and romanticized nostalgia associated with those products and activities. Further observation is needed to determine whether other nations and cultural groups selected different foodways activities to emphasize.

These groups affirmed the diversity as well as the individuality of US citizens—we could choose to connect with others who shared our interests, abilities, and tastes around baking. Not all of us were required to make bread; we could bake other items.

Not all of us had to acquire specialized skills to be part of the groups; "lurking" was, for the most part, permissible and accepted. This possibility for the performance of individuality challenges the sense of collective community that could have been possible during the pandemic and was hoped for by public health officials meekly requesting people to wear masks, social distance, and take other precautions for keeping the virus at bay. Even as of this writing in the summer of 2022, vaccinations were seen as a personal choice, an assertion of the rights of the individual over the rights of the collective that threatens the health of the entire nation. There is a long history of this phenomenon in the US (Leask 2020). The wide range of groups that emerged around baking reflects the basic American ethos of individualism and illustrates smaller collectives based on personal preferences and identities.

There also were many for whom the pandemic caused economic, social, and emotional hardships that could not be easily assuaged by spending an afternoon kneading dough and watching it rise. The turn to baking could be seen as a reflection of privilege and the groups developing around it as elitist and self-indulgent, dismissive or unaware of the realities of other people's lives. The emphasis on what is usually considered artisanal baking in the US was interpreted in this way by some, partly because of the associations of such baking with foodies, sophistication, and money.[24] While some individuals approached baking as cultural capital and were able to participate in these communities because of economic or social privilege, motivations for participating in specific practices and groups can be multiple and complex. The need to belong seems to be a universal of human behavior, and the pandemic accentuated that need. Also, some of these groups did go out of their way not only to make members feel welcome but to also contribute to the broader community. Postings in one virtual baking group, for example, told of donating their excess baked goods to food pantries, neighbors who might be in need, or to free community meals. Such offerings can be seen as a reaching out to expand the community of bakers.

Will these baking-focused "communities" continue after the pandemic? Folk groups that develop a range of traditions and expressive forms tend to last longer, so those that were based only on one aspect of bread making and did not allow for other interactions were probably not as strong. Geographic and physical proximity may contribute also, since there is then more potential for informal and unplanned interactions. It remains to be seen, then, whether or not the virtual baking groups will fade over time as individuals get back to routine life.[25] The knowledge gained will continue, as will memories of shared experiences during the pandemic. Those memories can remind individuals of the sense of community, whether or not the group itself continues. Furthermore, secondary commonalities may bring former group members together, so that baking during the pandemic will add a topic of conversation and a layer of connectedness between those individuals.

CRAFTSMANSHIP

The pandemic was—and still is—a time of uncertainty. COVID-19 disrupted daily routines and challenged the usual strategies for keeping oneself safe. It also threatened livelihoods and disrupted plans for the future. It is logical, then, that one of the things people seemed to seek during this time was a sense of their own agency and efficacy in controlling what was happening in their lives.

Baking offered an opportunity for that. Recipes and instructions could be followed; ingredients measured or tweaked; dough mixed and kneaded; oven times and temperatures adjusted. All of these activities were steps in the completion of the task, and if the results were unfavorable, the baker could then analyze where the process had failed and what needed to be done for the next attempt to be successful.

As the pandemic lingered on, individuals developed their baking skills—through classes, reading, watching videos, discussions in virtual groups, critiques by those consuming the final products, and trial and error.

The mastery of these skills was a matter of necessity for those who were dependent on their baking for meals and sustenance. Others enjoyed the mastery itself; it gave them a sense of competence and satisfaction. That mastery also tapped into the need to feel a sense of agency, to be able to control something from start to finish, to gain the satisfaction of successful achievement, or to experience full aesthetical engagement. Out of this mastery there also developed higher levels of critical assessment and evaluation of the final products. While the appreciation of quality baked goods can be seen as a sign of elitism, we suggest here that the drive to master baking skills is more accurately interpreted as a form of craftsmanship. That craftsmanship then fed into home baking as both comfort and community.

Craftsmanship is the mastery of skills, techniques, and tools needed to produce something. The term is most often used when its products are considered craft rather than art. Folklorists and other scholars have pointed out that the difference between the two is actually intent and use, and that these frequently overlap and can shift. Art has a primarily aesthetic and decorative function, while craft has a primarily practical and functional one (Pocius 2003, Vlach and Bronner 1986). Objects can be made for one purpose, however, but used for another; they can also serve both purposes simultaneously.

Home baking during the pandemic straddles this line between art and craft, challenging what can be understood as a specifically Eurocentric, American approach to creativity and production. As folklorist Henry Glassie points out: "Western definitions feature functions that separate art from utility and identify it with leisure, making art the province of the rich . . . The Turkish definition, centered existentially in performance, stresses the individual's passionate commitment to creation, despite differences of medium, function, and consumptions" (1999, 26). The bakers and eaters in our research and observations viewed these home-baked products with both a practical and aesthetic eye. They were making products that were meant to be consumed, but they also were critiquing their shape, color, texture, and taste, aspects irrelevant to the nutritional character of the bread or its potential to satisfy one's hunger. On the Facebook group Fiddle and Dough, for example, members frequently posted photographs of their productions, pointing out successes and failures in both artistic and functional qualities. Statements such as "It's not pretty, but it tastes wonderful" reflect this attitude toward their baking as simultaneously art and craft.

Discussions such as these illustrate the overlap of pragmatic function and aesthetic pleasure that was derived from home baking. They also suggest the fluidity of the meanings of home baking in that individuals could shift the purposes of the activity. There were times when the appearance of the bread did not matter, as long as it was tasty or served its purpose of feeding people. Also, individuals could choose the focus of their own baking. They could emphasize the technical challenges of baking bread, the aesthetic appearance of that bread, the nutritional content, or the taste as well as the social and cultural contexts surrounding it, and that emphasis could vary with different instances of baking. Their choice of focus might reflect personal interests, skills, available materials, circumstances, or other factors, and those choices could also determine which groups individuals chose to join and how they wanted to participate.

Folklore scholars have written extensively about the motivations and functions of craftsmanship (Glassie 1999; Jones 1995; Shukla 2008), and these are relevant to understanding home baking during the pandemic. Michael Owen Jones, for example, points out that "during an emotion-ally trying time, . . . one may turn to making things, finding the rhythmic motions soothing, the texture and colors and smells of materials a pleasant distraction, the preoccupation with ideas about form a needed diversion from personal problems, the association of the activity with other people and another time a source of strength, the successful completion of the object a concrete testimony to one's ability to restore order and to accom-plish something of value, and the public's reception of the object a rein-forcement of one's sense of self-esteem" (1995, 271).

Craftsmanship involves developing knowledge and skills in at least three areas involved in the actual making of an object: the materials going into it, the tools or equipment needed to execute the processes, and the techniques for using those tools on those specific materials. Each of these areas can be seen in home baking. Some forms of baking, however, require more specialized knowledge and skills and may take longer for individuals to master. Breads made with yeast, whether wild or commercially produced, frequently require a certain level of expertise, as do some other baked goods, and the craftsmanship needed to produce them was the subject of much discussion on social media.

Knowledge of the materials for home baking translates into familiarity with the ingredients. Different types of flours and even different brands tend to respond in their own ways and require different techniques for preparation. Also, knowledge of which flours work with each other and with other ingredients is needed in order to obtain the desired effect. Even the age of the flour makes a difference to the amount of liquid needed to make a pliable dough, something that many bakers claim can only be learned through experience and understanding the proper feel of a sufficiently but not overly hydrated dough. The shortages of white flour in mainstream supermarkets caused much dismay on social media and led to experimentation with other flours or brands. Similarly, cautions about going to the supermarket meant that many people dug into their stores of food supplies, relying on what they already had in stock. For some home bakers that meant using flours and grains they had been saving for special occasions or for specialized baking.

Lucy, for example, had a stash in her freezer of flours relatively unusual in mainstream American baking: teff, chestnut, cassava, yam, rye, soy, rice, and cornmeal—as well as miscellaneous grains and other things she frequently added to her baking—sorghum, millet, wheat berries, rye flakes, hominy grits, hemp seed, black walnuts, and dried goji berries. For sweetening, she had black strap molasses, sorghum molasses, cane syrup, and maple syrup. She had flaxseed meal that worked well as a substitute for eggs, although she did have friends who raised chickens and were sharing their eggs. She had no yeast but did have baking soda and baking powder to use as leavening agents. She did not want to venture into the stores for milk, but she did have several cartons of almond milk. This eclectic mixture of foodstuffs was not mentioned in most recipes, but she started experimenting with them, trying out various substitutions. She discovered that Irish soda bread could easily incorporate any of the flours available, and that buttermilk could be created with vinegar added to almond milk. Cornbread was similarly flexible, and could easily be turned into a cake with more eggs and sweeteners. She even found a recipe for a molasses cornmeal cake made with baking soda that was reminiscent of New England brown bread.

Necessity gave rise to this experimentation, but it was also a way to create something from the materials on hand, giving a sense of security in the knowledge that she could create tasty dishes from substitutions, a practice that came to be called by some people "Not this, that."[26] Music scholars Kate Galloway and Rachael Fuller point out that such substitutions can also be seen as improvisations, as intentionally creative productions based on a theme. In their study of "baker-listener-performers" who recorded their sourdough starters to determine their soundscape, they conclude, "Improvisation goes beyond music . . . It saturates our everyday lives. It is part of our social lives and during pandemic times, it has emerged in unexpected places" (2021, 1). Our observations of baking during the pandemic confirm that many individuals were "improvising" with whatever materials they could find.

Similarly, the basic materials needed to leaven baked goods became a prominent subject on social media, and those with knowledge of these rising agents oftentimes passed along their knowledge. Sourdough starters, along with instructions for caring for them, were frequently shared in social groups. Initially, it did not seem to be common knowledge that wild yeasts could be "caught," and posts began explaining how to do that.[27] Those familiar with the process seemed to revel in their knowledge as well as the public affirmation of their mastery of the materials. A number of posts on social media sites observed with bemusement the panic over the yeast shortage, revealing that their own craftsmanship in using other leavenings gave them a sense of security.

Familiarity with tools and equipment are also part of craftsmanship. American kitchens generally include an oven along with deep, rectangular pans and larger flat sheets. The common names of these pans suggest the fundamental role of baking in American food culture: loaf pans and cookie sheets. Discussions on social media, particularly after the pandemic was underway, oftentimes addressed specific types of equipment, with suggestions of brands to obtain or ways to adapt ones bakers already had. There also were instructions for matching specific pans with particular types of bread or pastry. Cast iron frying pans, for example, were suggested for cornbread, and covered Dutch ovens for sourdough bread.

Bakers also needed the technical skills to manipulate ingredients and tools. For those new to the craft, skills could be acquired from in-person demonstrations, online classes, cookbooks, baking blogs or vlogs, or instructional videos. The social media groups of which Lucy was a member usually included a great deal of discussion on specific skills, with individuals describing problems and others offering solutions. One obvious point from these interactions was that baking was a hands-on activity that required experiential knowledge to master. Successful bread bakers needed to be able to "feel" the texture of the dough when they were kneading it to know when to stop. They also needed to be able to judge doneness by sight and smell, skills that could be described by instructors but had to be experienced to master. An individual describes how they approached learning the craft—and the resulting satisfaction from mastery:

> One of the things I always do is I kind of set goals for myself, like I want to learn how to make whatever, and then I make it until I figure out how to make it, if it's something difficult. So like my husband and I every December make macarons, French macarons and I we, we started out being not so good at it, but, you know, we've gotten better at it over time. So anyway, one of the things I wanted to figure out how to make this summer was pizza, because . . . we've been making a lot of bread and things. And I'd made pizzas like a couple times in the past, but they were not highly successful. I mean, they were fine, but not great. And so every week

I've been making pizzas and I've got it and I have cracked the code. I can make a perfect pan pizza reliably. It's delicious. So this is my hashtag pandemic pizza. This is one of the things that I feel is now a triumph of this time. And I think that has definitely taken on significance because it feels very exciting to have a pizza because we can't you know, we're not buying anything from out. Normally, we would have always bought a pizza already made. So that's taken on some significance. (S.G., Comfort Foodways Oral History interview, Summer 2020)

The mastery of these skills and knowledge served a practical purpose in that it increased the likelihood of achieving the desired outcomes of the labor. One individual described his baking as a way to get certain products that he had previously only experienced during his travels:

I've started baking more . . . , including Parker House rolls and high-protein breads. One experiment I'm working on is getting the technique correct for using the New England bun pan from USA Pan to make the grillable buns for hot dog, lobster, and clam rolls, when those buns are unavailable in other locations. (D.L., Comfort Foodways Oral History interview, Summer 2020)

Mastery also satisfied emotional needs in that the experience of baking itself—as well as the eating that followed—seemed to bring comfort. The repetitiveness of kneading bread had a meditative quality for many (Siragusa 2021), and the process of creating something delicious arise from start to finish seemed to give a sense of efficacy: people could not do anything about the pandemic, but they could control the baking process. The activity of baking also brought an aesthetic engagement that fully engaged the senses and focused the mind on that engagement (Glassie 1986; Noyes 2014), distracting it from other concerns. One individual was delighted to find that she had the skills to be creative, mentioning that the results brought nostalgic memories as well as aesthetic pleasure:

There's a Jewish food noodle kugel. It's a noodle pudding like rice pudding. But instead of rice, you use egg noodles. It's got all these cheeses in it and it's really good. My husband loves it, and I do too, and I was like, well, I don't need a recipe. I'll just make this, and he was so happy. It was like, wow, we haven't had this in months, you know. It's like, wow, maybe we could live on this forever. You know, certainly as a kid, I grew up on it, you know, especially in the winter, having it once or twice a week, and it was a really nice welcome back to it. (H.G.S., Comfort Foodways Oral History interview, Summer 2020)

Developing skills in baking also fed into community. As individuals sought and offered information on the craft, they interacted, getting to know each other as well as shaping the identity of the larger group. Some groups, both virtual and real-life, seemed to focus on craftsmanship, while others emphasized the sociality, but in both cases, there was the potential for a community of insiders who now shared knowledge and experiences. An indication of the solidity of the group was the use of a common "work language," or vocabulary specific to the craft (McCarl 1986). This "jargon" referred to details of ingredients, tools, or technical skills involved in baking and was developed in order to communicate effectively about the processes and results. Its use demonstrated that individuals were part of the same reference group, of a folk group (Ben-Amos 1971). The nuances of coloration, form, texture, and flavor could be the source of endless conversations. Specialized vocabulary could also be used to signal membership in a group or hierarchies of mastery, as occurred in the example given earlier of the "poolish" comment in response to the joke about "biga."

Craftsmanship in baking could be interpreted as a sign of elitism and privilege. Artisanal breads and pastries in the US tend to carry those connotations. After all, time and material resources are necessary in order to develop those skills. Also, the attention to the aesthetics of the process as well as the appreciation of the sense of mastery gained from it do not seem to be part of the historical role of home baking as a functional, domestic chore. The rise of this craftsmanship, however, can also be seen as a vernacular response to the pandemic. This was not something suggested by policy makers or the medical establishment; it grew instead out of individuals' interests and needs as well as the public shortages and disruptions in the food system. It was a way for people to adapt, individually and collectively, to the circumstances. It arose organically through social media and social networks, borrowing at times from official "authorities," such as cookbooks or chef's instructional videos but, as individuals acquired more skills, the role of expert was passed around and shared. Hierarchies within the groups existed but seemed to be based on merit as well as an individual's willingness to be helpful in their critiques. It could be argued that the pandemic fostered a democratizing of baking craftsmanship in that it now seemed to be available to all—an apprenticeship in France or Italy, while still admirable, was not necessary to become a master. This vernacular craftsmanship, then, challenges the food industry's hold on baking in the US, while at the same time suppliers of baking ingredients have become more active in promoting and enabling at-home baking (Byron 2021).

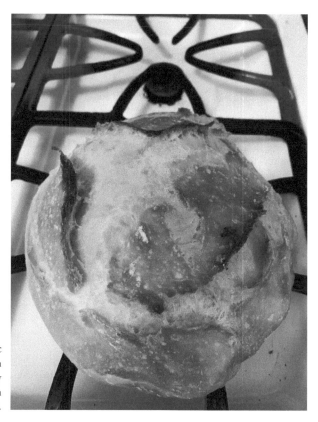

Figure 3.3. "Pandemic loaf" (sourdough boule), made by Theresa Vaughan in April 2020.

Not everyone who baked emphasized craftsmanship; for some, baking was an onerous obligation. Also, not everyone who appreciated the craftsmanship actually participated in baking. Eaters—and sometimes viewers—of the baked goods were part of the community of bakers as recipients of their labor. Some became more knowledgeable about baking through their consumption, and more adept at evaluating quality. They learned to detect nuances determined by differences in ingredients, tools, or techniques. They also frequently were exposed to a wider variety of baked products than previously. Their responses to a product could be taken as literal feedback to enable further development of craftsmanship. This perhaps challenges the assumptions about mainstream American food culture being made up of undiscriminating eaters who emphasize quantity and expense over quality and craftsmanship. Perhaps the pandemic is causing many more of us to become "foodies," making that the norm rather than what is usually perceived by cultural observers as an aberration.

Craftsmanship in vernacular baking is integrated with the other two themes we noticed, those of comfort and community. Mastery of skills and knowledge brought a sense of control, agency, and efficacy that was comforting on a psychological level. Many individuals also found communities in the process of gaining that mastery and then sharing it with others. This overlapping of these domains is a reflection of the complexity of lived realities that modern life has disguised. We tend to think of cooking and eating as separate from the initial growing of food, processing, and distribution of it. Similarly, we tend to think of our food choices as being up to the individual and separate from other aspects of life. Vernacular baking shows that these domains are all intermingled, that we as individuals are interconnected.

CONCLUSION

Home baking during the pandemic was a vernacular response to the events, conditions, and concerns created by the spread of the COVID-19 virus. While it served a practical function in providing food for sustenance, it also fulfilled a diverse range of needs—for comfort, community, and craftsmanship. While each of these needs was addressed at times by "official" culture (governmental groups, civic organizations, mass media), the emergence of vernacular practices oftentimes reflected an interplay with—and sometimes a challenge of—that official culture. Cookbooks, chefs, nutritional experts, and other food "pundits" seemed to be sources for inspiration, experimentation, and perhaps guidance, rather than the "final say" for evaluating quality and meaning.

For example, home baking was tied directly to the concept of comfort food, a category reflecting mainstream American moralities around food and eating that emphasize the impact of foods on physical appearance and health. The embracing of home baking and of home-baked goods, however, challenged that morality, asserting both that foods could be evaluated for reasons beyond their connection to body weight and that individuals who enjoyed such foods should not be shamed. Similarly, the idea of comfort food had been co-opted by the American food industry as a marketing category for certain dishes and cuisines, offering a definition that emphasized large quantities of salt, sugar, carbohydrates, and fats. The vernacular response allowed for each individual to find comfort in whichever foods "worked" for them. This "culinary relativism," as Lucy has called this elsewhere (Long et al. 2021), acknowledges that individuals have different memories attached to foods as well as different tastes, circumstances, and values that shape which foods are comforting to them. The vernacular response also meant that people could seek comfort from the processes and socializing around baking, not just the consumption of baked products. This shift from product to process could perhaps be seen as a challenge to the more usual consumerist ethos of mainstream American culture. While this turn to using home baking for comfort seemed initially to be a response to the food media's suggestions for ways to deal with the pandemic, it quickly was personalized and localized.

Vernacular responses can also be seen in the development of new communities around home baking as well as the re-envisioning or affirmation of previously established communities, particularly on social media. These groups shared skills and knowledge specific to baking, but they were also significant mediums for socializing and assuaging the isolation that many experienced during the pandemic. Perhaps because they were perceived as temporary and innovative, they tended to flexible and dynamic. Their different emphases allowed for varying interests, skills, personalities, and even values. For example, some groups focused on specific types of baking—sourdough, rye, bread in general, or any kind of pastries or desserts. The groups also took different approaches to the subject, with some emphasizing technical skills, others the sharing of recipes, and still others discussions of adaptations for health issues. This variety allowed individuals to find groups with which they felt compatible, increasing the likelihood that the group would develop into a community. This also allowed for communities to develop within larger groupings, making the smaller ones more expressive of specific localities and personalities.

These vernacular communities brought attention to individuals who might have been previously overlooked, allowing them to emerge as knowledge holders and authorities in the domain of home baking. For example, grandmothers and housewives became sources for information alongside, and perhaps replacing, trained nutritionists and professional chefs. The usual hierarchies of authority shifted through these groups, celebrating the value of lived experience and perhaps encouraging a democratization of roles.[28]

Similarly, the craftsmanship that developed around home baking was open to any individual who had the resources and interests.[29] The idea that anyone can master such skills without going through official culinary training challenges some of the popular perceptions of baking and of art in general. While inborn talent is recognized, the trends during the pandemic suggested that crafts can be learned through vernacular avenues, through imitative, hands-on experiences outside of formal institutions and from community members who are considered masters of those skills.

Furthermore, those trends also challenge the division between producers and consumers that tends to characterize our modern industrial-based society, demonstrating the interplay of those domains of activity. Baking offered an opportunity to follow a product from start to finish, giving a sense of connection between one's labor and the food eaten that is oftentimes not a part of contemporary eating.

A final pair of questions is why baking, and why bread? It is possible that Americans turned to them because of nostalgia around the foundational role of bread and other baked goods in historical and contemporary foodways, particularly in the idealized childhood and family life of the 1950s. As a staple of many everyday meals as well as an item frequently incorporated into celebratory and festive meals, bread offers continuity with a pre-COVID past. Those memories then gave hope for the future as well as comfort in the present (Sutton 2001). It is also possible that the symbolic meanings of bread as spiritual nourishment[30] spoke to people during this time of uncertainty and social isolation. Our own experiences, though, suggest that there is something about these objects and practices that makes them rich for expressive uses. Their very materiality engages all the senses, and the tangible nature of their preparation is "grounding" in a psychological sense. The physical efforts involved in kneading bread, rolling out pie crusts, or mixing cookie dough offer an interplay of physical and mental effort that is rewarding in itself. Also, the smelling, tasting, and eating of these foods brings together the individual and the community of others who supplied knowledge, encouragement, or even ingredients, making tangible the realities of those connections.

Home baking, as seen through the lenses of comfort, community, and craftsmanship, offers us an instructive and complex example of the resilience of vernacular culture. Vernacular culture has always been a framework within which individuals act, make meaning, and satisfy needs for aesthetic expression. By focusing on home baking, we have demonstrated that, despite the prevalence of various forms of media and the increased availability of expert instruction and information via the internet, robust vernacular expressions continue to arise in response to changing needs, both in the routines of daily life and in crises such as the COVID-19 pandemic.

NOTES

Lucy borrows the word *coroniverse* from a friend and mental health activist, Christen Giblin, who used it in a hometown newspaper, the Sentinel Tribune, in Bowling Green, Ohio. In her essay on "What have you learned in the coroniverse?" she states: "Yes, I did just coin a term to express how the coronavirus has transformed our entire world. At the same time it has changed each of our personal spheres, demanding adjustments and new behaviors." July 23, 2020 (https://www.sent-trib.com/community/what-have-you-learned-in-the-coroniverse/article_5db3dd42-ccc3-11ea-88b2-b3aa561ac99a.html). Folklore scholars will appreciate the word in the way it evokes the sense of liminality prevalent during this time.

1. Numerous journalists, cultural observers, and scholars from a wide variety of disciplines have noticed the rise of baking in the US and other nations during the pandemic. Not surprisingly, some of these share interpretations and conclusions similar to parts of our own work. We have tried to include citations for that scholarship throughout the chapter, but several that are closely aligned with our own folkloristic approach are Easterbrook-Smith 2020; Ocklenburg 2020; Siragusa 2021; and Sofo et al. 2021.

2. See Severson and Moskin 2020 for a newspaper report on these concerns in March 2020 at the beginning of the pandemic in the US.

3. Data is drawn from several sources. Our personal experiences are offered as auto-ethnographic accounts of the pandemic in the US, since we also were experiencing it. We recognize that our experiences are not necessarily representative of the living conditions and attitudes of other regions of the US. We are living in university towns, Lucy in Ohio and Theresa in Oklahoma, where the effects of the pandemic have been relatively restrained. Both of us are white, educated, middle class, and in established family and community social networks, so that we have a certain amount or privilege in not needing to worry about food security or economic stability. Both of us participated in social media and virtual groups that interacted around baking, and we both observed trends on various platforms and within our social universes. Also used are responses to a virtual oral history project on finding comfort/discomfort through foodways, directed by Lucy in the summer and fall of 2020 (Comfort Foodways Oral History), primarily in the US but also in six other countries (see www.foodandculture.org). Run through the nonprofit Center for Food and Culture, over sixty interviews were conducted by five graduate students. For further description of the project, see Long et al. 2021.

4. Often used to refer to material culture, the precise definition of *vernacular* changes somewhat from scholar to scholar and discipline to discipline. All uses, however, emphasize individual lives and works as lived; as such, they offer a more complete view of human creative endeavors than those that focus on the elite, or that relegate the "folk" to the rural, the unschooled, or the simple. Henry Glassie, for example, used the term in studying regional styles of architecture, focusing on buildings by those who had acquired housebuilding housebuilding skills through use of local materials and modular patterns of building design: "The term [vernacular] . . . marks the transition from the unknown to the known: we call buildings 'vernacular' because they embody values alien to those cherished in the academy. When we call buildings 'folk,' the implication was that they countered in commonness and tradition the pretense and progress that dominate simple academic schemes. Folk buildings contained a different virtue. The study of vernacular architecture, through its urge toward the comprehensive, accommodates cultural diversity. It welcomes the neglected into study in order to acknowledge the reality of difference and conflict" (1999, 230). For a more recent use of *vernacular*, see Diarmuid Ó Gilláin 2013.

5. The issue of privilege around baking was noted by other scholars and cultural observers, with some examining the racial disparities it represented. For example, see McCaugherty 2020; Mohabeer 2023; Somani 2021. I also discuss issues of privilege in reference to comfort food during the pandemic (Long et al. 2021; Long 2022).

6. The phrase was originally introduced to the public by a psychologist, Dr. Joyce Brothers, who heard it from clients as an explanation for their eating habits. She then used it to explain the obesity epidemic of the 1960s, but in recent years, the food industry has turned comfort food into a marketing category. That category includes commercially and heavily processed snack foods and calorie-laden desserts as well as dishes from certain food cultures—midwestern, southern, soul, and Jewish—that tend to emphasize large serving portions, frying (particularly deep frying), and quantities of salt, sugar, and fats that exceed the nutritionist-recommended amounts.

7. Recent work by humanities scholars has suggested additional needs, such as connectedness, efficacy, meaning, distraction, agency/control, and structure (Jones and Long 2017; Shen et al. 2020; Long et al. 2021). For overviews of the scholarship on comfort food, see Jones and Long 2017; and Spence 2017.

8. Gwen Easterbrook-Smith makes a similar point in an article in which she discusses bread baking during the pandemic as fulfilling three functions: "providing sustenance; filling newly available leisure time; and offering a way to demonstrate one's skill and activities on social media" (2021, 36).

9. For more on food and embodiment, see Heldke 1992 and Sutton 2010. Also, scholarship by folklorists addresses the full engagement of the senses that occurs with aesthetic experiences (Pocius 2003).

10. In fact, sensory pleasure and comfort were very much a part of pandemic baking. In a survey of New Zealanders (3,028 respondents, mostly female) by a team working in public health, the researchers expected to find an increase in healthy eating habits, focusing on fresh produce, as a means to mitigate COVID morbidity. Instead, they found a 41% increase in the consumption of sweet snacks, a 33% increase in the consumption of both salty snacks and alcohol, and a 20% increase in the consumption of sugary drinks (Gerritsen et al. 2021).

11. Nostalgia has been critiqued by many cultural scholars as a response to modernity and industrialization; however, folklore and other scholars have recently reevaluated it as a dynamic lens through which communities compare and define both their past and present. See Cashman 2006 for an overview of the scholarship and an illustration of this approach.

12. The usage of "proper" here refers to the Mary Douglas's work (1972) on implicit social meanings of food and her discussion of what constitutes meals in British food culture.

13. Bread is also a major staple food anywhere that wheat was grown as an early domesticated grain—in North Africa, West Asia, and Central Asia in addition to Europe. For an early influential study of the significance of bread, see Counihan 1984. Other materials—vegetables, grains, seeds, tubers, nuts—were also used to make baked foods throughout the world. The American usage of "bread" implies the norm of yeast breads made from wheat, frequently commercially made and store-bought. Other varieties and sources are usually clarified by grain (e.g., cornbread, rye bread) or rising agent (e.g., sourdough bread, soda bread) and also as bakery or home-produced.

14. For more specifics on class and gender issues around work during the pandemic, see the study released by the Pew Foundation on December 9, 2020, titled "How the Coronavirus Outbreak Has and Hasn't Changed the Way Americans Work," https://www.pewresearch .org/social-trends/2020/12/09/how-the-coronavirus-outbreak-has-and-hasnt-changed-the -way-americans-work/.

15. Lucy conducted interviews with individuals in northwest Ohio about how their living situations affected their ability to find comfort through foodways. Not surprisingly, those who were sharing small kitchen spaces with others tended to find it less convenient to

prepare baked goods, even though they were working at home and had the time to do so. See Long et al. 2021.

16. Louise O. Vasvári (2018) uses this phrase in her discussion of food memories among Jewish Hungarian survivors of the Holocaust.

17. Examples include the listservs and Facebook pages of two scholarly associations of which the authors are members, the American Folklore Society and the Association for the Study of Food and Society. The *New York Times* food section also began featuring recipes for comfort foods from individual chefs who came from diverse backgrounds.

18. Human Relations Area Files, "Craving Comfort: Bonding with Food across Cultures," https://hraf.yale.edu/craving-comfort-bonding-with-food-across-cultures/.

19. See, for example, work by sociologist Alice Julier (2013).

20. See, for example, Siragusa 2021.

21. One example, "Rye Revival," based in Madison, Wisconsin, "supports the expansion of ecological rye production; educates about rye for human, animal, and agricultural purposes; advances research on rye; and centers these efforts on the promotion of food equity, good food, and cultural heritage" (https://www.facebook.com/ryerevival.org/). The fledgling organization uses a variety of social media as well as socially distanced personal communication to promote the baking and consuming of rye bread to support rye production and preservation. The group was not developed specifically as a response to COVID-19, but during the pandemic, its in-person group activities had to be put on hold. It moved to Zoom meetings, which actually meant that it could cast a wider geographic net, attracting more members. Also, the leader had to travel for family reasons during the pandemic and took rye bread to people for tastings during these trips. Lucy was the fortunate recipient of some of these loaves and then shared them with a local group of friends that enjoyed tasting new foods. While this loose network of rye eaters would not be considered a folk group, it did broaden the rye "community" of those who appreciated the bread.

22. Facebook "communities" often have limited membership and can be moderated so that rules around subject matter and interactions can be enforced. This is different from Twitter, which is much more public and anonymous. Does Facebook, therefore, better mimic the actual structure of social relationships than do some other social media platforms? The same is true of Zoom meetings, which are invitation-only.

23. It is evident now that, while the virus itself jumps across various social divides specific populations are more vulnerable, particularly regarding the availability of high-quality medical care. The number of cases and deaths within Black and Native American communities has been much higher than among Whites, bringing attention to how race, ethnicity, and class are still factors in quality of life the US (Smith 2020; McLernon 2021).

24. One individual participating in the oral history on comfort/discomfort foods pointed out that the shortages of yeast and flour affected only a part of the American population and also tended to be seen primarily in the industrial food system and mainstream food culture. "Ethnic" groceries did not have shortages, even of items like flour (H.G.S., Comfort Foodways Oral History, Summer 2020).

25. There is evidence that after two years into the pandemic, interest in virtual baking groups faded. Part of that is due to "Zoom fatigue," exhaustion from sitting in front of a computer, but other factors were also at play, such as people going back to work outside the home and having more face-to-face interactions. Some posts on social media attribute fading interest to the weight gain resulting from so much baking.

26. Thanks to Diane Goldstein for pointing out this phrase. She recounts how a hostess gift was "not this, that" bags filled with newly discovered products and recipes created by forced substitutions due to the pandemic.

27. One group that emerged on Facebook is the Sourdough Bread Support Group, which developed a web page giving directions for how to make a wild starter: https://sourdough-breadsupportgroup.com/making-a-sourdough-starter/. This is just a single example of many.

28. We recognize that there is a paradox here. If we are looking primarily at communities mediated through social media, Zoom, or other forms of electronic facilitation—which we tend to think of as anonymizing—we can return to a more "traditional" style of learning from family or friends rather than through the Food Network, celebrity chefs, or other institutions that teach culinary skills. Social media itself is simultaneously supportive of "expert" teaching and democratizing, because individual voices can still be heard. Popular culture scholar Henry Jenkins (2008) describes this paradox as characteristic of the "convergence culture" resulting from the emergence of new media that allows viewers to participate in the creation of productions and encourages them to find connections between various media products.

29. Resources are obviously shaped by sociocultural and historical factors that reflect racial, class, and gender inequalities. Demographic studies of who exactly was involved in home baking during the pandemic is needed. See, for example, Faludi and Crosby 2021. Geographic location, urban or rural, and type of living circumstances also impact individuals' abilities to follow their interests.

30. Bread plays a significant role in religious rituals in Christian cultures, metaphorically—and for some literally—standing in for the body of Christ during Communion services. It is significant in a broader cultural sense, however, as implied when bread is referred to as the "staff of life," the higher wage earner in a family is called the "breadwinner," or when people refer to a job that is not their first choice as what they do for their "bread and butter." For more on bread's symbolism from a global perspective, see Lewis 2017 and Matvejević 2020.

REFERENCES

Bauman, Richard. 1972. "Differential Identity and the Social Base of Folklore." In *Towards New Perspectives in Folklore*, edited by Americo Paredes and Richard Bauman, 31–41. Austin: University of Texas Press.

Belasco, Warren J. (1993) 2014. *Appetite for Change: How the Counterculture Took on the Food Industry*. Ithaca, NY: Cornell University Press.

Ben-Amos, Dan. 1971. "Toward a Definition of Folklore in Context." *Journal of American Folklore* 84 (331): 3–15.

Byron, Ellen. 2021. "Is Baking's Pandemic Popularity Just a Flash in the Pan?" *Wall Street Journal*, May 25. https://www.wsj.com/articles/is-bakings-pandemic-popularity-just-a-flash-in-the-pan-11621951200.

Cashman, Ray. 2006. "Critical Nostalgia and Material Culture in Northern Ireland." *Journal of American Folklore* 119 (472): 137–60.

Castrodale, Jelisa. 2020. "Our Pandemic Baking Binges Are Causing a Yeast Shortage." *Food and Wine*, April 16. https://www.foodandwine.com/news/yeast-supply-shortage-coronavirus.

Comfort Foodways Oral History. 2020. Center for Food and Culture. www.foodandculture .org and https://comfortfoodwaysexhibit.wordpress.com. (Directed by Lucy Long.)

Counihan, Carole. 1984. "Bread as World: Food Habits and Social Relations in Modernizing Sardinia." *Anthropological Quarterly* 57 (2): 47–59.

Dadalt, Audrey. 2021. "Why Is My Boule Black?" *Audrey Dadalt* (blog). https://audrey-dadalt.com/2021/08/18/why-is-my-boule-black/.

Delap, Josie. 2020. "Why Sourdough Went Viral: Wild Yeast Has Become Domesticated during the Pandemic." *Economist*, August 4. https://www.economist.com/1843/2020 /08/04/why-sourdough-went-viral.

Deutsch, Tracey. 2019. "Home, Cooking: Women's Place and Women's History in Local Foods Discourse." In *Food Fights: How the Past Matters in Contemporary Food Debates*, edited by Charles C. Ludington and Matthew Morse Booker, 208–29. Chapel Hill: University of North Carolina Press.

Douglas, Mary. 1972. "Deciphering a Meal." *Daedalus* 101 (1): 61–81.

Dutch, Jennifer Rachel. 2018. *Look Who's Cooking: The Rhetoric of American Home Cooking Traditions in the Twenty-First Century*. Jackson: University Press of Mississippi.

Easterbrook-Smith, Gwen. 2021. "By Bread Alone: Baking as Leisure, Performance, Sustenance, during the COVID-19 Crisis." *Leisure Sciences* 43 (1–2): 36–42.

Faludi, Julianna, and Michelle Crosby. 2021. "The Digital Economy of the Sourdough: Housewifisation in the Time of COVID-19." *Triple C* 19 (1): 113–24.

Galloway, Kate, and Rachael Fuller. 2021. "'Unmute' Bread: Listening, Improvising, and Performing with Sourdough in Quarantine." *Critical Studies in Improvisation/Études critiques en improvisation* 14 (2–3).

Gerritsen, Sarah, Victoria Egli, Rajshri Roy, Jill Haszard, Charlotte De Backer, Lauranna Teunissen, Isabelle Cuykx, Paulien Decorte, Sara Pabian Pabian, Kathleen Van Royen, and Lisa Te Morenga (Ngapuhi, Ngāti Whātua, Te Uri o Hua, Te Rarawa). 2021. "Seven Weeks of Home-Cooked Meals: Changes to New Zealanders' Grocery Shopping, Cooking and Eating during the COVID-19 Lockdown." *Journal of the Royal Society of New Zealand* 51 (supplement 1): S4–S22.

Giorgis, Hannah. 2020. "Foodie Culture as We Know It Is Over." *Atlantic*, May 5. https:// www.theatlantic.com/culture/archive/2020/05/foodiness-isnt-about-snobbery -anymore/611080/.

Glassie, Henry. 1986. "The Idea of Folk Art." In *Folk Art and Art Worlds*, edited by John Michael Vlach and Simon J. Bronner, 269–74. Ann Arbor: University of Michigan.

Glassie, Henry. 1999. *Material Culture*. Bloomington: Indiana University Press.

Goldberg, Emma. 2020. "Disordered Eating in a Disordered Time." *New York Times*, June 5. https://nyti.ms/2Y48XMH.

Güler, Ozan, and Murat Ismet Haseki. 2021. "Positive Psychological Impacts of Cooking during the COVID-19 Lockdown Period." *Frontiers in Psychology* 12 (635957).

Heldke, Lisa M. 1992. "Foodmaking as a Thoughtful Practice." In *Cooking, Eating, Thinking: Transformative Philosophies of Food*, edited by Deane W. Curtin and Lisa M. Heldke, 203–29. Bloomington: Indiana University Press.

Human Relations Area Files. 2023. "Craving Comfort: Bonding with Food across Cultures." Yale University. https://hraf.yale.edu/craving-comfort-bonding-with-food -across-cultures/.

Jenkins, Henry. 2008. *Convergence Culture: Where Old and New Media Collide*. New York: New York University Press.

Jones, Michael Owen. 1995. "Why Make (Folk) Art?" *Western Folklore* 54 (4): 253–76.

Jones, Michael Owen. 2017. "'Stressed' Spelled Backwards Is 'Desserts': Self-Medicating Moods with Foods." In *Comfort Food Meanings and Memories*, edited by Michael Owen Jones and Lucy M. Long, 17–41. Oxford: University of Mississippi Press.

Jones, Michael Owen, and Lucy M. Long. 2017. Introduction to *Comfort Food Meanings and Memories*, edited by Michael Owen Jones and Lucy M. Long, 3–16. Oxford: University of Mississippi Press.

Julier, Alice P. 2013. *Eating Together: Food, Friendship and Inequality*. Urbana: University of Illinois Press.

Koenig, Debbie. 2020. "The Pandemic Diet: How to Lose the 'Quarantine 15.'" *WebMD*. www.webmd.com/lung/news/20201029/pandemic-diet-how-to-lose-the-quarantine-15.

Lantis, Margaret. 1988. "Defining the Nature of Vernacular." *Material Culture* 20 (2–3): 1–8.

Leask, Julie. 2020. "Vaccines—Lessons from Three Centuries of Protest." *Nature* 585:499–501. https://www.nature.com/articles/d41586-020-02671-0.

Levenstein, Harvey. 1988. *Revolution at the Table: The Transformation of the American Diet*. New York: Oxford University Press.

Lewis, Hilda. 2017. *Bread: Consumption, Cultural Significance and Health Effects*. Hauppauge, NY: Nova Science.

Locher, Julie L. 2002. "Comfort Food." In *Encyclopedia of Food and Culture*, edited by Solomon H. Katz, 442–43. New York: Charles Scribner's Sons.

Locher, Julie L., William C. Yoels, Donna Maurer, and Jillian Van Ells. 2005. "Comfort Foods: An Exploratory Journey into the Social and Emotional Significance of Food." *Food and Foodways* 13:273–97.

Long, Lucy M. 2015. "Introduction to Part II." In *Food and Folklore: A Reader*, edited by Lucy M. Long, 51–59. London: Bloomsbury.

Long, Lucy M. 2020. *Finding Comfort/Discomfort through Foodways during the COVID-19 Pandemic*. Website and online exhibit. Center for Food and Culture. www.foodandculture.org.

Long, Lucy M. 2022. "How the Pandemic Redefined Comfort Food: American Individualism, Culinary Relativism, and Shifting Moralities." *Popular Culture Studies Journal* 10 (1): 1–18.

Long, Lucy M., Jerry Lee Reed III, John Broadwell, Quinlan Day Odum, Hannah M. Santino, and Minglei Zhang. 2021. "Finding Comfort and Discomfort through Foodways Practices during the COVID-19 Pandemic: A Public Folklore Project." *Digest* 8 (2). https://scholarworks.iu.edu/journals/index.php/digest/article/view/33644.

Mak, Aaron. 2020. "The Yeast Supply Chain Can't Just Activate Itself: There's a Reason the Ingredient Is Still Missing from the Stores." *Slate*, April 15. https://slate.com/business/2020/04/yeast-shortage-supermarkets-coronavirus.html.

Marvar, Alexandra. 2020. "Stress Baking More Than Usual? Confined to Their Homes, Americans Are Kneading Dough." *New York Times*, March 30. https://www.nytimes.com/2020/03/30/style/bread-baking-coronavirus.html.

Matvejević, Predrag. 2020. *Our Daily Bread: A Meditation on the Cultural and Symbolic Significance of Bread throughout History*. London: Istros Books.

McCarl, Robert. 1986. "Occupational Folklore." In *Folk Groups and Folklore Genres: An Introduction*, edited by Elliott Oring, 71–89. Logan: Utah State University Press.

McCaugherty, Stephen. 2020. "Caren White: New Jersey Woman's 'Stop Baking Bread' Medium Post Goes Viral." *Heavy*, May 3. https://heavy.com/news/2020/05/caren-white-stop-baking-bread/.

McLernon, Lianna Matt. 2021. "Reports Detail High COVID-19 Burden among Native Americans." *CIDRAP News* (Center for Infectious Disease Research and Policy), April 9. https://www.cidrap.umn.edu/news-perspective/2021/04/reports-detail-high-covid-19-burden-native-americans.

Mohabeer, Ravindra N. 2023. "COVID Bread-Porn: Social Stratification through Displays of Self-Management." In *The Cultural Politics of COVID-19*, edited by John Nguyet Erni and Ted Striphas, ch. 16. New York: Routledge.

Mull, Amanda. 2020. "Americans Have Baked All the Flour Away: The Pandemic Is Reintroducing the Nation to Its Kitchens." *Atlantic*, May 12. https://www.theatlantic .com/health/archive/2020/05/why-theres-no-flour-during-coronavirus/611527/.

Noyes, Dorothy. 2003. "Group." In *Eight Words for the Study of Expressive Culture*, edited by Burt Feintuch, 7–41. Urbana: University of Illinois Press.

Noyes, Dorothy. 2014. "Aesthetic Is the Opposite of Anaesthetic: On Tradition and Attention." *Journal of Folklore Research* 55 (2): 125–75.

Ocklenburg, Sebastian. 2020. "Distractibaking: A Note on the Psychology of Baking in Times of the COVID-19 Crisis." *Gastronomica* 20 (3): 5–6.

O'Connell, Kaete. 2021. "Breadlines and Banana Bread: Rethinking Our Relationship with Food in the Age of COVID-19." *Diplomatic History* 45 (3): 556–63.

Ó Giolláin, Diarmuid. 2013. "Myths of Nation? Vernacular Traditions in Modernity." *Nordic Irish Studies* 12:79–94.

Oleschuk, Merin, Josée Johnston, and Shyon Baumann. 2021. "Foodie Tensions in Tough Times." *Footnotes: A Publication of the American Sociological Association* 49 (1). https:// www.asanet.org/news-events/footnotes/jan-feb-mar-2021/features/foodie-tensions -tough-times.

Pew Foundation. 2020. "How the Coronavirus Outbreak Has and Hasn't Changed the Way Americans Work." December 9. https://www.pewresearch.org/social-trends/2020 /12/09/how-the-coronavirus-outbreak-has-and-hasnt-changed-the-way-americans -work/.

Pocius, Gerald. 2003. "Art." In *Eight Words for the Study of Expressive Culture*, edited by Burt Feintuch, 42–68. Urbana: University of Illinois Press.

Primiano, Leonard Norman. 1995. "Vernacular Religion and the Search for Method in Religious Folklife." *Western Folklore* 54 (1): 37–56.

Severson, Kim, and Julia Moskin. 2020. "Food, a Basic Pleasure, Is Suddenly Fraught." *New York Times*, March 17.

Shen, Wan, Lucy M. Long, Chia-Hao Shih, and Mary-Jon Ludy. 2020. "A Humanities-Based Explanation for the Effects of Emotional Eating and Perceived Stress on Food Choice Motives during the COVID-19 Pandemic." *Nutrients* 12 (2712).

Shukla, Pravina. 2008. "Evaluating Saris: Social Tension and Aesthetic Complexity in the Textile of Modern India." *Western Folklore* 67 (2–3): 163–78.

Sims, Martha C., and Martine Stephens. 2005. *Living Folklore: An Introduction to the Study of People and Their Traditions*. Logan: Utah State University Press.

Siragusa, Laura. 2021. "Reflection: Making Kin with Sourdough during a Pandemic." *Food and Foodways* 29 (1): 87–96.

Smith, Timothy M. 2020. "Why COVID-19 Is Decimating Some Native American Communities." *AMA Online*, May 13. https://www.ama-assn.org/delivering-care /population-care/why-covid-19-decimating-some-native-american-communities.

Sofo, Adriano, Annamaria Galluzzi, and Francesca Zito. 2021. "A Modest Suggestion: Baking Using Sourdough—a Sustainable, Slow-Paced, Traditional and Beneficial Remedy against Stress during the COVID-19 Lockdown." *Human Ecology* 49 (1): 99–105.

Somani, Reena. 2021. "Good Taste: White People's Sourdough Craze Highlights Colonization." *Daily Trojan*, October 11. https://dailytrojan.com/2021/10/11/good -taste-white-peoples-fermentation-colonization/.

Spence, Charles. 2017. "Comfort Food: A Review." *International Journal of Gastronomy and Food Science* 9:105–9.

Sutton, David E. 2001. *Remembrance of Repasts: An Anthropology of Food and Memory.* New York: Berg.

Sutton, David E. 2010. "Food and the Senses." *Annual Review of Anthropology* 39:209–23.

Troisi, Jordan D., and Shira Gabriel. 2011. "Chicken Soup Really Is Good for the Soul: 'Comfort Food' Fulfills the Need to Belong." *Psychological Science* 22:747–53.

Troisi, Jordan D., Shira Gabriel, and Jaye L. Derrick. 2015. "Threatened Belonging and Preference for Comfort Food among the Securely Attached." *Appetite* 90:58–64. https://doi.org/10.1016/j.appet.2015.02.029.

Vasvári, Louise O. 2018. "Identity and Intergenerational Remembrance through Traumatic Culinary Nostalgia: Three Generations of Hungarians of Jewish Origin." *Hungarian Cultural Studies* 11:57–77.

Vlach, John Michael, and Simon J. Bronner, eds. 1986. *Folk Art and Art Worlds.* Ann Arbor: University of Michigan Press.

Wallach, Jennifer Jensen. 2013. *How America Eats: A Social History of US Food and Culture.* New York: Rowman & Littlefield.

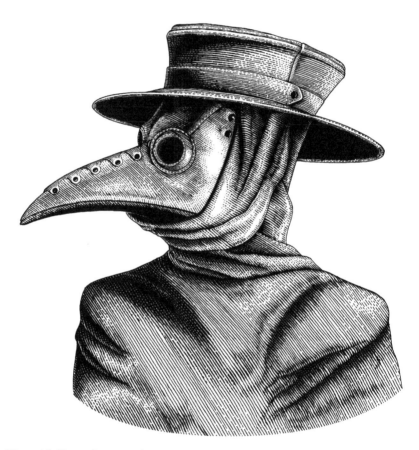

Figure 4.0. Plague doctor mask.

Section II
The Failure of Experts and the Rise of Vernacular Expertise

THE RESPONSE TO THE COVID-19 PANDEMIC, ESPECIALLY IN the US, has been referred to as a master class in government and scientific failure—including failures in planning, preparation, communication, and implementation—with leadership and coordination in nearly every sector clearly lacking. As scientific and governmental agencies failed to adequately address the needs and concerns of a worried and dismayed public, the resulting information and leadership vacuum left room for unconventional voices to intervene. This resulted in what Steven Epstein referred to in relation to HIV as the "public negotiation of a credibility crisis" in which "boundaries around scientific institutions become more porous, more open to the intervention of outsiders."[1] In other words, as experts failed, vernacular culture expanded to fill the needs of communities.

As is so often the case when new diseases arise, the community turned to matters of disease origin, transmission, and treatment in an attempt to exert epistemological and discursive control over the rapidly deteriorating health situation. The three chapters in this section focus on emerging patterns in the way communities digest and shape information when credible messaging from leadership is lacking. Through explorations of vernacular narrative and action surrounding lay approaches to transmission, vaccine rollout, and animal origins, this section focuses on vernacular responses to the void in information, leadership, and trust.

NOTE

1. Steven Epstein, "Democracy, Expertise, and AIDS Treatment Activism," in *Science, Technology, and Democracy*, ed. Daniel Lee Kleinman, 15–32 (Albany: State University Press of New York, 2000).

https://doi.org/10.7330/9781646424818.p002

4

Beyond the Deliberate Infector
Emergent Categories of Infector Narratives during COVID-19

Sheila Bock

INTRODUCTION

As the novel coronavirus took shape in US public consciousness in March 2020 as an *immediate* threat, not as something that was understood as affecting "others" in some distant location, the emerging stories that took shape about the transmission of the virus followed some very familiar patterns. This is not surprising, of course. In times of widespread disruption, stories work powerfully to help people grapple with anxiety, uncertainty, and fear. Sharing and consuming stories that are not only familiar but that make "good cultural sense" (Goldstein 2004, 115), in turn, help transform the unknown into something that is legible, something that maps onto people's understandings of the world.

The sudden emergence of the COVID-19 crisis laid bare, and in fact intensified, ruptures in the broader social contexts within which stories about the transmission of the new virus circulated. Take, for example, the meanings attached to face masks.[1] Early on in the pandemic, public health officials in the United States actively discouraged people in the general public from wearing masks, but as scientific understandings of the virus developed, along with increasing recognition of the prevalence of airborne transmission, public health messaging shifted in early April 2020 and began to highlight the importance of wearing masks in containing the spread of the virus. Coinciding with this shift in messaging was an increased voicing of frustration with the lockdown restrictions in place that many people, particularly those who identified on the right end of the political spectrum, felt infringed on their rights and personal freedoms. This frustration culminated in right-wing protests in April to reopen businesses that were deemed

https://doi.org/10.7330/9781646424818.c004

nonessential (bars, hair salons, and the like). Similar sentiments informed the so-called Costco "Mask Wars" in early May 2020, as Costco became one of the first businesses to require customers to wear masks, and highly publicized confrontations broke out between store employees trying to enforce the policy and customers refusing to comply. As masks became embroiled in what the *Guardian* termed the "US culture war" (Noor 2020), both wearing and *not* wearing masks took on heightened partisan meanings, acting as visible markers of where one sat on the increasingly polarized political spectrum.

While many in the US dismissed the threat of the novel coronavirus, describing it as "no worse than the flu" or framing it as a hoax manufactured by the mainstream media to hurt the reelection efforts of then president Donald Trump, many others were frightened and took active steps to minimize their risk of infection (such as wearing masks and keeping physical distance from others). The anxieties of people in the latter category surrounding the risks both of getting infected and of passing the virus on to someone else were exacerbated by the invisibility of the virus, particularly in the case of asymptomatic carriers. This fraught social context set the stage for emergent narrative patterns offering multiple constellations of intent, consequence, and blame. This chapter identifies these emergent narrative patterns as well as the ways in which they align with and diverge from the familiar "deliberate infector narratives" documented during earlier epidemics. In the process, it considers how the patterns speak to broader social contexts shaped by invisible threats and the destabilization of clear-cut categories of culpability.

NEW VIRUS, FAMILIAR STORIES: FEAR, CONTAMINATION, AND DELIBERATE INFECTION

In early April 2020, not long after the abrupt shutdown of nonessential businesses, schools, and other public spaces to help slow the spread of COVID-19, a grocery store employee in Las Vegas recounted the following exchange she had with her coworker.[2]

> This morning, I said hi to one of my coworkers in the produce section, and we were talking about the coronavirus crisis. He said, "This is crazy—how people are lining up for food. I've never seen anything like this before."
>
> I said, "Yeah, I've worked here for fourteen years and I've never seen this ever."

He said, "All the stocking up and panic buying, especially when all of this is happening . . . and there's these stupid, crazy people going around coughing on produce and licking ice cream tubs. We already have problems with stock not coming in. I heard they had to throw thousands of dollars of produce out."

I said, "Why would people do something like this, when we should be conserving the food?"

And he said, "Has to be totally irresponsible."

We just agreed that I guess people like that exist in the world. What can we do about it?

This exchange offers a glimpse into what was happening at that point in time, including the widespread panic buying of food and other supplies at grocery stores, the felt experience of the unprecedented nature of that moment in people's lifetimes, and the sharing of stories—or rather, in this case, brief references to stories in circulation, stories featuring themes that are very familiar to folklorists.

The stories invoked in the exchange recounted above feature one of the most common themes in rumors and contemporary legends more broadly and in health-related rumors/legends in particular: *contamination* (see Goldstein 2004; Kitta 2019; Turner 1993). Reports here of people "licking ice cream tubs" referenced the trending #IceCreamChallenge that gained popularity in July 2019: individuals would contaminate packages of ice cream with their bodily fluids (such as spit or urine) before returning the package to the freezer for another unsuspecting customer to purchase and consume. While initial outraged responses to these intentional acts of contamination focused on how disgusting they were, the emergence and quick spread of the novel coronavirus reframed the act as one of potential (and likely) contagion, as we can see in the following examples of posts on Twitter:

"what if the corona virus came from the weirdos that would lick ice cream and drink mouth wash and put it back . . . or did we just forget that happened?" (@_milfshake_, Twitter, April 11, 2020)

"The icecream lick challenge started corona" (@Gablorin, Twitter, May 17, 2020)

The exchange among coworkers recounted above also references a number of news reports emerging in different geographical locations, both inside and outside the United States, in the preceding weeks, stories featuring customers who deliberately coughed or spit on produce in grocery stores. In the case of one Pennsylvania woman who, in the words of local police, "intentionally contaminated" produce and other food items, the store ended up throwing out $35,000 worth of food for safety reasons (*ABC7News* 2020a).

To my knowledge, there were no reported cases of this behavior where I live in Las Vegas (and where these grocery store employees were working), though the widespread nature of the news reports and the ease with which one *could* contaminate food in a store without being noticed made it feel like a real possibility. And for folklorists who study contemporary legends and related genres, the emergence and circulation of stories featuring contamination in general—and contaminated food in particular—is in no way surprising. The link between contaminated food and contaminated bodies already has a precedent in the stories circulating in the midst of frightening epidemics, so they not only seem very much within the realm of possibility, they also feel very familiar.

As the two grocery store workers talked about "stupid, crazy people going around coughing on produce and licking ice cream tubs," there is little indication that they saw these people as particularly dangerous, that is, as a threat to public health. Rather, they voiced the most concern over the fact that these actions of contamination led to the waste of a substantial amount of food during a time where food shortages were a very real concern. The actions were characterized as "stupid" and "irresponsible," but not necessarily *dangerous*. And some of the news stories about people coughing or spitting on produce did identify these actions as "pranks," framing them more as mischievous acts than as serious public health threats.

In this same time period, though, there emerged a large number of news reports that attributed more nefarious purposes to the act of coughing in public. These stories feature not just acts of contamination but claims of *deliberate infection*, another theme that is well documented in the study of contemporary legends and related genres. The *New York Post*, for example, reported a story about a man in California who purposefully coughed on a gas pump handle at a gas station and said, "This is how you get coronavirus" (Miller 2020). The *Philly Voice* reported on a slew of incidents in which individuals deliberately coughed directly onto other people. One woman in New Jersey, "belligerent and uncooperative" after a minor car crash while driving intoxicated, reportedly coughed on police officers who came to the scene, saying she was "happy" to spread the coronavirus. In another incident in New Jersey, a man reportedly coughed on and laughed at a grocery store employee who asked him to move away from her because he was standing too close. And in yet another incident, in Pennsylvania, a man reportedly coughed on an elderly shopper who was wearing a face mask and gloves, claiming he had the coronavirus (Streva 2020).

Reports of deliberate infection during this time period were not limited to the United States. A *Newsweek* article shared the story of a man in Australia who, in the midst of restrictions put in place due to the panic buying that accompanied the COVID-19 outbreak, tried to purchase more than the two packets of noodles allowed. When approached by store employees, the man reportedly coughed on the packets he was not allowed to buy. According to the news report, "During the supermarket encounter, after coughing, the suspect allegedly told a member of staff that they were also now infected with the novel coronavirus" (Murdock 2020).

Clear contaminating actions such as licking, spitting, and (most often) coughing are perhaps the most recurring visible marker of the deliberate infector in the stories circulating at the beginning of the coronavirus pandemic, though there were instances in which the culprit was marked in other ways. According to several news sources in March 2020, for example, an asymptomatic man in Japan whose parents had both contracted COVID-19 tested positive for the disease. Though he was told to wait at home until a medical facility could be found for him, he instead reportedly told a family member, "I am going to spread the virus" before visiting two different bars.

Reports of this man's actions circulated widely, and the way he is characterized in these various reports clearly illustrates a phenomenon that has been studied extensively by folklorists (see Frank 2000, 2013; Goldstein 2004)—namely, in the words of Rachel Hopkin, that "media stories are often informed by traditional narrative patterns, becoming overdetermined in their development as a result. In other words, such inconvenient matters as facts do not prevent mediatic descriptions of newsworthy people and events from conforming with pre-existing patterns" (2019, 149). In the case of the man in Japan, he is a priori taken to be a villainous character, and the details of the story take shape in a way to support that characterization.

For example, one story, leading with the headline "COVID-19: Infected Man in Revenge Mode, Spreads Virus in Bars" (Sikander 2020), foregrounded *revenge* as the key motivation for his actions (a motif that has been documented in earlier disease outbreaks, including the plague in medieval Europe),[3] though no details presented in the story itself directly supported this explanation. Another version of this story stated, "According to some reports, he even told others that he had tested positive at each establishment. After smacking his lips on tasty finger-foods and knocking back a few drinks, *which in all likelihood resulted in him using the restroom and not properly washing his hands several times*, the man finally went home" (SoraNews24 2020; emphasis added). The italicized text, purely speculative in nature, envisions a character whom read-ers would view with disgust independently of his infected status, and reso-nates with other stories of contamination that feature body fluids.

Deliberate infection is a recurring, well-documented motif in narratives that circulate in the midst of disease outbreaks, ranging from the plague to HIV/AIDS, and now to COVID-19 (Bird 1996; Brunvand 1989; Goldstein 2004; Kitta 2019; Lee 2014; Mayor 1995; Smith 1990). In addition to giving voice to broader anxieties about contamination and one's own susceptibility to infection, stories about the intentional weaponization of a deadly disease, as transmitted through the body (or bodily fluids) of infected individuals, work in powerful ways to designate scapegoats, assign blame, and to rein-force boundaries between self and other, the dominant and the marginal-ized. As tales of morality that clearly identify distinctions between right and wrong, acceptable and unacceptable behavior, they shed insight into broader social and cultural values.

In the examples above featuring individuals who explicitly declare an intent to spread the coronavirus, as in previous outbreaks, the details of the story reinforce the idea that these are *bad* people. They are people who fail to follow laws and agreed-upon social conventions—people who drive under the influence of alcohol, people who are not respecting restric-tions to ensure that everyone has access to food items, people who do not wash their hands after using the bathroom. And when they are identified in these stories, the victims of these malicious acts, in stark contrast, are at the opposite end of the spectrum: a police officer seeking to uphold the law and protect the public; a grocery store employee (that is, an essential worker) invoking public health safety recommendations; an elderly person wearing a mask and gloves—that is, someone in a high-risk category *and* actively trying to protect herself.

Fears about deliberate infection in the United States during this time were further heightened by reports of white racially motivated violent extremists (WRMVEs) encouraging people to weaponize the virus as a form of bioterrorism against law enforcement and people of color. First reported in *YahooNews* (Walker and Winter 2020) and then in *Rolling Stone* (Wade 2020), the story highlighted an intelligence brief distributed by the Federal Protective Service, part of the US Department of Homeland Security, on February 17, 2020. The brief included, among other things, a list of recommended methods shared by WRMVEs for spreading the virus:

- Spend as much time as possible in public places with their "enemies"

- Visit local FBI offices and leave saliva on door handles
- Spray saliva from spray bottles on the faces of law enforcement
- Commit crimes such as arson of [*sic*] a shooting and leave coronavirus laced items at the scene for detectives to find
- Spit on elevator buttons
- Spread coronavirus germs in non-white neighborhoods. (Wade 2020; Walker and Winter 2020)

Rather than focusing on specific individuals, as the examples above do, these news reports attributed the act of deliberate infection to a generalized group of deplorable individuals, individuals that easily fit within the category of "bad guys"—neo-Nazis and white supremacists.[4]

These early characterizations of deliberate infectors as unapologetic racists invoked a recognizable stock character in the popular imagination (Pardo 2013, 65), invocations that were present in several stories I saw on my Facebook feed in March 2020. For example, on March 23, one day after the publication of the *Rolling Stone* article, a Facebook friend of mine shared a personal narrative that was initially posted on Twitter by Asian American author and cultural critic Jeff Yang (@originalspin), accompanied by her commentary: "This is the second report I've seen about white supremacists using COVID-19 as biological warfare." The story she shared read: "So I had my first 'breathing while Asian' moment. Went out for groceries and an older masked white woman passing by the line shouted 'FUCK YOU!' at me for no apparent reason. As I stared at her, she pulled off her mask, coughed directly at me, turned on her heel and walked off." Framing the story as one recounting his first " 'breathing while Asian' moment," Yang invoked the phrase "breathing while Black," which functions as a gloss of sorts in stories shared by and about Black people to highlight the excessive levels of profiling and policing Black people encounter while going about their daily lives. The racist motivations of his attacker, as recounted in this personal narrative, were further emphasized by how he established a stark contrast between the white woman's unprovoked acts of aggression (shouting an obscenity and pulling down her mask to cough directly at him) and his passivity in the face of this aggression. The narrative itself offers no assessment of the actual danger Yang felt he was in, though when this story was passed along by my friend on Facebook, she added her own interpretation of the events that unfolded in the story, characterizing it as a clear act of a white supremacist weaponizing COVID-19 and targeting people of color, in essence carrying out biological warfare, categorizing it squarely within the tradition of deliberate infector narratives.

The deliberate infector motif found in stories circulating in the wake of COVID-19, as in previous disease outbreaks, assigned clear blame to individuals who embody recognizable character traits of "bad people." And as in previous disease outbreaks, these narrative constructions worked effectively to externalize blame and, in turn, reinforce a schema for localizing danger that makes "good cultural sense" (Goldstein 2004, 115). In addition to clear examples of deliberate infector narratives, though, related categories of narratives emerged in the midst of the novel coronavirus pandemic, narratives that similarly spoke to widespread fears about the spread of the virus from person to person, but where the linking of intent and culpability is not so clear-cut. It is to these stories that I will now direct my attention.

BEYOND THE DELIBERATE INFECTOR: DIFFERENT CONSTELLATIONS OF INTENT, CONSEQUENCE, AND BLAME

Unintentional Infector Narratives

As deliberate infector narratives circulated early in the pandemic, another category of story emerged: the *unintentional infector* narrative. While deliberate infector narratives are set in public places and involve interactions between strangers, unintentional infector narratives are set in more "private" spaces among people who know and care about one another. Another recurring theme in this category is a tragic outcome, marked by a strikingly high number of COVID-19 diagnoses and/or the death(s) of a friend or family member. Indeed, a key distinction between unintentional infector narratives is that they focus less on dramatizing the moment of contact between people and more on the *consequences* of that contact.

In the US, an early iteration of this story that received widespread attention in the media featured a church choir, composed mostly of elderly members, that gathered in the state of Washington in early March to practice. Of the sixty-one people who gathered, fifty-two were later diagnosed with COVID-19, and two ultimately died from the disease. As news of this tragic event spread in late March 2020 on social media, the media framings of the story, as well as the commentary people added as they shared news reports on social media, tended to focus not on the fault of the person who infected their friends but rather the tragic consequences.

A *Los Angeles Times* report published on March 29, 2020, for example, described this localized outbreak of airborne transmission as something that "stunned public health officials" and included details that worked to mitigate the blame assigned to the individuals who chose to attend the choir practice. It emphasized how the county where this event took place had not had any reported cases, and that the choir met *before* large gatherings had been prohibited. It also highlighted the actions people took in response to news of the virus: "A greeter offered hand sanitizer at the door, and members refrained from the usual hugs and handshakes . . . Everybody came with their own sheet music and avoided direct physical contact" (Read 2020). In addition to highlighting the steps individuals took to prevent the spread of the virus, the *Los Angeles Times* story framed the gathering as helping people deal with the anxieties surrounding the new virus, describing the choir as a "centralizing force" in the participants' lives. This was not a morality tale, casting blame on the person who infected such a large group of their friends. It was a tale of tragedy about the scale of damage that could be done before people knew better. In other words, it highlighted the insidiousness of the virus, not the recklessness of the people who facilitated its spread. As public health understandings of the virus were growing more sophisticated, this tragic story served as a warning to a general public still trying to grasp the scale of the danger associated with the virus: you see no visible signs of danger, interact with "low-risk" people you know, take preventative measures such as keeping distance and using hand sanitizer, yet the disease will still spread and people will die.

As the initial lockdown measures began to relax in late spring and early summer, more stories about gatherings among family and friends turning deadly began to circulate, though they took on decidedly more moral tones. In these stories, individuals who contracted the virus during these gatherings were not framed in a sympathetic light. The key takeaway from them is that the people in attendance should have known better, and they have only themselves to blame. A vivid example of this emerging moral slant is a story shared by the online news platform *BGR* on July 4, 2020, entitled "How an Asymptomatic Coronavirus Carrier Infected a Dozen People, Killing One" (Smith 2020). The story is about a fifty-one-year-old man who attended a party in California, and soon after was diagnosed with COVID-19 (along with several other people who had been at the event). Within a week of his diagnosis, he was dead. The day before he died, he reportedly shared a message on Facebook: "I went out a couple of weeks ago . . . because of my stupidity, I put my mom and sisters and my family's health in jeopardy . . . This has been a very painful experience. This is no joke. If you have to go out, wear a mask, and practice social distancing . . . Hopefully, with God's help, I'll be able to survive this."

One thing that distinguishes this event from others is that the individual who spread the virus knew he had tested positive for COVID-19, but did not realize he could spread the virus because he was asymptomatic. The *BGR* story includes a quote from the brother-in-law of the man who died, who explained: "Our understanding is that a gentleman had called him and said, 'hey I was at the party, I knew I was positive. I didn't tell anybody.' I think the gentleman was regretting not telling everybody, and he was calling people who were at the party to recommend they get tested."

Unlike stories in the narrative tradition of the deliberate infector, where the infector communicates with the newly infected after the moment of infection (for example, "Welcome to the world of AIDS," "Now you have the coronavirus"), this act of communication is presented as being born out of regret and a sincere desire to help. In other words, the story is not about assigning blame to this individual. In fact, immediately following this quote, the news story reoriented the blame away from him, noting that the man who ultimately died "was upset but *blamed himself* for the error in judgment" (emphasis added). And the final line of the story reinforced this idea that the "patient zero" at the party should not be viewed as a villain, highlighting his intent (or rather his lack of intent) to absolve him from being characterized as the villain of the story: "He didn't mean to infect anyone, but he'll live for the rest of his life knowing that he was likely responsible for his friend's death."

Indeed, unlike deliberate infector narratives, this corpus of stories does not depend on clear-cut binaries between the guilty and the innocent, villain and victim. By choosing to attend social gatherings, the victims could just as easily have been in the position of asymptomatically infecting others. Within these stories, there is little to morally differentiate those who infect and those who are infected. All are culpable.

Deliberate Exposure Narratives

The blame attached to those who attend social gatherings and ultimately pay the price (by either dying themselves or passing the virus along to unsuspecting loved ones at home) inspired a related corpus of stories and rumors, *deliberate exposure* narratives that feature people intentionally trying to expose themselves to the virus by attending so-called COVID parties.[5] In April 2020, for example, an epidemiologist published an op-ed in the *New York Times* offering "seven reasons your 'coronavirus party' is a bad idea," referencing unspecified "rumblings" that these parties were taking place (Bauer 2020). The presumed motive for these parties was that people thought they would be better off if they contracted the antibodies for COVID-19. In early May, a more specific variant of this rumor emerged in Walla Walla, Washington. In news reports of this iteration, a public health official claimed to know of at least two patients who had attended COVID parties in order to "get it over with," a claim that was verified by the local police chief. Two days later the public health official announced that she had been wrong: "We have discovered that there were not intentional Covid parties . . . just innocent endeavors" (Edelman 2020a).

In late June and early July, more dramatic variants of the story emerged as news outlets, including ABC News, Associated Press, and CNN, began reporting on dangerously reckless behavior among students in Alabama: "Officials in Tuscaloosa, Alabama say some students are throwing parties, competing to see who can catch COVID-19 first. Tuscaloosa Fire Chief Randy Smith spoke about this during a city council meeting . . . confirming the parties" (*ABC7News* 2020b). Students attending these parties were reportedly taking "snot shots" and pooling money to be given to the first party attendee to be diagnosed. Like the Walla Walla reports, this story was soon debunked. Follow-up reports found that what actually happened was that "several college students, who were aware they had tested positive for the coronavirus, attended parties around Tuscaloosa" (Helean and Mapp 2020).

Then, in mid-July, yet another version of the story was widely circulated. In this version, as reported in the *Verge*, "a 30-year-old man attended a 'COVID party,' where people gathered with someone who tested positive for COVID-19 to test whether the virus is 'real.' The man believed it was a hoax until he contracted it and died in the hospital" (Robertson 2020).

In all these iterations, the act of intentional exposure was debunked (or at least not able to be verified). This, of course, raises the question of why this type of story—where people attend social gatherings for the express purpose of exposing themselves to the virus—was so tellable. One factor is that there are narrative precursors that make this storyline look very familiar. In the past, for example, some parents have intentionally exposed their children to chicken pox at events called "pox parties" so they could "get it over with" (Biss 2015). And during the H1N1 pandemic in 2009, rumors about people hosting "swine flu parties" circulated widely in the media. Outside of the realm of disease outbreaks, there are also narrative precursors featuring young people deliberately engaging in reckless behavior, including the legend cycles about "rainbow parties" in the early 2000s and "pharm parties" in the mid-2000s, as well as the moral panic surrounding the "Tide Pod Challenge" in 2018.

In the context of COVID-19 in particular, it is particularly striking how these stories simultaneously invoke *and* establish distance between both the typical deliberate infector narratives and unintentional infector narratives described above. Consider, for example, the version featuring students in Tuscaloosa, Alabama, where the actual facts could have lent themselves quite easily to a classic deliberate infector story. Instead of morally vilifying the people who knew they were infected and still attended parties, the act of deliberate infection (and the negative character traits such an act connotes) was narratively transferred to the people exposing themselves to the virus by attending the parties. Aligning with the moral framework set up within the category of unintentional infector narratives, this corpus of narratives clearly places blame on the people exposed to the virus. At the same time, the *intentionality* of the dangerous behavior in these stories is a key element to constructing the people who attended these parties as decidedly unsympathetic figures. For example, when the rumors about COVID parties in Walla Walla were debunked, a public health official distinguished "intentional Covid parties" from "just innocent endeavors" (Edelman 2020a). This binary between intentionality and innocence, voiced explicitly here, functions implicitly in the stories about people seeking out infection, adding extra weight to the idea that the people infected while attending these social gatherings brought it upon themselves.

This framing, in turn, also perhaps worked to create moral distance between the teller and the characters in the story. As unintentional infector narratives, and their moral implications for the people who caught the virus, increasingly spread, it is likely that they caused discomfort among people who generally tried to avoid risky behaviors but who were tiring of life in lockdown and yearning to return to some kind of normalcy. And as the pandemic wore on, even people who were trying to be as safe as possible were likely to find slippages between what they knew they were supposed to do and what they were actually doing in their day-to-day lives. These slippages, in fact, were so prevalent that they became the subject of satire on comedy shows like *Saturday Night Live* (*Saturday Night Live* 2021) and in the *New Yorker*, which featured a spoof of a mother exhorting her adult children to come home for Thanksgiving by assuring them of how safe she was being in relation to the virus while actually revealing the numerous ways in which she was being decidedly unsafe.

> I promise I'm taking this very seriously. Unlike your cousin Kevin. You won't believe what Kevin did. He went to some kind of crazy sex party or concert or something in a warehouse on Staten Island. Your Aunt Susan

said that he came home covered in glitter—lips and chin, too, so you know he wasn't wearing a mask. Can you believe how irresponsible that is? Behaving like that when he lives with his sixty-five-year-old mother? So dangerous! I said to her, "You have to tell Kevin to be more careful. This *covid* stuff is serious!" Yes, I said exactly that when she came over yesterday to watch "The Crown." I'm not messing around with this stuff. (Wolff 2020)

So many of the characters in the unintentional infector stories, characters who ultimately died or spread the virus to people they cared about, similarly asserted that they had been so careful, that they had done everything "right" up to that point. For people who could see themselves as a potential character in those tragic events, stories featuring irresponsible characters taking "snot shots" and gleefully seeking out exposure created opportunities for moral distancing: "I may not be following all public health recommendations to the letter, but I'm not being so reckless as *those* people."

AMBIGUOUS INFECTOR NARRATIVES

Ambiguous infector narratives constitute another emergent narrative category that grappled with issues of intent during the COVID-19 pandemic. I use this term to refer to stories featuring people whose actions, while interpreted as dangerous to those who came in contact with them, were not easy to categorize as overtly threatening. These stories, which I heard often in the early days of mask-wearing in my informal encounters with friends and family members, share similarities with deliberate infector narratives and rumors of deliberate exposure in that they dramatize the moment of contact between people rather than the consequences of that contact (which is more of the focus of unintentional infector narratives). Here is one representative example of this type of story, a personal narrative shared on Facebook in early May 2020 by a friend of mine, a white woman in her early sixties living in a midwestern city.[6]

I've been thinking about this experience for a few days and realized it has been bugging me more than I thought, so I thought I'd share it to see what you thought. I was in CVS buying a few essential drug store things. I was wearing a mask. At the checkout, I noticed the clerk, who was also wearing a mask, look up sharply, over my shoulder, with a surprised expression in her eyes. I turned slightly and saw a man about two feet behind me, not wearing a mask. I was a little startled, because he was even closer than someone would typically stand in a store line. He and I appeared to be the only customers in the store. He smiled and said, "Hi" with a big grin. I quickly finished the transaction and stepped toward the door sideways so I could avoid the guy. Then he leaned in just a few inches from me, kind of laughed, and said loudly, "You have a nice day now!" I stepped back, fast, and left. The rational part of me wants to believe he was just some weird oblivious person, but the anxious part of me thinks he was being obnoxious because of my mask. I hope I'm being paranoid.

The narrator begins by characterizing herself as someone doing things "right" in terms of public health recommendations: being out in public for the purpose of buying *essential* things, wearing a mask, and trying to keep distance from others (creating a stark contrast between her and the antagonist in the story). She also positions the checkout clerk as a witness to her account equally taken aback by the invasive man in the story (in effect validating her responses in the moment).

Notably, while the man in line with her is engaging in "bad" behaviors for public health purposes—he is not wearing a mask and is not keeping six feet apart—his interactions with her feature actions that, under other circumstances, might be interpreted as friendly: smiling, greeting her, saying "Have a nice day." In other words, unlike stories featuring a verbal assertion of intention and/or a manufactured cough, there is a sense of plausible deniability here. Although engaging in dangerous health behaviors, the man in her personal narrative may not be mean-spirited but rather "weird" or "oblivious" or just trying to be friendly. Unlike in the "breathing while Asian" story presented earlier, where the events in the story were characterized as a deliberate act with a clear intent to do harm, the narrator of this story does not have such a clear-cut evaluation to offer. Indeed, she ends her story with the possibility that she is "being paranoid" and that her embodied response in the moment was a misinterpretation.

This feeling of potentially "being paranoid" while acutely experiencing feelings of discomfort is not limited to navigating physical and social interactions in the time of COVID-19. Independently of the virus, women consistently have to deal with men who invasively engage with them in public, physically (through unwanted touching) and verbally (catcalls, telling women to smile). People who are part of marginalized groups consistently encounter micro-aggressions in their daily lives ("Where you are from? No, where are you *really* from?" "You speak English so well!" "You are so articulate," "You are the whitest Black person I know"). These experiences with micro-aggressions, while not overtly threatening, reinforce the idea that people from marginalized groups don't really belong, that any sense of belonging is contingent. And when marginalized people try to call out

micro-aggressions, they are often met with gaslighting ("You are too sensi-
tive," "You are just looking for problems that aren't there") and defensive
assertions of intention ("I was just trying to compliment you," "It was just
a joke. I wasn't being serious"), so that harmful actions are couched in deniability. This creates broader cultural norms where women, people of color,
and other marginalized groups might recognize an experience as part of a
pattern of behavior but don't feel equipped or justified to call it out as such,
leading to the questioning of one's own ability to interpret the situation
fairly (as the narrator here does in suggesting possible paranoia). And as the
CVS story shows us, these issues are exacerbated amid the uncertain social
contexts created by the coronavirus pandemic.

Responses to this narrator's story from her Facebook friends were
mixed. One of the commenters on the post attributed the man's actions to
his being a "weird guy" and "maybe isolating too much," though the vast
majority of responders agreed that he was being obnoxious at her expense,
with assertions such as "That was deliberate" and "I think he acted with
intention because you wore a mask. smh [shaking my head]." Notably,
intentionality is important for this narrator and those who responded to her
post in determining how to attribute meaning to the story. If the man in line
was intentionally *not* following public health recommendations and engaging with her so invasively because she *was*, then she was the victim of a
malicious act. If the man could be characterized as "just some weird oblivious person" who had not yet figured out how to interact with other people
in public in the midst of the new normal of pandemic life, the encounter
would be experienced as far less disturbing.

CONCLUSION

The different categories of COVID-19 narratives I have described in this
chapter—deliberate infector narratives, unintentional infector narratives,
deliberate exposure narratives, and ambiguous infector narratives—all
coexisted with one another in the discursive landscape of the pandemic.
Bringing them together and attending to the ways in which these stories
are constructed in dialogue with one another reveals a kind of grappling
with intent as a marker of blame. The deliberate infector narratives in the
time of COVID-19—dramatizing scenarios where clearly identifiable bad
people engage in clearly identifiable dangerous actions for the clear purpose
of doing harm to others—remain quite consistent with the deliberate infector narratives documented during earlier disease outbreaks. The unintentional infector narratives, however, decouple intent and culpability so that

blame is narratively attached to actions, not intentions. At the same time, the motif strikingly makes its way back into the parallel category of deliberate exposure narratives, where intent is the means by which *true* guilt is determined, an idea echoed in the evaluation of the man's actions in the line at CVS in the ambiguous infector narrative above. The different framings of intent in these separate though related categories—ones that destabilize intent and ones that reassert intent as a marker of blame—were both eminently tellable as people grappled with the need to make sense of the risks involved in interacting with people during a pandemic. Ultimately, even as the clear-cut lines between "bad guys" and "good guys" become troubled in this larger corpus of stories, the motif of intent remained a mechanism for externalizing blame and risk perception.

ACKNOWLEDGMENTS

The ideas presented in this chapter began to take shape during conversations with Savannah D'cruz in the late spring and summer of 2020. Once these initial ideas were translated into a messy draft, Kate Horigan played a key role in helping me articulate my key arguments. Finally, I owe thanks to my colleagues in the UNLV Department of Interdisciplinary, Gender, and Ethnic Studies and to the volume editors for their thoughtful feedback at different stages in the writing process.

NOTES

1. See Bock 2020 for further consideration of the different meanings attached to face masks.

2. This recounting was shared with me in early April 2020 by a former undergraduate student who had been in my Interpreting Illness honors seminar the previous semester. In that class, we talked extensively about the familiar narrative patterns that emerge during disease outbreaks, and she shared her mother's account with me because of its resonance with topics we had addressed in that class. She has given me permission to include it in this chapter.

3. See, for example, Fine 1987 and Goldstein 2004.

4. One of the online comments on the *Rolling Stone* article featured a variant that illustrates a phenomenon identified initially by Patricia Turner (1993) and elaborated on by Gary Alan Fine and Patricia Turner (2001), where key details (in this case the race of the villain and the victim) shift depending on who is sharing the story: "Yeah you can find a few whites on Telegram joking about it. But I am on Twitter right now and I can see at least 2 dozen blacks and asians at this very moment laughing about giving white people the virus, coughing on them, and taking revenge" (RedCorn, March 23, 2020).

5. While the stories I have discussed thus far contain motifs commonly found in contemporary legends, this category of stories aligns with this genre more broadly, in that the authority of the stories is based on unverified secondhand reports of the events under

question (a narrative device contemporary legend scholars refer to as FOAF, an acronym for "Friend of a Friend"), often including warnings shared by people in authoritative positions (such as medical professionals, law enforcement officials, governmental officials). My thinking about the ways in which this category of stories exemplifies recurring patterns found in the genre of contemporary legend more broadly was heavily informed by insights shared by folklorist Merrill Kaplan (2020) in on online discussion on social media. See also Edelman 2020a, 2020b and Robertson 2020.

6. This personal narrative is shared here with permission.

REFERENCES

ABC7News. 2020a. "14-Year-Old Boy Charged After Coughing on Produce as Prank, Sheriff Says." March 29. https://abc7news.com/coronavirus-prank-teen-coughs-on -produce-cough-update/6061177/.

ABC7News. 2020b. "Students Throw COVID-19 Parties to Bet on Who Will Catch Virus First." July 3. https://abc7ny.com/alabama-students-having-covid-19-parties-to-see -who-gets-it-first-pandemic-coronavirus/6291801/.

Bauer, Greta. 2020. "Opinion: Please, Don't Intentionally Infect Yourself. Signed, an Epidemiologist." *New York Times*. https://www.nytimes.com/2020/04/08/opinion /coronavirus-parties-herd-immunity.html.

Bird, S. Elizabeth. 1996. "CJ's Revenge: Media, Folklore, and the Cultural Constructions of Contemporary Deviants." *Contemporary Legend* 1:107–21.

Biss, Eula. 2015. *On Immunity: An Inoculation*. Minneapolis: Graywolf.

Bock, Sheila. 2020. "Masks On." *Nevada Humanities Heart to Heart*, August 17. https://www .nevadahumanities.org/heart-to-heart/2020/8/17/masks-on.

Brunvand, Jan Harold. 1989. *Curses! Broiled Again! The Hottest Urban Legends Going!* New York: Norton.

Edelman, Gilad. 2020a. " 'Covid Parties' Are Not a Thing." *Wired*, July 2. https://www .wired.com/story/covid-parties-are-not-a-thing/.

Edelman, Gilad. 2020b. "The Latest Covid Party Story Gets a Twist." *Wired*, July 14. https://www.wired.com/story/the-latest-covid-party-story-gets-a-twist/.

Fine, Gary Alan. 1987. "Welcome to the World of AIDS: Fantasies of Female Revenge." *Western Folklore* 46 (3): 192–97.

Fine, Gary Alan, and Patricia A. Turner. 2001. *Whispers on the Color Line: Rumor and Race in America*. Berkeley: University of California Press.

Frank, Russell. 2000. "The Making and Unmaking of a Folk Hero: The Ellie Nesler Story." *Western Folklore* 59 (3–4): 197–214.

Frank, Russell. 2013. "Covering Captain Cool: The 'Miracle on the Hudson' as a Hero Tale." *Western Folklore* 72 (1): 59–81.

Goldstein, Diane. 2004. *Once upon a Virus: AIDS Legends and Vernacular Risk Perception*. Logan: Utah State University Press.

Helean, Jack, and Annie Mapp. 2020. "Tuscaloosa Students Who Knew They Had COVID-19 Attended Parties." *ABC3340News*, June 30. https://abc3340.com/news /local/university-of-alabama-students-who-knew-they-had-covid-19-attended-parties.

Hopkin, Rachel. 2019. "Villainy, Mental Health, Folklore, and the Mediatic Literature." *Journal of Literary and Cultural Disability Studies* 13 (2): 141–58.

Kaplan, Merrill. 2020. Personal communication, July 2.

Kitta, Andrea. 2019. *The Kiss of Death: Contagion, Contamination, and Folklore*. Logan: Utah State University Press.

Lee, Jon D. 2014. *An Epidemic of Rumors: How Stories Shape Our Perception of Disease.* Logan: Utah State University Press.

Mayor, Adrienne. 1995. "The Nessus Shirt in the New World: Smallpox Blankets in History and Legend." *Journal of American Folklore* 108 (427): 54–77.

Miller, Joshua Rhett. 2020. "Man Intentionally Coughs on Gas Pump Handle, Mentions Coronavirus: Cops." *New York Post*, April 6. https://nypost.com/2020/04/06 /arizona-cops-bust-man-for-coughing-on-gas-pump-handle/.

Murdock, Jason. 2020. "Man Charged After Allegedly Coughing on Packets of Noodles Refused Due to Coronavirus Purchase Limits." *Newsweek*, March 31. https://www .newsweek.com/australia-police-charge-man-cough-noodles-coronavirus-covid19 -food-limits-1495221.

Noor, Poppy. 2020. "No Masks Allowed: Stores Turn Customers Away in US Culture War." *Guardian*, May 22. https://www.theguardian.com/us-news/2020/may/22/us -stores-against-face-masks.

Pardo, Rebecca. 2013. "Reality Television and the Metapragmatics of Racism." *Journal of Linguistic Anthropology* 23 (1): 65–81.

Read, Rickard. 2020. "A Choir Decided to Go Ahead with Rehearsal. Now Dozens of Members Have COVID-19 and Two Are Dead." *Los Angeles Times*, March 29. https:// www.latimes.com/world-nation/story/2020-03-29/coronavirus-choir-outbreak.

Robertson, Adi. 2020. "'COVID Parties' Are a Pandemic Urban Legend That Won't Go Away." *Verge*, July 22. https://www.theverge.com/21324034/covid-party -coronavirus-intentional-infection-not-real-alabama-washington-texas.

Saturday Night Live. 2021. "Super Bowl Pod—*SNL*." Streamed live on YouTube, February 6. https://www.youtube.com/watch?v=-8p0iDjAiwE.

Sikander, Sana. 2020. "COVID-19: Infected Man in Revenge Mode, Spreads Virus in Bars." *Siasat Daily.* March 9. https://www.siasat.com/covid-19-infected-man-revenge -mode-spreads-virus-bars-1850857/.

Smith, Chris. 2020. "How an Asymptomatic Coronavirus Carrier Infected a Dozen People, Killing One." *BGR*, July 4. https://bgr.com/2020/07/04/coronavirus-symptoms -not-necessary-to-spread-covid-19-asymptomatic-contagious/.

Smith, Paul. 1990. "'AIDS—Don't Die of Ignorance': Exploring the Cultural Complex." In *A Nest of Vipers: Perspectives on Contemporary Legend*, vol. 5, edited by Gillian Bennett and Paul Smith, 113–41. Sheffield, UK: Sheffield Academic Press.

SoraNews24. 2020. "Confirmed Coronavirus Patient in Aichi Told to Go Home, Goes Bar Hopping Instead." *Japan Today*, March 7. https://japantoday.com/category/national /Confirmed-coronavirus-patient-in-Aichi-told-to-go-home-goes-bar-hopping-instead.

Streva, Virginia. 2020. "South Jersey Woman Allegedly Coughs on Police, Says She's 'Happy' to Spread COVID-19." *Philly Voice*, April 8. https://www.phillyvoice.com /intentional-coughing-coronavirus-police-assault-new-jersey-woman-covid-19/.

Turner, Patricia A. 1993. *I Heard It through the Grapevine: Rumor in African-American Culture.* Berkeley: University of California Press.

Wade, Peter. 2020. "Just When You Thought Things Couldn't Get Worse, Neo-Nazis Are Trying to Weaponize Coronavirus." *Rolling Stone*, March 22. https://www.rolling-stone.com/politics/politics-news/neo-nazis-are-trying-to-weaponize-the -coronavirus-971002/.

Walker, Hunter, and Jana Winter. 2020. "Federal Law Enforcement Document Reveals White Supremacists Discussed Using Coronavirus as a Bioweapon." *Yahoo News*, March 21. https://news.yahoo.com/federal-law-enforcement-document-reveals -white-supremacists-discussed-using-coronavirus-as-a-bioweapon-212031308.html.

Wolff, Susanna. 2020. "We're Being So Safe." *New Yorker.* November 25. https://www .newyorker.com/humor/daily-shouts/were-being-so-safe.

5

Fake Grannies, Extra Doses, and the One Hundred
COVID-19 Vaccine Hunting and Accessibility

Andrea Kitta

MISUNDERSTANDINGS, ACCESSIBILITY, AND MANY OTHER issues plagued the COVID-19 vaccine rollout across the United States. As states followed different schedules and established different interpretations of priorities, what might be true in one state was not guaranteed to be true in another, causing confusion. In late January 2021, articles started appearing all over social media about lucky people being vaccinated ahead of their cohort and rich people taking vaccines from poor people. These stories complicated the experience of receiving the vaccine: notions of "fairness" meant people did not want to appear to be vaccinated out of turn, but they also wanted to celebrate their decision and the process to encourage others to vaccinate.

My friends who were vaccinated quickly stopped telling others based on the reactions they faced. One colleague reported multiple people telling her she didn't deserve the vaccine and that she had taken it from someone else who needed it more, even though she received vaccines that would have spoiled otherwise. I too had an early first dose (as I describe below), and I received hate mail and offensive responses on Twitter, accusing me of stealing or using my privileged position to get a vaccine I didn't deserve. When I asked if I was supposed to let the vaccine go to waste instead, I was told that surely someone more deserving than myself could have received it. I queried colleagues working in vaccination centers, and they reported that they had diligently contacted others, including essential workers in public-facing jobs, first. It was only out of desperation that they would contact anyone they knew personally. One nurse reported to me:

https://doi.org/10.7330/9781646424818.c005

Last week, we had a bunch of people not show, but we had to use the vaccines, so we called the sheriff's office and had a bunch of them come out. They took up most of them, but when they arrived, we asked them to contact their colleagues not working that day and we got a few more [from the sheriff's office] in. One guy asked if he could call his wife—she works in a grocery store and takes care of her elderly mother—so we got her too. But then we all ran out of people to call, so we had to start calling anyone we knew, anyone who might be home in the middle of a Wednesday that could get there in fifteen minutes. We were almost out of time, started vaccinating the people who worked in the building, grabbing anyone we could. I got a hotel worker. A few friends of people showed up, but we still probably had to dump three doses and that just killed me. A friend showed up ten minutes after we had to dump them and we were all devastated. She would have made it too, but she got stopped by a train. I told her I'd call her again if it happened again. It's rough, so many of the elderly don't have transportation, so they make the appointment, but then they can't get here or their ride arrives late—we do what we can, but it's an issue. (Interview with author, January 30, 2021)

All of the people I spoke to were talking about the Pfizer vaccine, which has to be stored at −80 to −60 degrees Celsius and cannot be refrozen once it has been thawed. After the vaccine has been thawed and diluted, it must be used within six hours if stored between 2 and 25 degrees Celsius. (Undiluted vials are good at room temperature only for two hours.) There are approximately six doses per vial, but some vials contain more doses. However, each dose, which is 0.3 milliliters, has to come from the same vial—you cannot combine doses from other vials, which means that there could be more left in the vial that isn't being used if it doesn't constitute a full dose (Food and Drug Administration 2021). This waste, especially of such a precious commodity, bothered many of the vaccination center workers I spoke to, even though they knew there was no way around it. Their knowledge of vaccine waste, however unavoidable, may be a contributing factor in their persistent efforts to find people to vaccinate when in possession of full extra doses.

UNUSED DOSES AND THE ONE HUNDRED

My own experience with receiving the COVID-19 vaccine began the morning of January 26 at 9:05 a.m. when I received a text from a close friend consisting simply of a link and the words "Vaccine appointments!!!!" I immediately clicked on the link, which said that all East Carolina University employees were now eligible for vaccination, whereas before, following the state's guidelines, only those over sixty-five were. This sudden change was due to the lack of scheduled appointments by those who qualified, and concerns that the vaccine would have to be discarded if it wasn't used. I signed up for an appointment at the first available time, 2 p.m., while my friend who texted me was scheduled for an 11:30 a.m. appointment. I was surprised that appointments were even available, as previously I had only heard of last-minute calls for extra doses or people being in the right place at the right time. I was also surprised that I found out via this friend, another ECU professor—who, in turn, had been told by a colleague unknown to me in the Public Health Department—because I had previously assumed that if there were any chance of me getting the vaccine early, it would come via my connections through my husband, a critical care (ICU) doctor and pulmonologist, or via my colleagues in Public Health.

I quickly posted this exciting news to Facebook so my friends and colleagues could also benefit from this sudden change in fortune. All morning I fielded questions about this change in policy, issues with the scheduling website, and other queries. Many people had trouble with the link, but others were able to register for appointments that day, later in the week, and even up to a month later. We could hardly believe our good luck: friends asked me to text once I was vaccinated to make sure it was real. My friend sent me a picture of her vaccine card shortly after her shot, and emails and texts poured in from friends and colleagues with the dates of their appointments. There was so much press about how many of the vials of the Pfizer vaccine had an expected extra dose or more (see Weiland et al. 2021), and that vaccines were being wasted because of appointments not taken by those eligible that we all assumed that explained the situation—we were lucky *and* we were helping by using vaccines that were otherwise going to be thrown out, not that we were taking them away from anyone else. I was vaccinated that day and given an appointment for my second dose.

The following day, none of the vaccine appointments were honored. The day after that, the provost sent out an email stating that there were no more vaccine appointments available except for Groups 1 (healthcare workers, long-term care staff, and residents) and 2 (adults over sixty-five) and that there was a vaccine shortage (see Romero and del Rio Giulia McDonnell 2021). Another flurry of emails and texts followed from people more confused than ever. Were they supposed to cancel their appointments or not? What if appointments were for weeks from now when Group 3 (teachers[1] and frontline essential workers) was potentially eligible? Did the provost's email refer to appointments for the extra doses? Professors and staff were all confused about what was happening—we had been told we were taking extra doses, not doses that were slated for others. People were racked with guilt, myself included. Had we just taken a dose from another person or not? Was this a failure of the university system? A failure at the state or federal level? A failure of the vaccine manufacturer or distributor? Shouldn't people be unable to register if they weren't in the proper group? Was anyone actually tracking or paying attention to any of this?

On January 27, 2021, a friend in another state told me she too had received a text from a friend telling her to rush over to the vaccine distribution center because there were extra vaccine doses. She hurried to the site only to be told that they were out, but an individual grabbed her and sent her to another person to take her information so she could be a part of "the one hundred" tomorrow. She gave her information and was told she would be contacted the next day. The next day she received a call giving her a time and location, including a specific door, where she would be vaccinated. She was told the vaccines were opened in packs of six and they needed to be used within two hours, so my friend wondered if "the one hundred" referred to a set that was taken out of the specialized cold storage and had to be used. She was told to arrive fifteen minutes before her given time so she wouldn't be in a line of a hundred people. As my friend was keeping me updated before the scheduled time, she stated that the whole situation felt clandestine and she wondered if she was really going to receive a vaccine. In the end she was vaccinated and given an appointment for her second dose.

VACCINE HUNTERS

Shortly after the news broke about the extra vaccines, rumors—and, later news stories—about vaccine hunters began to emerge. Vaccine hunters were, at best, portrayed as people concerned about vaccines going to waste, but most often they were seen as opportunistic, privileged people with abundant time and resources trying to get a vaccine before they were eligible. Vaccine hunting differed from the fortuitous opportunity of being offered an extra dose; it involved the overt seeking of extra doses, which could involve stalking vaccination centers. The website vaccinehunter.org (which originally began on Reddit) directly states that vaccine hunting is about making sure vaccines are not going to waste:

> Due to the intricacies around the extremely cold storage that the COVID vaccines require, there are rare occasions where "spare doses" may go unused & should be made available to anyone. When a distribution site defrosts a tray with 100s of vials, they must use all the doses between 5

and 24 hours (depending on the manufacturer)—before, according to their protocol, the remaining doses must be thrown out. When there are no shows at the end of the day, some providers will start letting anyone they can find through the door to have their first shot. We aim to help connect and crowdsource information about vaccine distribution sites that have expiring doses with the goal of getting ANYONE that's mobile and ready their first dose. (Vaccine Hunter 2021)

They compare what they're doing to a single-rider line at an amusement park, which fills in the spaces left by uneven groups (Vaccine Hunter 2021). While this website represented the largest group of vaccine hunters, mostly a place to organize smaller, local groups and help them connect to others, there are certainly other such sources, such as vaccine.sexy, VaxStandBy, VaxxPaxx, and TurboVax. Vaccine Hunter and some of the other sites have an area for vaccine providers to alert people if they find themselves with extra vaccines. However, not all vaccine providers see this as a welcome service. One public health department posted on Twitter, "We've been very busy helping vaccinate those in Dane [County, Wisconsin] who are eligible for the COVID vaccine, & we use every dose allotted to us. We plan this out very carefully so all doses are used. Please do not show up at our vaccination site at the end of the day hoping you can get vaccinated" (PublicHealthMDC 2021). Nevertheless, people were still encouraged by the CDC to take the vaccine if possible, especially if it was a dose that might otherwise spoil.

VACCINE HELPERS

For many people, the purportedly straightforward process of registering for an appointment through official channels was arduous at best. I heard from colleagues, friends, and loved ones about their experiences booking appointments for themselves or others, and all of the stories were negative. Most people experienced long wait times for phone booking, constant refreshing and waiting for online booking, and overall general frustration with the process itself, including downed websites, inefficient systems, and dropped calls/internet service. Very few if any appointments were open, and times were not always convenient for individuals. Often, if a vaccine date had to be changed, there was only the option for canceling, not rescheduling, so that people had to begin the entire process all over again. I came across many people who just gave up and decided to wait because they did not have the time or energy to devote to getting a vaccine. This was especially true for older workers who were unable to take the time to get an appointment because they were at work. Overall, those who received appointments the fastest were people who were already retired, had help with scheduling, or otherwise had the time to sit on the internet or on hold. This generally meant that essential workers outside of the medical field, while crucial to infrastructure and one of the most vulnerable groups, rarely received their vaccinations as soon as they were available.

Services emerged during the early days of the rollout, such as groups dedicated to getting appointments for those eligible for the vaccine. One example was LA County COVID-19 VaxForce, self-described as a "small but mighty group of tech-savvy millennials helping eligible folks schedule COVID-19 vaccine appointments. We'll post info when appointments become available and if needed, directly book appointments for you" (LA County VaxForce 2021). Folklorist Luisa Del Giudice first told me about VaxForce and encouraged me to use the service after I expressed frustration on social media at the difficulty in using the online registration systems for my eligible family members. Even though I was trying to get appointments in southwestern Pennsylvania, Gracie, the founder of VaxForce, was able to get vaccine appointments for several of my family members, and encouraged me to pass on the information to others. VaxForce became so popular that the site had to be paused several times while volunteers caught up with those who had already applied.

I spoke to Gracie in July 2021, when vaccine appointments were readily available and her services were no longer needed. Like many people, she first experienced frustration with getting her own family members vaccinated, and realized that others facing the same difficulty might need help. She saw a disconnect between how public health information was communicated, typically via social media like Twitter, and how those over sixty-five searched for that information, usually by calling or looking at the websites of organizations. Gracie was astonished by the number of people who volunteered after a news article featured VaxForce: she immediately had around a hundred new volunteers as well as others who offered to donate money to the cause. Using Slack, a friend helped her organize the team by state so volunteers could immediately go to work scheduling appointments. Gracie mentioned that while she's glad volunteers are no longer needed, she did enjoy helping others and doing something that made a difference during the pandemic. The knowledge that she could be saving lives kept her motivated, as she sometimes went without sleep so she could book more appointments. We discussed how amazing it was to see so many people working together to contribute to a single goal, negotiating the complexity of the issue in order to alleviate suffering.

Although the vaccine rollout was flawed when it came to access and scheduling, many people reported overwhelmingly positive experiences while receiving their vaccines. Locally in Greenville, North Carolina, the site at the convention center was heralded as efficient. Many people commented positively on the live music (typically a single masked violinist or cellist) and the selfie station encouraging people to post their vaccination selfie to show others the process was effective and safe. My friends and family in other areas reported similar positive experiences, including efficient systems that allowed them to get their vaccines quickly and safely and providers who were willing to come out to the car to vaccinate a person with mobility issues. Nevertheless, although the actual process of vaccination was safe and effective, there remained clear access issues when it came to scheduling.

VACCINE ACCESS IN EASTERN NORTH CAROLINA

Volunteer-driven organizations like VaxForce could not single-handedly redress systemic problems with the rollout. Access was a major issue, especially in many rural areas, including where I live in Eastern North Carolina. Locally, a group known as CAREE (Citizens Advocating for Racial Equity and Equality) organized "vaccine events" for those who qualified but had difficulty registering for vaccine appointments and/or had issues with mobility (Saunders 2021). I attended one of these vaccine administration events where I spoke to some of the volunteers. There were several factors that made vaccine accessibility difficult in Eastern North Carolina.

Appointments could only be booked online, and a significant number of people over sixty-five did not have the technology to register for them. Many of those who came in that day to be vaccinated did not have smart phones or computers, internet access, the knowledge of where or how to register, or the ability to spend hours attempting to get a vaccine appointment. In some cases, this was a matter of affordability, but in other cases, it was that internet services weren't available in rural areas.[2]

Many people over sixty-five no longer drove: they relied on others for their transportation, whether friends or family members, or taxi services and rideshares. Even in non-pandemic times, keeping a specific medical appointment time was always laborious, contingent as they were on the schedules of others and a wealth of circumstances beyond their control. This is especially true regarding individuals with mobility issues, if special vehicles or services are required, but the pandemic introduced a host of complications that made established strategies impossible. A standard solution, chartering buses, was not feasible since people had to be socially distanced, and would still have been an impediment to people with mobility issues.

Other forms of transportation were also difficult, given that it was winter and social distancing was in place. People were not supposed to be inside a car with anyone outside of their household, and cold weather prevented them from circulating fresh air by opening windows. Taxi use was limited, and carpooling was restricted. At best, if adult children were part of the bubble, the task of driving would fall on family members, pending their availability during appointment hours. And in circumstances where specialized transportation would normally have been arranged for those with accessibility issues, many people were afraid to touch others in order to help them in and out of vehicles.

Finally, many rural people and the elderly did not have access to masks; mask supplies were particularly limited at the time. Additionally, because they rarely wore masks, they had difficulty wearing one, keeping it on, and hearing others who were wearing masks.

Overall, it would have been much easier to bring vaccines to people instead of bringing people to the vaccines, but since the Pfizer vaccine, with its requirements for cold storage, was all that was available, that was not possible. The CAREE volunteers were dedicated to their mission, figuring out transportation and scheduling all of the appointments with the closest vaccine center, located at the Health Department in Greenville, North Carolina. The event was so successful that CAREE organized additional events to help both the Black community and, in conjunction with the Association of Mexicans in North Carolina, the local Latinx population receive vaccines (Joseph 2021).

VACCINE FRAUD, VACCINE TOURISM

Unfortunately, for every piece of good news about the vaccine rollout, there were more and more instances of systemic failure. Reports of people unable to get appointments or spending all day booking appointments were everywhere, and it seemed that every day there was a new story about people trying to be vaccinated before their scheduled time. Perhaps the most widely known case of the latter involved two women in Florida, Olga Monroy-Ramirez, forty-four, and Martha Vivian Monroy, thirty-four, who were caught dressing as "grannies" to receive their second COVID-19 shot (Deliso 2021). It was later discovered that the two received their first vaccine at a local vaccine center, but it is unknown how they passed as over sixty-five, especially since their appointments and vaccine cards were in their actual names (Cutway 2021). On body camera video, the women were called "selfish" by local deputies, with one stating, "You've stolen a vaccine from someone that needs it more than you" (Kornfield 2021).

This was far from the only case of vaccine-related fraud in the United States. Former paramedic of the year Joshua Colon was arrested and charged in Polk County, Florida, for helping a fire-rescue captain steal vaccine doses meant for first responders to give the vaccine to his mother (Blest 2021). In Houston, Dr. Hasan Gokal administered at least eight vaccine shots to otherwise ineligible people, including his wife. Gokal stated that the vaccines were going to expire and he was just trying to use them before then. He was charged with misdemeanor theft and fired, but the case was thrown out by the judge (Debenedetto 2021). Dr. Claude Varner, a physician in Memphis, Tennessee, stole five vaccines in total on two different occasions for his wife, friends, and daughter-in-law. He was fined $1,500 and told to take a medical ethics class within the year (Cook 2021). An unnamed nurse in Detroit was caught stealing two doses of the Moderna vaccine as she was leaving the vaccination center (Dupnack and Ainsworth 2021). Additionally, there were vaccine cards being sold on Facebook, Twitter, Etsy, and eBay from $20 to $60 each: some of these cards were stolen while others were forged. People were later prosecuted for everything from petit larceny and criminal possession of a forged instrument to a felony count of grand theft (Durkee 2021; Paybarah 2021). Lastly, pharmacist Steven Brandenburg of Wisconsin ruined 570 doses of the Moderna vaccine because he thought vaccination was unsafe. An additional fifty-seven people were injected with ruined vaccines and had to be alerted that they might not have immunity (Romo 2021). Brandenburg was sentenced to three years in prison (Associated Press 2021).

COVID cases and deaths were directly tied to inequality (Qureshi 2020; Van Beusekom 2021). The wealthiest people significantly increased their wealth during the pandemic while continuing to vacation, eat indoors, and enjoy their lives while inequality grew (Elbaum 2021; Jamieson 2021; Peterson-Withorn 2021; Picchi 2021). Concierge physicians, doctors who charge an upfront fee for upgraded service and patient access, report that they have often been offered bribes for vaccines, and it was discovered that MorseLife Health System in Florida and three separate health systems in Washington State gave vaccines to their donors, foundation members, and supporters (Hauck 2021). Some of the wealthy, like casino executive Rodney Baker and his wife, actress Ekaterina Baker, went so far as to steal vaccines from those most at risk. The couple chartered a plane to a remote Indigenous community, the White River First Nation, in Beaver

Creek, Yukon, Canada. The Bakers pretended to be local motel employees to receive their vaccines. They were fined $2,300 CAD for breaking quarantine (Farzan 2021; Hauck 2021).

The wealthy also engaged in vaccine tourism. Florida, which relies on travel as a major part of its economy, offered to vaccinate anyone in the currently eligible group, regardless of whether they were from Florida. Many from Latin American countries flew to the US for vaccines, and places such as New York responded by placing vaccine centers near tourist attractions (Rebaza 2021). Vacation and vaccination packages became popular in many countries, with offers to get "vaccinated on the beach" in the Maldives and Bali. In January 2021, while the UK was still in lockdown, the Knightsbridge Circle offered a £25,000-a-year private members' club. This club, for an additional fee, could provide "first-class or private jet flights, accommodation for up to one month while you wait for your second dose, and a private vaccination. Trips can cost around $55,000 (£40,000). Currently, the options on offer are either Dubai, which now has private appointments for the Pfizer jab, or the Oxford/AstraZeneca vaccine in India, which is being sold at 1,000 rupees (£10) on the private market" (Robson 2021). In 2021, travel to the US is common as vaccines are plentiful, even if only 49.2 percent of the population is fully vaccinated to date (Carlsen et al. 2021). Simply put, if you were wealthy enough, vaccines were available.

Despite all the evidence, there are still some that insist viruses don't discriminate. While this might be technically true, healthcare systems and other institutions do discriminate. Throughout the pandemic, we have seen one example after another of how class, race, gender, ethnicity, and many other factors put certain individuals at risk. People of color are hospitalized and die at much higher rates than their White counterparts (Centers for Disease Control and Prevention 2021). There has been an increased negative outlook on transgendered and nonbinary healthcare, with patients seeking out healthcare less than ever and suffering from worse mental health issues during the pandemic (Woulfe and Wald 2020). While more men than women tend to die of COVID, women seem to have worse issues with long COVID (Chinnappan 2021), are disproportionately leaving the work force to homeschool and act as caregivers (Hsu 2021; Rothwell and Saad 2021), and are suffering more from domestic violence (Evans et al. 2020).

VACCINE REFUSAL AND HESITANCY

While many people were eager to receive the COVID-19 vaccine, vaccination itself is still a polarized issue that falls along a variety of political ideologies and belief systems. To say that this issue is only political would be to understate complex individual belief systems and ignore many of those who do not fit into specific groups generally associated with vaccine refusal. Just as there is no one profile of someone eager to receive the vaccine, there is also no one profile of a vaccine refuser or someone who is vaccine hesitant. More recently, especially in the media, vaccine refusers have been characterized by political affiliation, religion, and tendency to believe in conspiracy theories, with some of the more subtle media criticisms concerning marginalized groups and the history of violence against them. However, as I've written previously, I believe that privilege has more to do with vaccine refusal than other factors (Kitta and Goldberg 2017). At the core of vaccine refusal is the firm belief that the individual either knows better than experts or that they are privy to additional information that subverts the dominant narrative. Vaccine hesitancy, which is completely different and where we should put our efforts, is more complex, involving the personal experience and belief of the individual. Those who are vaccine hesitant are questioning vaccination, not outright refusing it, and are often actively searching for answers and reassurance that they are making the right decision. When the media focuses on vaccine refusers, or another group, which I have started to call the vaccine hostile (Kitta 2023), it feeds the narrative, giving the group more power, and disenfranchising those who are vaccine hesitant and have real questions and concerns about vaccination. Additionally, focusing on the vaccine hostile and vaccine refusers negatively affects the mental health of frontline workers, who are already overtaxed, and all of those involved in the creation, manufacturing, distribution, and study of vaccination. Until worldwide issues of access have been solved, it is best to put our efforts into persuading the vaccine hesitant and disregard the vaccine hostile. It would also behoove us as academics to give vaccine acceptors more press and more attention, as they are the much larger group, while the vaccine hostile are a small minority who receive undue attention, making them look like the more dominant group.

VACCINE PERCEPTION AND POPULARITY

Another aspect of vaccine acceptance and refusal is the idea that some vaccines are better than others. TikTok user Idrinkurmilkshake (2021) declared, "Um, only hot people get the Pfizer vaccine. If you got Moderna then, I don't know what to tell you, queen. This message is brought to you by Pfizer gang." This was one of many popular videos, memes, and other forms of vernacular culture surrounding the idea of "vaccine teams" or "vaccine rivalries." Although most people were not given a choice in what vaccine they received, many had preferences of what vaccine they wanted. One friend commented, "It's like wanting a boy or a girl—you get what you get and you're not upset about it. You're happy either way, but deep inside you do have a preference." Many people I knew expressed hope that they would be on "Team Pfizer" or "Team Moderna," while a few of my family members were hoping for Johnson & Johnson because it was "one and done" and they were concerned about the side effects of the second shot being worse. Vaccines were given their Hogwarts houses by Harry Potter fans, and impressions about each vaccine became an ongoing joke, with some seriousness, as people posted and reshared memes about their vaccine status. Pfizer became the "it" vaccine, perhaps because it was first, had a high level of efficacy, and excellent marketing (Schwedel 2021).

This clearly demonstrates that there is a vernacular association with the vaccines, and it shows a vernacular understanding of science. The various vaccines being associated with popular culture to create "houses" or "teams" with value associated with each one demonstrates the acceptance of the vaccine and its incorporation into already established folkloric perceptions of identity. As mentioned above, assigning Hogwarts houses to vaccines (in the type of interplay we see constantly between folklore and popular culture) is a way to make the vaccines part of one's identity. As posts circulated, some people argued that certain vaccines were sorted into the wrong house or made comments comparing those against vaccines to Muggles (those without magic). Anti-vax Harry Potter fans replied with comments about how they wanted to be called "Purebloods" instead, referencing a group in the series that did not want wizards and Muggles to intermarry, leading to further debates and both groups calling each other Nazis. A vernacular understanding of science was also part of these discussions, with people quoting vaccine effectiveness statistics to prove their vaccine was "better" or mentioning the mRNA technology as proof of why a vaccine might be more "Ravenclaw" than "Hufflepuff." In an era when the media and scientists bemoan the lack of scientific knowledge, these examples may be underestimated as vernacular understandings of science.

While the status of most preferred vaccine hovered between Pfizer and Moderna, I knew the day the Johnson & Johnson vaccine was announced that it was doomed to become the less desirable vaccine. As soon as I heard the announcement of its launch, I felt relief, because the vaccine didn't require cold storage, a major barrier to access, but I was also unsettled by the knowledge that the Johnson & Johnson vaccine would be less desirable to many because it was designed to work in rural and poorer areas.

Journalist Kaitlyn Tiffany (2021) also wrote about this issue, stating, "The CDC reported last week that many public-health departments have been using Johnson & Johnson specifically for homeless people, as well as those who are homebound or incarcerated. Meanwhile, public-health leaders have struggled to avoid portraying the Johnson & Johnson vaccine, which is also targeted to rural and migrant populations, as a second-class option."

People were excited to display their vaccine status: manufacturers and creators cashed in on T-shirts and other items declaring that one was vaccinated, with everything from *Hamilton* parodies (declaring that one "wasn't going to throw away their shot"), logos that said, "Thanks Science!" and tributes to Dolly Parton and her contribution to vaccine efforts. One example of the latter was a parody of Parton's song "Jolene" replacing the title character's name with "Vaccine"—a joke that even Parton participated in, singing it while she was being vaccinated and posting it as a PSA on her Instagram (Parton 2021). The summer of 2021 became known as "Shot Girl Summer" (parodying "Hot Girl Summer") or "Hot Vaxxed Summer," with "Vaxed and Waxed" being declared the motto of summer 2021 (Gallucci 2021).

It's difficult to know if these vaccine rivalries had any effect on vaccine uptake, but it's unlikely: the people who were the most excited to declare their vaccine status were also the most likely to get vaccinated in the first place. Peer pressure overall may have influenced some people to get the COVID vaccine, and the idea of choice in what vaccine you could get might influence some people. One source of hesitation I heard from friends and family was that there was no real way to know what vaccine you would get when you showed up for your appointment. Vaccine choice (or even the illusion of choice) could convince some to vaccinate; however, since worldwide access to the vaccine is still an issue, this seems unrealistic.

In spite of a rocky start and clear issues with access, the COVID-19 vaccine rollout has become a streamlined process that most participants have found to be safe and easy. However, inequalities still abound in our healthcare system that have a long-term effect on every aspect of American life and health. These issues were always present; the pandemic just made them more obvious. Additionally, vaccine hesitancy is still a crucial issue that must be addressed, and the most effective way to do that is via individual conversations with those who have questions about vaccines (Kitta 2019, 2012; Kitta and Goldberg 2017). Vaccine refusal and vaccine hostility have resulted in a low uptake in the COVID-19 vaccine so far, with just under half (49.2 percent) of the US population vaccinated as of July 30, 2021, in spite of the relative accessibility of vaccines (Carlsen et al. 2021). Clearly, there is more work to be done to ensure healthcare access and equity in the United States, and those doing this work should look to folklore and vernacular understandings of science to aid them in this pursuit.

NOTES

1. There was mixed information about whether or not professors were going to be considered teachers. In the end, they were not and placed in group 5 (everyone who wants a vaccine). See Kaplan and Lazano 2021 and North Carolina Department of Health and Human Services 2021 for more details.

2. This also proved true with teaching online—many people simply weren't able to get internet access at home, so wireless hotspots were purchased by many schools and offered to students so they could complete their coursework.

REFERENCES

Associated Press. 2021. "A Pharmacist Who Deliberately Ruined COVID Vaccine Doses Is Going to Prison." *National Public Radio*, June 8. https://www.npr.org/2021/06/08/1004585024/the-pharmacist-who-deliberately-ruined-covid-vaccine-doses-is-going-to-prison.

Blest, Paul. 2021. "So Now People Are Stealing COVID-19 Vaccines." *Vice*, January 27. https://www.vice.com/en/article/akdaej/so-people-are-now-stealing-covid-vaccines.

Carlsen, Audrey, Pien Huang, Connie Hanzhang Jin, Zach Levitt, and Daniel Wood. 2021. "How Is the COVID-19 Vaccination Campaign Going in Your State?" *National Public Radio*, July 16. https://www.npr.org/sections/health-shots/2021/01/28/960901166/how-is-the-covid-19-vaccination-campaign-going-in-your-state.

Centers for Disease Control and Prevention. 2021. "Risk for COVID-19 Infection, Hospitalization, and Death by Race/Ethnicity." *CDC.gov*, July 16. https://www.cdc.gov/coronavirus/2019-ncov/covid-data/investigations-discovery/hospitalization-death-by-race-ethnicity.html.

Chinnappan, Shivani. 2021. "Long COVID: The Impact on Women and Ongoing Research." *Society for Women's Health Research*, March 18. https://swhr.org/long-covid-the-impact-on-women-and-ongoing-research/.

Cook, Kelli. 2021. "Memphis Doctor Fined for Stealing Vaccines to Give to Friends and Family." *WMC5 News*, June 15. https://www.wmcactionnews5.com/2021/06/16/memphis-doctor-fined-stealing-vaccines-give-friends-family/.

Cutway, Adrienne. 2021. "Those Fake Florida Grannies Got Their First COVID-19 Vaccine Doses After All." *Click Orlando*, February 23. https://www.clickorlando.com/news/local/2021/02/23/those-fake-florida-grannies-got-their-first-covid-19-vaccine-doses-after-all/.

Debenedetto, Paul. 2021. "Judge Throws out Case against Harris County Doctor Accused of Stealing Vaccines." *Houston Public Media*, January 25. https://www.houstonpublicmedia.org/articles/news/harris-county/2021/01/25/390064/judge-throws-out-case-against-harris-county-doctor-accused-of-stealing-vaccines/.

Deliso, Meredith. 2021. "Two Women Dressed as 'Grannies' to Get COVID Vaccine, Florida Officials Say." *ABC News*, February 19. https://abcnews.go.com/US/women-20s-dressed-grannies-covid-19-vaccine-florida/story?id=75984671.

Dupnack, Jessica, and Amber Ainsworth. 2021. "Detroit Officials: Nurse Caught Stealing COVID-19 Vaccines from TCF Center." *Fox 2 Detroit*, March 16. https://www.fox2detroit.com/news/detroit-police-nurse-caught-stealing-covid-19-vaccines-from-tcf-center.

Durkee, Alison. 2021. "Fake Vaccine Cards on the Rise: CVS Employee Arrested for Stealing Them." *Forbes*, May 14. https://www.forbes.com/sites/alisondurkee/2021/05/14/fake-vaccine-cards-on-the-rise-cvs-employee-arrested-for-stealing-them/?sh=35ce6d564a71.

Elbaum, Rachel. 2021. "World's Richest Become Wealthier during Covid Pandemic as Inequality Grows." *NBC News*, January 25. https://www.nbcnews.com/news/world/world-s-richest-become-wealthier-during-covid-pandemic-inequality-grows-n1255506.

Evans, Megan L., Margo Lindauer, and Maureen E. Farrell. 2020. "A Pandemic within a Pandemic—Intimate Partner Violence during Covid-19." *New England Journal of Medicine* 383:2302–4. https://www.nejm.org/doi/full/10.1056/NEJMp2024046.

Farzan, Antonia Noori. 2021. "Wealthy Couple Chartered a Plane to the Yukon, Took Vaccines Doses Meant for Indigenous Elders, Authorities Said." *Washington Post*, January 26. https://www.washingtonpost.com/nation/2021/01/26/yukon-vaccine-couple-ekaterina-baker/.

Food and Drug Administration. 2021. "Pfizer COVID-19 Vaccine EUA Fact Sheet for Healthcare Providers Administering Vaccine (Vaccination Providers. FDA)." *FDA.gov*. https://www.fda.gov/media/144413/download.

Gallucci, Nicole. 2021. "The People have Spoken: 'Vaxed and Waxed' Is the Summer 2021 Motto." *Mashable*, April 19. https://mashable.com/article/vaxed-waxed-hot-girl-summer-meme.

Jamieson, Amber. 2021. "'Rich People Gonna Rich People': People Say Their Wealthy Friends Disappointed Them during the Pandemic." *BuzzFeed News*, May 27. https://www.buzzfeednews.com/article/amberjamieson/pandemic-exposed-the-rich.

Joseph, Amber. 2021. "Association of Mexicans Hosts COVID-19 Vaccination Event." *WNCT*, February 20. https://www.wnct.com/top-stories/association-of-mexicans-hosts-covid-19-vaccination-event/.

Hauck, Grace. 2021. "Cutting, Bribing, Stealing: Some People Get COVID-19 Vaccines Before It's Their Turn." *USA Today*, February 3. https://www.usatoday.com/story/news/health/2021/02/03/covid-vaccine-some-people-cutting-bribing-before-their-turn/4308915001/.

Hsu, Andrea. 2021. "Millions of Women Haven't Rejoined the Workforce—and May Not Anytime Soon." *National Public Radio*, June 4. https://www.npr.org/2021/06/03/1002402802/there-are-complex-forces-keeping-women-from-coming-back-to-work.

Idrinkurmilkshake. 2021. "Um, only hot people get the Pfizer vaccine. If you got Moderna then, I don't know what to tell you, queen. This message is brought to you by Pfizer gang." TikTok, April 1.

Kaplan, Jonah, and Michael Lazano. 2021. "Teachers Can Get Vaccinated in Late February, Essential Workers in March, Gov. Cooper Announces." *ABC 11 News Raleigh*, February 10. https://abc11.com/covid-vaccine-nc-phase-3-group-walgreens/10326497/.

Kitta, Andrea. 2012. *Vaccinations and Public Concern in History: Legend, Rumor, and Risk Perception*. New York: Routledge.

Kitta, Andrea. 2019. *The Kiss of Death: Contagion, Contamination, and Folklore*. Logan: Utah State University Press.

Kitta, Andrea. 2023. "God Is My Vaccine: Religious Belief and COVID in the United States." *Cultural Analysis*.

Kitta, Andrea, and Daniel S. Goldberg. 2017. "The Significance of Folklore for Vaccine Policy: Discarding the Deficit Model." *Critical Public Health* 27 (4): 506–14.

Kornfield, Meryl. 2021. "Video Shows Deputies Confronting Young Women Who Dressed as 'Grannies' for Coronavirus Vaccines." *Washington Post*, February 19. https://www .washingtonpost.com/nation/2021/02/18/florida-women-dress-elderly-vaccine/.

LA County VaxForce. 2021. "About Us Facebook Page." Facebook. https://www.facebook .com/groups/lacountycovidvaccine.

North Carolina Department of Health and Human Services. 2021. "Deeper Dive: Group 3—Frontline Essential Workers (School and Childcare)." *NCDHHS*, February 10. https://files.nc.gov/covid/documents/vaccines/Deeper-Dive-Moving-to-Group-3 .pdf.

Parton, Dolly. 2021. "Dolly gets a dose of her own medicine @vanderbilthealth." Instagram, March 2. https://www.instagram.com/tv/CL7o1CaDMH0.

Paybarah, Azi. 2021. "A Nevada Man Is Charged in the Theft of More Than 500 Blank Vaccine Cards in Los Angeles." *New York Times*, June 9. https://www.nytimes.com /2021/06/09/world/covid-vaccine-card-theft.html.

Peterson-Withorn, Chase. 2021. "How Much Money America's Billionaires Have Made during the Covid-19 Pandemic." *Forbes*, April 30. https://www.forbes.com/sites /chasewithorn/2021/04/30/american-billionaires-have-gotten-12-trillion-richer -during-the-pandemic/?sh=6509004cf557.

Picchi, Aimee. 2021. "Billionaires Got 54% Richer during Pandemic, Sparking Calls for 'Wealth Tax.'" *CBS News*, March 31. https://www.cbsnews.com/news/billionaire -wealth-covid-pandemic-12-trillion-jeff-bezos-wealth-tax/.

PublicHealthMDC. 2021. "We've been very busy helping vaccinate those in Dane Co who are eligible for the COVID vaccine, & we use every dose allotted to us. We plan this out very carefully so all doses are used. Please do not show up at our vaccination site at the end of the day hoping you can get vaccinated." Twitter, February 2.

Qureshi, Zia. 2020. "Tackling the Inequality Pandemic: Is There a Cure?" *The Brookings Institute*, November 17. https://www.brookings.edu/research/tackling-the-inequality -pandemic-is-there-a-cure/.

Rebaza, Claudia. 2021. "Vaccine Tourists Are Coming to America." *CNN*, May 26. https://www.cnn.com/2021/05/26/americas/vaccine-tourism-usa-latam-intl/index .html.

Robson, Michele. 2021. "Vaccine Vacations—Getting a Private COVID-19 Shot Abroad." *Forbes*, January 17. https://www.forbes.com/sites/michelerobson/2021/01/17 /vaccine-vaccationsgetting-a-private-covid-shot-abroad/?sh=165df52076be.

Romero, Simon, and Nieto del Rio Giulia McDonnell. 2021. "New Pandemic Plight: Hospitals Are Running out of Vaccines." *New York Times*, January 22. https://www .proquest.com/newspapers/new-pandemic-plight-hospitals-are-running-out /docview/2479921923/se-2?accountid=10639.

Romo, Vanessa. 2021. "Pharmacist Who Spoiled More Than 500 Vaccine Doses Said He Thought They Were 'Unsafe.'" *National Public Radio*, January 4. https://www.npr .org/2021/01/04/953348619/pharmacist-who-spoiled-more-than-500-vaccine -doses-said-he-thought-they-were-uns.

Rothwell, Jonathan, and Lydia Saad. 2021. "How Have U.S. Working Women Fared during the Pandemic?" *The Gallup Poll*, March 8. https://news.gallup.com/poll/330533 /working-women-fared-during-pandemic.aspx.

Saunders, Ford. 2021. "Special COVID-19 Vaccine Event Held for Marginalized Communities." *WNCT*, January 30. https://www.wnct.com/health/coronavirus /special-covid-vaccination-event-held-for-marginalized-communities/.

Schwedel, Heather. 2021. "How Pfizer Became the Status Vax." *Slate*, April 17. https:// slate.com/human-interest/2021/04/best-vaccine-choice-pfizer-joke.html.

Tiffany, Kaitlyn. 2021. "The Hot Person Vaccine." *Atlantic*, April 30. https://www.the atlantic.com/technology/archive/2021/04/pfizer-gang-and-sadness-vaccine -culture/618755/.

Vaccine Hunter. 2021. "Vaccine Hunter." https://www.vaccinehunter.org/.

Van Beusekom, Mary. 2021. "Income Inequality Tied to More COVID-19 Cases, Deaths." Center for Infectious Disease Research and Policy, May 4. https://www.cidrap .umn.edu/news-perspective/2021/05/income-inequality-tied-more-covid-19-cases -deaths.

Weiland, Noah, Katie Thomas, and Sharon LaFraniere. 2021. "Pfizer Will Ship Fewer Vaccine Vials to Account for 'Extra' Doses." *New York Times*, January 24. https:// www.proquest.com/newspapers/pfizer-will-ship-fewer-vaccine-vials-account /docview/2480547724/se-2?accountid=10639.

Woulfe, Julie, and Melina Wald. 2020. "The Impact of the COVID-19 Pandemic on the Transgender and Non-binary Community." *Columbia Psychiatry*, September 22. https://www.columbiapsychiatry.org/news/impact-covid-19-pandemic-transgender -and-non-binary-community.

6

Beyond Bat-Eating
Digital Discourses of Zoonotic Disease in the COVID-19 Era

Julianne Graper

> *Content warning: This chapter mentions anti-Asian violence,*
> *including racial epithets, as well as cruelty to animals.*

> Now, a lot of people blame bats for the coronavirus. But imagine how they
> feel about that. I mean, first Ben Affleck is cast as Batman and now this.
>
> —Peter Sagal, *Wait Wait Don't Tell Me*, June 20, 2020

> That song is catchier than SARS—in a good way.
>
> John Oliver, *Last Week Tonight*, February 15, 2021

INTRODUCTION: "NORM MACDONALD'S BAT SONG"

ON MARCH 29, 2020, CONSERVATIVE COMEDIAN Norm Macdonald posted a video to YouTube in which he feigned making a sandwich out of bat meat. The black-and-white video, overlaid with an original song by comedian Josh Gardner, echoed the controversial claim that bushmeat consumption in China instigated the first spillover of COVID-19 from bats to humans. With lyrics lauding conservative bluegrass great Lester Flatt, paired with racializing substitutions such as "Once you go bat, you never go back," Macdonald's video does more than simply highlight the visibility of Trump-era politics surrounding the COVID-19 pandemic:[1] it underscores crucial conversations about the relationship between race, zoonoses, and pandemic disease.

In the chapter that follows, I will examine how songs about bat consumption like Norm Macdonald's emerge from disputes over zoonotic disease narrativity, especially scapegoating bats as a cause of COVID-19.

https://doi.org/10.7330/9781646424818.c006

Engaging with theoretical interventions from cultural geography (Elder et al. 1998), science and technology studies (Crosson 2016), and critical-animal studies (Kim 2015), I claim that disease narratives materialize from power struggles between social groups in ways that illuminate structural hierarchies. In the case of COVID-19, conflicts over appropriate consumption and treatment of wild animals thinly mask racist assumptions that become validated through the misinterpretation of scientific findings by mass media. Musical performances like Norm Macdonald's not only disseminate misinformation, they also actively engage with it in ways that serve to naturalize and normalize racist ideologies. I offer "bat soup" songs like Norm Macdonald's both as evidence of prevalent attitudes about bats during the COVID-19 pandemic and as a way of unveiling the connection between species narratives and ideologies of race.

Situating my claims in past zoonotic epidemics, including the 2014 Ebola epidemic, the 2002–4 SARS pandemic, and the rise of rabies (Messenger et al. 2003; Tuttle 2017, 2020b), I argue that scientific approaches to disease are key players in the naturalization of racist narratives. Examining critiques of scientific practice and popular discourse made by bat conservationists, I demonstrate the ways in which scientific practices are deeply affected by existing anti-bat narratives, which then become legitimized through scientific data. That data then becomes the basis not only for public policy but also for racist actions perpetrated by individuals, including acts of anti-Asian violence that proliferated in 2020 and 2021. While news media have thoroughly discussed both the scapegoating of bats and the rise of anti-Asian hate during the pandemic, I claim that these two issues are deeply interrelated in vernacular discussions of disease.

Second, I address how critiques of food practices, including the consumption of bushmeat, serve as a tool of cultural imperialism geared toward placing blame on China for the COVID-19 pandemic. I examine the origins of the internet rumor that "bat soup" caused the first spillover of COVID-19 from bats to humans. I then situate this rumor in historical narratives about Chinese food and disease.

Finally, I examine the transfer of the "bat soup" rumor into a musical genre, which I dub bat soup songs. Unlike musical interventions documented in previous pandemics (Rivera 2017; Stone 2017; Tucker 2014), bat soup songs sit in an uncomfortable place between disease prevention and political scapegoating. Whether or not they offer advice about hygienic cultural practices, bat soup songs serve as tools for mobilizing racist actions against Asians and Asian Americans.

Fully understanding the dynamics of pandemic narratives involves a serious consideration of the landscape of human personhood. Zoonotic diseases—passed from nonhumans to humans—irreparably trouble the existence of species boundaries, a lacuna filled by speculation, paranoia, and anxious negotiation of social categories. Diane Goldstein argues that questions of disease origin necessarily involve "the transgression of alien substances (the virus) across categorical boundaries," a "contamination" that "threaten[s] cultural norms and encourage[s] the expression of opinions, variants and negotiated facts. Under these conditions, the contemporary legend is inevitable" (2004, 79). In other words, viral crossover inherently threatens "the human" as a social category, necessitating the renegotiation of social norms through discursive means. This is as evident during COVID-19 as it has been in previous epidemics: heightened anxieties about viral transmission make materially evident the tensions between human social groups as well as the contested boundaries of humanity. The transmission of viral bodies from animals to humans is linked to ideologies of social categorization.

The global scale of the COVID-19 pandemic and its attendant alterations to human mobility demonstrate that interspecies relations are everywhere. In fact, we can understand the blurred boundaries between humans and nonhumans as not simply incidental to the COVID-19 pandemic, but as its defining feature. The significance of human-nonhuman relations during the COVID-19 pandemic are evident in the discourses we mobilize to understand the disease and its origins, as well as the ways we demarcate the line between persons and nonpersons.

HOW SCIENTIFIC PRACTICES LEGITIMIZE BAT-BASED RACISM

By now, the myth of COVID-19's potential origin in a wet market in Wuhan, China is well known. As anthropologist Lyle Fearnley (2020) describes it, stall owners at the Huanan Seafood Wholesale Market in Wuhan fell ill with severe cases of pneumonia in late 2019. Following the report of the incident to the World Health Organization (WHO), the international media gradually revealed the presence of wild animals for sale at the market, much as they did during the 2002 SARS epidemic. Scientists at the Wuhan Institute of Virology announced that the virus they had isolated from the market had a high genetic resemblance to SARS, as well as another coronavirus previously isolated in bats. Finally, the Chinese Center for Disease Control and Prevention (China CDC) reported having isolated COVID-19 viral genes from samples taken at the Huanan Seafood Market, declaring the wild animals sold there to be the cause (Fearnley 2020, 210).

News media began rapidly proliferating the theory, with headlines like "Infectious Coronaviruses 'Circulating in Bats for Decades'" (Briggs 2020) and "Bats: The Mystery behind COVID-19" (CNN Press Room 2020).[2] Though many news outlets have since nuanced their claims regarding the relationship between bats and COVID-19 transmission, these assertions were initially taken so seriously in the United States that they led to the suspension of bat-related research activities for fear of viral transmission. In an online post, conservationist Merlin Tuttle (2020a) pointed out, "Public overreaction to hypothetical threats of disease from bat droppings, or even bat breath, could prove disastrous, leading to intolerance and widespread killing of bats. Media speculation has already caused harm that could last for decades."

In many countries around the world, the consequences for bats were indeed dire: large colonies of bats were "culled," or killed out of fear that they would pass viruses to nearby human populations (Bittel 2020; Goyal 2020; Tsang 2020). News media reported large-scale culling of bat colonies in Indonesia (Tsang 2020), Peru (*Phys.org* 2020), Cuba (*ADNCUBA* 2020), Rwanda (Bittel 2020), and India (Goyal 2020).[3] While culling animals suspected to be vectors of zoonotic disease has been a key feature of management strategy in several large-scale epidemics (Zhan 2005, 36; Fearnley 2020, 69), biologists claim that the practice is largely ineffective (Erickson 2013). Amy Fraenkel (2020), executive secretary of the United Nations' Convention on the Conservation of Migratory Species of Wild Animals, wrote:

> First, let's look at what we know. Bats do not spread COVID-19. COVID-19 is being transmitted from humans to other humans. Virologists are in total agreement that the spread of the virus across the planet has been due to human to human rather than animal to human contact. Moreover, there is no evidence that bats infected humans with COVID-19 to begin with. Inaccurate reports suggesting otherwise may be contributing to the ill-advised killing of bats.

Regardless of whether bats instigated the first zoonotic spillover to humans, claims Fraenkel, disease management should be focused on human-human contact. Or, as author Jason Bittel (2020) wrote, "Lighting [bats] on fire . . . will not help save anyone."

The rise in bat culling led to an outpouring of such opinion pieces by conservationists in an effort to change governmental policy and public opinion by pointing out the research inconsistencies responsible for the widespread assumption that bats cause human diseases (Tuttle 2020b). Because bats were blamed for dieases ranging from Ebola, SARS, MERS, rabies, Nipah virus, and Hanta virus, conservationists claim that bats are often selected as case studies for zoonotic disease simply due to the precedent provided by existing research. For example, a review article about the zoonotic origins of SARS (Wang and Eaton 2007) claimed that because two independent research studies demonstrated that bats in the genus *Rhinolophus* are "natural reservoirs of SARS-like viruses," they necessarily "provid[ed] evidence that SARS-CoV is indeed a new zoonotic virus with a wildlife origin" (326). During COVID-19, "a virus related to SARS-CoV-2, called RatG2013, was isolated from an intermediate horseshoe bat from China in 2013, and that led to suggestions that perhaps the bat virus jumped from bats to people. There has been a flurry of research since, and now we know this is extremely unlikely," states biologist Tigga Kingston (2020). In other words, because bats *can* host coronaviruses, scientific studies assumed that they *did*, even without more than circumstantial evidence.

That scientists like Amy Fraenkel and Tigga Kingston are speaking up to reinterpret such findings for the broader public demonstrates what scholar J. Brent Crosson (2016) has configured as the difference between "evidence" and "proof." An extensive literature in science and technology studies has been devoted to this question, which essentially destabilizes the commonsense interpretation of scientific findings as "facts." It also calls into question claims about scientific reification of objectivity: for example, in Bruno Latour's *On the Modern Cult of the Factish Gods* (2010 [1996]). Rather, within the sciences, findings are presented as evidence in support of or against a particular claim, yet they can never be naturalized as objective truth. It is popular media intervention that reinterprets scientific findings in this way, running the risk of validating dangerous and tentative claims.

As scholar Jon Lee has pointed out, theories become facts when they are translated from specialist circles for the general public via mass media. "The media, which has arguably . . . simple[r] language . . . is the main source of communication between the scientific and lay communities . . . considerable loss of nuance and meaning results from such pairing, a consequence that can result in miscommunication and misunderstanding" (2014, 10). The media's depiction of expert opinion—including the propagation of rumors—contributes not only to individual opinion but to the actions of governments: for example, in halting bat-based research in the US or in the widespread culling of bat colonies. In this case, the hypothetical possibility of bats as a viral reservoir for COVID-19 was based on the existence of the *possibility* that bats can harbor coronaviruses, yet it was quickly established as the definitive paradigm for understanding the virus's origins. While more recent media has nuanced its claims in regard to the bat-based origins of COVID-19, bats nonetheless remain deeply associated in the public consciousness with the propagation of the disease.

Yet bats have been debunked as potential causes of outbreaks of several of these diseases. For example, a 1976 Ebola outbreak in Sudan blamed bats purely on circumstantial evidence, and more recent outbreaks of Ebola have been attributed to the virus's ability to remain undetected in a human host for more than five years (Messenger et al. 2003, 628; Grady 2021). Additionally, research since the time of the first SARS epidemic has confirmed that bats were not the origin of the SARS spillover to humans, and that some studies sampled bats nearly twice as often as other species, leading to skewed statistics (Kuzmin et al. 2011, 4; Tuttle 2020b). The number of epidemiological studies on bats thus propagates exponentially, as scientists seek out species that they think are likely to transmit disease based on the results of previous studies, reproducing faulty data.

In addition to faulty methodologies, the scapegoating of bats as disease reservoirs is linked to the fundamental assumption that bats can be asymptomatic carriers of disease. Yet this assumption is derived from a faulty study conducted in the 1950s that examined rabies transmission from infected bats to mice. It was later uncovered that the bats used in the study had not had rabies at all, but rather a kind of Rio Bravo virus that is deadly to mice but harmless to both bats and humans (Messenger et al. 2003, 664–65). The assumption—based on this erroneous study—that bats can be asymptomatic carriers of diseases like rabies has led to speculation about why bats can carry diseases like coronaviruses without getting sick, some scientists claiming that differences in their physiology and/or a history of coevolution with viruses helps them to combat disease more effectively than humans (Kuzmin et al. 2011, 7; Messenger et al. 2003, 627). During COVID-19, the claim that there are fundamental physical characteristics of bats that predispose them to be asymptomatic disease carriers became a key talking point in discussions of the disease, as we shall see momentarily.

Claims about bats' ability to act as asymptomatic carriers are both highly debated in scientific circles and bespeak an ongoing politics of the outbreak narrative, as theorized by Priscilla Wald (2008). Focusing her efforts on the concept of a carrier—first through the figure of Typhoid Mary, then through patient zero of the AIDS epidemic—Wald demonstrates how outbreak narratives place blame on individuals classified as foreign, un-American, or otherwise transgressive, positioning scientists as the heroes who will contain the deadly disease. These narratives proliferated particularly during the Cold War and form the basis for concepts of collective American identity, which resists the invasive influence of foreign nationals through emergent disease. In other words, the concept of a carrier harboring an unseen and undetectable disease bespeaks a deep-seated political alignment focused on differentiating between the heroic "us" and the invasive "them." Wald claims that these cultural assumptions then become validated through scientific channels of communication, even when they are culturally inflected, not empirically irrefutable. In the case of COVID-19, bats came to serve as a stand-in for racialized Others, a tool for negotiating collective identity based on the scapegoating of Chinese citizens.

CONSUMING BATS

The link between scapegoating bats and anti-Asian racism results from disputes about the ethical treatment of animals. Cultural geographers Glen Elder, Jennifer Wolch, and Jody Emel have demonstrated how "conflicts over animal practices, rooted in deep-seated cultural beliefs and social norms, fuel ongoing efforts to racialize and devalue certain groups of immigrants" (Elder et al. 1998, 73) in a range of case studies. Similarly, political scientist Claire Jean Kim (2015) offers a nuanced perspective on how conflicting cultural perceptions of harm played out in politics surrounding live animal markets in San Francisco. By the same token, pandemic diseases have often deployed animal scapegoats in ways that place blame on specific cultural groups: the "green monkey" theory of AIDS (Goldstein 2004) and the palm civet link to SARS (Lee 2014; Zhan 2005) are but a few examples. In each of these cases, as in COVID-19, animals have acted as tools for the negotiation of human social groups in ways that serve to naturalize racist attitudes.

Sarah Monson (2017) has written how Ebola, another disease mistakenly attributed to consumption of bats, was manipulated in mainstream media to reflect and encourage otherized thinking about Africans, particularly through accusations about eating bats. The Ebola epidemic demonstrated a cultural double standard that led to racial blaming of Africans as the cause of the epidemic because of "backwards" management of human-animal relations. Monson cites a cover story in *Newsweek* that portrays smuggled "African bushmeat" as a potential Ebola carrier and a threat to the United States. It was criticized "for both its racializing association of primates with

Africans, and its depiction of bushmeat, a West African delicacy, which the article calls a cultural touchstone." Monson claims, "Americans also consume bushmeat but call it venison . . . and game. Referring to the consumption of bushmeat as cultural but framing as exotic, dirty, devious, and 'other' perpetuates the 'Dark Continent Myth' of Africa . . . and reinforces xenophobia toward Africans and African immigrants" (13). In early 2021, a fresh outbreak of Ebola in Guinea, likely caused by transmission from someone who had been sick during the 2012–14 Ebola outbreak, suggested that the disease might not have come from an animal reservoir at all.[4]

Such claims were reiterated with the emergence of monkeypox as a global health emergency in 2022. In addition to similarly false assumptions about monkeys as the main reservoir for the virus (leading to the stoning of wild primates), scientists suggested that the common name for the virus evoked excessive and unrealistic associations with Africa. Noting that many articles about the virus used misleading imagery that claimed that the virus was "endemic" to Africa, as well as the treacherous stereotype of African people and members of the African diaspora as similar to monkeys, scientists across the African continent suggested that the name "monkeypox" be changed to avoid the dangerous repetition of racist stereotypes (Jacobs 2022).

These examples demonstrate selective decision making surrounding the narrativization of animals as the source of disease, a topic that gained currency in popular media as the COVID-19 pandemic wore on. Comedian John Oliver pointed out in a news spot in early 2021 that contrary to the suppositions that China and/or Africa are hotspots for zoonotic spillover, many contagious diseases have spread in the United States due to phenomena like state fairs and the exotic pet trade (*Last Week Tonight* 2021). That news media focused exclusively on the "foreignness" of bushmeat consumption practices in the COVID-19 origin story speaks to long-standing patterns of racist scapegoating during disease epidemics (Kraut 1994, 2).

Mei Zhan (2005) encapsulates this claim in her discussion of "unruly" human-animal relations during the SARS epidemic. She writes, "The story of the 'zoonotic origin' [of SARS] did not blame nature itself for the SARS outbreak; what went wrong was the Chinese people's uncanny affinity with the nonhuman and the wild" (37). In other words, narrativizing pandemic outbreaks as a result of human-animal relations—and more specifically wet markets, which are not the only sites of human-animal interchange in China or any other locality—suggests a racist optic that has more to do with the limitations of acceptable behavior according to globalized publics than with factual evidence about the spread of disease.

BAT SOUP SONGS

It was not simply human-animal interactions that were targeted during the COVID-19 pandemic but, more specifically, culinary practices that were misread in order to serve a broader imperialist narrative. This is evident in the case of travel blogger Wang Mengyun. A video of Wang eating a fruit bat in a bowl of soup surfaced during the pandemic, in which she picked up a whole bat with chopsticks and bit into its wing. UK gossip rag the *Daily Mail* called the footage "revolting" in an article that was shared 352,000 times and received over a thousand comments, ranging from "disgusting," "revolting," "barbaric," and "proud to be an American" (Thomson 2020). One user commented "There needs to be a massive public health campaign in China about the risks of eating wildlife. Now there's panic in Wuhan and everyone is desperate to avoid the Coronavirus. The outbreaks will continue if nothing changes because some animals are natural carriers and hosts for these pathogens." Another stated, "I've lived in China for 30+ years . . . and I still can't understand how or why they eat the foods they do. There is no part of any animal they don't consider food. Not surprised this is now going to become a major world epidemic." Similar reporting from the *U.S. Sun* tabloid referred to the footage as "gruesome," and included a graphic that explicitly linked bat soup to the spread of COVID-19 (Mullin 2020; Knox 2020).

Wang's original video prompted such outrage that she was forced to offer a public apology. " 'You should go to hell. You should be killed in the evening. You're abnormal. You're disgusting. Why haven't you died?' These are the messages I just received today," Wang stated, following with an explanation that she was unaware of the connection between bats and COVID-19 at the time the video was filmed (O'Neill 2020). In fact, Wang's footage was filmed several years prior to the start of the pandemic, in the Pacific Island nation of Palau, where bat soup is a traditional food (Gaynor 2020). That viewers of the video assumed that the Chinese woman in the video was eating bushmeat from her own country speaks to a double standard that forbids Asians from engaging in cultural crossover, while American travel bloggers often consume foods perceived as exotic without repercussions.

Claims that Chinese people will eat anything—especially animal products that Westerners will not touch—underline assumptions of Chinese cruelty and question their humanity (Kim 2015, 56–57). Yet far from representing traditional modes of consumption that need to be "modernized," consumption of exotic bushmeat has more to do with the rising middle class. Mei Zhan suggests that consumptive excess in China is a response to the privation of the Mao era, noting that "visceral practices of consumption" like eating exotic animals indicate shifting economic realities in China (2005, 38). Scholar Michelle King furthers this claim:

> Other animal species are much more likely to be consumed in China as delicacies (e.g., sharks, masked palm civet, sika deer), used in Traditional Chinese Medicine (e.g., pangolin scales, tiger bones, bear bile, antelope horns), or purchased as status symbols, either as fashion, decor, or exotic pets (e.g., elephant ivory, crocodile skin, various rare birds) . . . Most importantly, despite references to the use of wild animals in historic texts on Chinese medicine, today's wildlife trade in China does not reflect traditional patterns of consumption so much as it reflects the rapid development of China's reform era economy and the growth of its industrialized agriculture. (2020, 242)

Thus, the consumption of bat meat in China has more to do with the wealthy in search of culinary thrills than traditional food practices. The misplaced assumptions about Wang's bat soup video therefore suggest a willful misread of Chinese culture based on historical assumptions about food.

The bat soup narrative has nonetheless become so pervasive that it spawned a rash of responses on the internet, including responses from musicians. Canadian singer Bryan Adams wrote on his social media, "Tonight was supposed to be the beginning of a tenancy of gigs at the @royalalberthall, but thanks to some f——bat eating, wet market animal selling, virus making greedy bastards, the whole world is now on hold, not to mention the thousands that have suffered or died from this virus" (Aviles 2020).[5] Adams's rant used the bat soup narrative as a platform for promoting veganism, arguing that bushmeat consumption was evidence of Chinese degeneracy. Paul McCartney made a similar claim, describing Chinese wet markets as "medieval," comparing them to slavery, and claiming "they might as well be letting off atomic bombs because it's affecting the whole world" in an interview with Howard Sterne (Greatrex 2020; Blisten 2020; Beaumont-Thomas 2020). Musicians, the sounds they produce, and the bodies they inhabit thus became entangled with nonhuman animals through racist negotiations over the ethics of consumption.

Additionally, many people responded by writing and posting songs about bat consumption to social media. Tucker (2014) has classified songs written in Africa during the Ebola epidemic based on their function in sensitization/education, memorial/dedication, or politics; "bat soup" songs, I argue, tread a narrow line between education and politics. While education songs offer prescriptive activities to warn listeners about the dangers of disease transmission, such as washing hands and avoiding the bodily fluids of infected individuals, they also sometimes include prohibitions on bushmeat consumption. For example, Rivera (2017) has written about two songs, "Ebola Song" and "Ebola in Town," which both include prohibitions against bat-eating as advice for mitigating the spread of disease (66, 72). Bat consumption prohibitions are situated in a longer litany of behaviors designed to protect individual listeners from viral transmission. Bat soup songs during COVID-19, however, mobilize narratives about bushmeat consumption in service of anti-China politics rather than as protection from virological harm. Bat soup songs sit in an uncomfortable categorical space in which activities allegedly geared toward pandemic management actually serve the function of racialized scapegoating.

Bat soup songs' function in scapegoating results in part because they are largely composed by individuals and showcased on the internet, not part of a government-formulated campaign or based on advice from the CDC. Some notable examples include a song by parodist Carlos Chavira, "No Coman Murciélago,"[6] which articulates a variety of "acceptable" foods to be eaten instead of bats; hip-hop track "Bat Soup" by Shawty Gawd, featuring Nada 5150, BB Sun, and Astral Tap; a *Bat Soup* musical performed live in New South Wales, Australia; and musicalized memes, including at least one mashed up with clips of dancing Ghanaian coffin dancers (*El Universal* 2020; Shawty Gawd 2020; McKnight 2020; WhirlwindGaming 2020). Many explicitly use the bat soup narrative in service of conservative politics—for example, the album *Bat Soup* by John Ward (2020) includes tracks titled "M.A.G.A Kid" and "Don't Trust China," discursively linking support of Donald Trump with scapegoating of Chinese citizens. As such, bat soup songs act primarily in the service of political scapegoating rather than disseminating health information.

The link between bats and anti-China, pro-Trump politics is particularly visible in the Deplorable Choir's "Bat Soup Song." The group, which consists of three women from Houston, appropriates a term used by Hillary Clinton in 2016 to describe Trump supporters. Their musical oeuvre cuts across many conservative topics, including pro-life legislation, anti-masking, and rejection of gun control.

Following on the heels of their first album, *Real Women Vote for Trump*, the women posted a series of songs regarding the experience of quarantine. In "Bat Soup Song," the Deplorable Choir mobilize the bat soup narrative to push racist claims about China, repeatedly intimating, "I don't trust the Chinese, do you?" The almost ten-minute livestream opens with two women making an "AOC margarita," referencing a video of Congresswoman

Alexandria Ocasio-Cortez from a few days prior (Fearnow 2020) and is peppered with statements about hydroxychloroquine and silver as potential cures for COVID-19 (LoneStar CJaye 2020).

Interestingly, while "bat soup" remains the song's hook, the group actually shies away from claims that Chinese wet markets are to blame for the COVID-19 pandemic, instead pushing a theory put forth by President Trump that the virus originated in the lab of Shi Zhengli, principal investigator at the Wuhan Institute of Virology (Areddy 2020).[7] Listing statistics "straight from Wikipedia," the women detail alleged "deaths by communism" from various countries around the world, shifting the coronavirus narrative to one focused on foreign relations and international politics (LoneStar CJaye 2020). Thus, narratives about disease, animal consumption, and politics become entangled while nonetheless maintaining a clear message: China is to blame for the COVID-19 pandemic.

Comments by listeners to bat soup songs on the internet further support the intersection of bat narrative and anti-China sentiment. One user commenting on "Norm Macdonald's Bat Song" wrote: "Wow, 'Chinese virus' is extremely offensive and racist. Even the GOP will tell you that the correct term is 'Kung Flu,' although Rudy Giuliani prefers 'Mulan Cooties.'" This comment received sixty-eight likes, followed by a list of other racist puns on COVID-19, including "slantAIDS," referencing stereotypes of Asian eye shape; "CCPvirus," in reference to the Chinese Communist Party; "Yellow Fever 2: Epidemic Boogaloo," referencing the racist stereotype of Asian skin color as yellow; "the Chinese sneeze"; and the "Shanghai Shivers." Some users also wrote their own additional verses to the song, some of which made the racist Chinese-bat parallel even more apparent. One wrote: "I like to eat bat in a stew with dog meat, now that's a combination that's impossible to beat. Anger is spreading like a global shockwave, but here in Wuhan it's just the chicken of the cave," mentioning the racist stereotype that Chinese people eat dogs (Macdonald 2020).

Such racist nomenclature was even more evident in President Trump's use of the term "Chinese virus," against advice from the CDC and the World Health Organization. News opinion pieces published in 2020 interpreted the term in light of the "Yellow Peril" politics of the nineteenth century (Chiu 2020; Itkowitz 2020; Zhou 2020; Zhang 2020), pointing out its historical basis in stereotypes about Chinese peoples' propagation of disease. Not only were Chinese immigrants blamed for outbreaks of syphilis, smallpox, and bubonic plague in California (Shah 2001, 89), a pamphlet from 1880 linked their alleged degeneracy with a distinctly anti-American political stance. The pamphlet suggested that if Chinese American people in San Francisco "should so perniciously and willfully disregard our sanitary laws . . . so maliciously pursue that course of conduct which they know is bringing distress upon our city, by destroying the lives of our citizens . . . [their actions] can only be accounted for on the supposition that they are enemies of our race and people" (Workingman's Committee of California 1880, 5–6), despite the fact that the conditions leading to poverty were a direct result of exclusionary practices (Kim 2015, 54).

President Trump's use of the term "Chinese virus" reflects a long precedent of typifying viruses themselves as racialized invaders. At the end of the nineteenth century, tuberculosis was referred to as the "Jewish disease" (Kraut 1994, 155); while syphilis was variously referred to as the "French pox," "*morbus Germanicus*," "the Naples sickness," and "the Chinese disease," depending on the nationality of the accuser (Sontag 2001, 136). Even microbes themselves have been anthropomorphized along nationalist lines: "Asian cholera" bacilli were described in 1926 as "puny but terrible little murderers from the Orient" (Wald 2008, 171), and medical texts have historically metaphorized cellular function according to an invasion narrative. One text stated, "It can be as difficult for our immune system to detect foreignness as it would be for a Caucasian to pick out a particular Chinese interloper at a crowded ceremony in Peking's main square," suggesting not just that certain nationalities were more likely to be carriers of particular viruses, but that the microbes themselves were agents of a foreign maliciousness (Martin [1990] 1999, 362). We find ourselves embroiled in a mess of significations in which animals are used as the justification for blaming Chinese people for viral infection, but at the same time, the viral infections are metaphorized as Chinese subjects.

Racist name-calling is more than discursive, however; news media reported extreme increases in hate crimes against Asian Americans in 2020. As of late April 2020, *NBC News* reported on a poll showing that 30 percent of Americans had witnessed "someone blaming Asian people for the coronavirus pandemic"; that statistic jumped to 60 percent when surveying Asian Americans who had observed the behavior (Ellerbeck 2020). A few months later, on July 2, *CBS News* reported 2,120 anti-Asian hate incidents, most occurring in California. The incidents ranged from verbal abuse to physical assault (Donaghue 2020). As of February 2021, reports tallied "2,808 firsthand accounts of anti-Asian hate from 47 states and the District of Columbia" (Chen 2021). Particularly gruesome incidents included victims Noel Quintana, a sixty-one-year-old who was slashed with a box cutter in New York City, and a ninety-omme-year-old man who was shoved to the ground in Oakland, California, both in February 2021 (Chen 2021). In a report from ABC, a professor at the University of Pennsylvania is quoted as saying, "We didn't see the spike in anti-Asian violence, until President Trump started saying Wuhan virus, China virus" (Han 2020).[8] Reporter Jennifer Chen, writing for *Oprah* magazine, stated that when she had written about why the term "kung flu" was racist in 2020, readers responded by telling her that it wasn't "real" racism (2021).

The blaming of China as a source of the novel coronavirus has been made more than evident in recent news media. What has been less often discussed is the use of bat consumption practices not only as evidence of allegedly backward cultural practices in China, but as scientific "proof" of China's guilt in causing the COVID-19 pandemic. As we have seen, not only are claims about bats as originators of COVID-19 scientifically suspect at best, they are rooted in long-standing cultural discourses about bats as disease carriers and as analogous to racial others. The scapegoating of bats as a part of anti-China rhetoric during the pandemic is not accidental; it demonstrates how racialized narratives persist through time in a combination of oblique and overt representations.

CONCLUSIONS: MULTISPECIES ETHNOGRAPHY IN THE ERA OF ZOONOTIC DISEASE

The COVID-19 pandemic makes evident that to ignore nonhumans in analyses of social formulations is to grossly misunderstand the position of humanity in the broader ecological world. Viruses that allegedly jump from one species to another call into question the validity of species boundaries. Furthermore, the narrativization of that jump via scientific publications, news, and social media speaks to ongoing efforts to stabilize group identity through aggressive demarcation of boundaries. That nonhuman animals act as tools for the crystallization of human social groups is increasingly evident in the ongoing struggle to regain control over a world beset with viral contagion.

This chapter has brought together some of the disparate threads present in popular discourse surrounding the causes of the COVID-19 pandemic. In discussing the scientific history of bats in epidemic research, I have sought to demonstrate the pathways by which scientific theories—designed by cultural individuals operating in a subjective world—become normalized as objective facts when translated via the media. The translation of scientific theory to objective fact is not a neutral transition; it serves as the basis for validating racialized categories under the aegis of "truth."

Norm Macdonald, the Deplorable Choir, and other online media users' mobilization of the bat soup narrative evidence the deep entanglement of bats, scientists, journalists, and other animal and technological bodies during COVID-19. Yet they also speak to deep-seated prejudices in US culture surrounding the acceptability of certain food products and the entitlement of certain citizens to make moral judgments about others' cultural practices. The rise in anti-Asian violence during the COVID-19 pandemic is not an isolated incident, therefore, but one rooted in much deeper and more insidious cultural histories and practices.

NOTES

1. Macdonald's politics have been lauded by conservative news outlet the *Federalist*, which called his lampooning of political correctness "brave." The *Federalist* cited his criticism of the #MeToo movement, his ability to mock while simultaneously supporting conservative politicians like Bob Dole, and his support of the George W. Bush administration's stance on the Iraq War (Capshaw 2018). His statements about President Donald Trump have been mixed, however: in 2015, he described Trump as a "fascist" in an interview with the *Hollywood Reporter*; in 2018, in an interview with the same reporter, he claimed that the Trump presidency had not been as bad as he expected (Abramovitch 2015, 2018).

2. Imagery depicted in such news media often showed very different species of bat, but rarely the horseshoe bat (*Rhinopholous* spp.) allegedly sold at the Wuhan market.

3. Local experts blamed culling in Rajasthan on both the COVID-19 pandemic and a "number of myths that bats are inauspicious in family life if seen near the domicile" (Goyal 2020). To ensure protections for the bats, the Karnataka and then the Rajathan governments' wildlife warden issued a warning under the 1972 Wildlife Act leading to potential "legal action" against citizens found to harm bats (Goyal 2020).

4. The new outbreak evidenced the longest period of time that someone who had previously had the disease was known to have harbored it in their tissues—more than five years, where previously the record had been five hundred days. Reporters summarized the issue in the following way: "People recover from Ebola when their immune systems wipe out the virus. But certain parts of the body, including the eyes, the central nervous system and the testes are so-called privileged sites, beyond the reach of the immune system. The virus can sometimes hide in those spots. But no one knew it could hide out for so long" (Grady 2021). In the same article, Thomas Skinner, CDC spokesperson, stated: "This suggests that the outbreak was likely started from a persistent infection, a survivor, and not a new introduction of the virus from an animal reservoir."

5. Shortly after, the singer was pressured to offer an apology and change the post.

6. This song was later reproduced by Mexican singer Thalía as well as others across the internet. Many thanks to the student who pointed out this example to me.

7. In a briefing on April 30, President Trump answered in the affirmative as to whether he had seen convincing evidence that the Wuhan Institute of Virology was the source of the virus but declined to offer what that evidence was (CNBC Television 2020). Dr. Shi, on the other hand, wrote in Wuhan's main Communist Party newspaper in February that she could "guarantee on my life" that the virus hadn't come from her lab. She continued to "advise those who believe and spread malicious rumors to close their stinky mouths," as she mostly does genetic sequencing with computers, and when she used samples from bats to culture

viruses, she didn't use the COVID-19 virus (Areddy 2020). The paper that initially suggested the virus came from Dr. Shi's lab was withdrawn after its "speculation" caught international attention.

8. The racism was not confined to the United States, as evidenced by the emergence of the #Jenesuispasunvirus ("I am not a virus") hashtag in France in February (*NBC News* 2020).

REFERENCES

Abramovitch, Seth. 2015. "Norm Macdonald: A Raw and Uncensored Interview." *Hollywood Reporter*, September 1. https://www.hollywoodreporter.com/tv/tv-news /norm-macdonald-a-raw-uncensored-819420/.

Abramovitch, Seth. 2018. "Norm Macdonald Won't Go Pundit on His Netflix Talk Show." *Hollywood Reporter*, September 11. https://www.hollywoodreporter.com/news /general-news/why-norm-macdonalds-new-talk-show-wont-target-trump-1141832/.

ADNCUBA. 2020. "Exterminan colonias de murciélagos en Cuba por temor al coronavirus." April 8. https://adncuba.com/noticias-de-cuba/exterminan-colonias -de-murcielagos-en-cuba-por-temor-al-coronavirus?fbclid=IwAR00CX2jebE_Y _x0bMEGHtw1NNx9bcax183ZBZ8X2Ze3bYZkbzY9QHrPh0M.

Areddy, James T. 2020. "China Bat Expert Says Her Wuhan Lab Wasn't Source of New Coronavirus." *Wall Street Journal*, April 21. https://www.wsj.com/articles/chinas-bats -expert-says-her-wuhan-lab-wasnt-source-of-new-coronavirus-11587463204?mod= searchresults&page=1&pos=2.

Aviles, Gwen. 2020. "Singer Bryan Adams Slammed for Blaming 'Bat Eating' People for Coronavirus." *NBC News*, May 12. https://www.nbcnews.com/pop-culture/pop -culture-news/singer-bryan-adams-slammed-racist-post-blaming-bat-eating-people -n1205166.

Beaumont-Thomas, Ben. 2020. "Paul McCartney Calls for 'Medieval' Chinese Markets to Be Banned over Coronavirus." *Guardian*, April 14. https://www.theguardian.com /music/2020/apr/14/paul-mccartney-calls-for-medieval-chinese-markets-to-be -banned-over-coronavirus.

Bittel, Jason. 2020. "Experts Urge People All over the World to Stop Killing Bats out of Fears of Coronavirus." *Natural Resources Defense Council*, June 2. https://www .nrdc.org/stories/experts-urge-people-all-over-world-stop-killing-bats-out-fears -coronavirus.

Blisten, Jon. 2020. "Paul McCartney Calls for an End to China's 'Wet Markets.'" *Rolling Stone*, April 14. https://www.rollingstone.com/music/music-news/paul-mccartney -china-wet-market-coronavirus-983463/.

Briggs, Helen. 2020. "Covid-19: Infectious Coronaviruses 'Circulating in Bats for Decades.'" *BBC News*, July 29. https://www.bbc.com/news/science-environment -53584936.

Capshaw, Ron. 2018. "Norm Macdonald Is Conservative and Brave, a Rarity among Comedians." *Federalist*, September 14. https://thefederalist.com/2018/09/14/norm -macdonald-is-conservative-and-brave-a-rarity-among-comedians/.

Chen, Jennifer. 2021. "How You Can Join the Stop Asian Hate Movement." *Oprah Magazine*, February 23. https://www.oprahdaily.com/life/a35604044/what-is-stop -asian-hate-movement-join/.

Chiu, Allyson. 2020. "Trump Has No Qualms about Calling Coronavirus the 'Chinese Virus.' That's a Dangerous Attitude, Experts Say." *Washington Post*, March 20.

https://www.washingtonpost.com/nation/2020/03/20/coronavirus-trump-chinese
-virus/.

CNBC Television. 2020. "President Trump Delivers Remarks on Protecting America's
Seniors—4/30/2020." Streamed live on YouTube, April 30. https://www.youtube
.com/watch?v=mtTYAZXTsTU.

CNN Press Room. 2020. "CNN to Air Special on the Connection between Bats and
COVID-19." June 9. https://cnnpressroom.blogs.cnn.com/2020/06/09/cnn-to-air
-special-on-the-connection-between-bats-and-covid-19/.

Crosson, J. Brent. 2016. "Oil, Obeah, and Science." *Cosmologics.* http://cosmologicsmag
azine.com/brent-crosson-oil-obeah-and-science/.

Donaghue, Erin. 2020. "2,120 Hate Incidents against Asian Americans Reported during
Coronavirus Pandemic." *CBS News,* July 2. https://www.cbsnews.com/news/anti
-asian-american-hate-incidents-up-racism/.

Elder, Glen, Jennifer Wolch, and Jody Emel, eds. 1998. *Animal Geographies: Place, Politics, and
Identity in the Nature-Culture Borderlands.* London: Verso.

Ellerbeck, Alex. 2020. "Over 30 Percent of Americans Have Witnessed COVID-19 Bias
against Asians, Poll Says." *NBC News,* April 28. https://www.nbcnews.com/news
/asian-america/over-30-americans-have-witnessed-covid-19-bias-against-asians
-n1193901.

El Universal. 2020. "'No coman murciélago, coman pollito . . .': Thalía." May 5. https://www
.eluniversal.com.mx/espectaculos/musica/no-coman-murcielago-coman-pollito-thalia.

Erickson, Jim. 2013. "Culling Vampire Bats to Stem Rabies in Latin America Can
Backfire." *University of Michigan News,* December 2. https://news.umich.edu/culling
-vampire-bats-to-stem-rabies-in-latin-america-can-backfire/.

Fearnley, Lyle. 2020. *Virulent Zones: Animal Disease and Global Health at China's Pandemic
Epicenter.* Durham: Duke University Press.

Fearnow, Benjamin. 2020. "AOC Calls U.S. 'Brutal Society' in Video While Making
Margarita, Conservative Critics Mock Coronavirus Message." *Newsweek,* April 4.
https://www.newsweek.com/aoc-calls-us-brutal-society-video-while-making
-margarita-conservative-critics-mock-1496145.

Fraenkel, Amy. 2020. "Opinion: Far from Being Our Enemies, Bats Need Protection Now
More Than Ever." *Convention on the Conservation of Migratory Species of Wild Animals,*
July 22. https://www.cms.int/en/news/opinion-far-being-our-enemies-bats-need
-protection-now-more-ever.

Gaynor, Gerren Keith. 2020. "Coronavirus: Outrage over Chinese Eating 'Bat Soup'
Sparks Apology." *Fox News,* January 28. https://www.foxnews.com/food-drink
/coronavirus-chinese-blogger-eats-bat-soup.

Goldstein, Diane E. 2004. "What Exactly Did They Do with That Monkey, Anyway?
Contemporary Legend, Scientific Speculation, and the Politics of Blame in the
Search for AIDS Origins." In *Once upon a Virus: AIDS Legends and Vernacular Risk
Perception,* 77–99. Logan: Utah State University Press.

Goyal, Yash. 2020. "More Than 150 Bats Killed in Rajasthan Owing to Fear of COVID-19
Spread." *Tribune India,* May 7. https://www.tribuneindia.com/news/nation/more-than
-150-bats-killed-in-rajasthan-owing-to-fear-of-covid-19-spread-81668?fbclid=IwAR0y
8PXDD7tMzTGtqQWw0RPJI2e6JutlSVI1eDDAfNhYuRoRYnDNP5DMdr4.

Grady, Denise. 2021. "Ebola Survivor Infected Years Ago May Have Started New
Outbreak." *New York Times,* March 12. https://www.nytimes.com/2021/03/12
/health/ebola-old-infection-new-outbreak.html.

Greatrex, Jack. 2020. "From Bat Soup to Bean Sprouts: Coronavirus Food Fears in
Historical Perspective." *Somatosphere,* July 20. http://somatosphere.net/2020/corona
virus-food-fears.html/.

Han, Nydia. 2020. "The Virus of Hate: COVID's Impact on Asian Americans." *ABC*, May 21. https://6abc.com/coronavirus-backlash-covid-19-asian-american-hate -crimes/6201660/.

Itkowitz, Colby. 2020. "CDC Director Rejects Label 'Chinese Virus' After Trump, McCarthy Tweets." *Washington Post*, March 10. https://www.washingtonpost.com /politics/cdc-director-rejects-label-chinese-virus-after-trump-mccarthy-tweets/2020 /03/10/58bd086c-62e5-11ea-b3fc-7841686c5c57_story.html.

Jacobs, Andrew. 2022. "Why Experts Want to Rename Monkeypox." *New York Times*, August 23. https://www.nytimes.com/2022/08/23/health/monkeypox-name -stigma.html.

Kim, Claire Jean. 2015. *Dangerous Crossings: Race, Species, and Nature in a Multicultural Age*. New York: Cambridge University Press.

King, Michelle T. 2020. "Say No to Bat Fried Rice: Changing the Narrative of Coronavirus and Chinese Food." *Food and Foodways: Explorations in the History and Culture of Human Nourishment* 23 (3): 237–49.

Kingston, Tigga. 2020. "Bats Have Earned an Unwarranted Reputation as Disease Spreaders since the Covid-19 Outbreak. With April 17 Marking World Bat Appreciation Day, Dr Tigga Kingston Sets out to Provide the Full Picture on the Misunderstood Mammals." *Austin Bat Refuge*, April 17. https://austinbatrefuge.org/author/leemack/.

Knox, Patrick. 2020. "Bat Sip Crazy: Who Is Bat Soup Influencer Wang Mengyun?" *U.S. Sun*, January 28. https://www.the-sun.com/news/322002/who-is-bat-soup-influ encer-wang-mengyun/.

Kraut, Alan M. 1994. *Silent Travelers: Germs, Genes, and the "Immigrant Menace."* Baltimore: Johns Hopkins University Press.

Kuzmin, Ivan V., Brooke Bozick, Sarah A. Guagliardo, Rebekahh Kunkel, Joshua R. Shak, Suxiang Tong, and Charles E. Rupprecht. 2011. "Bats, Emerging Infections Diseases, and the Rabies Paradigm Revisited." *Emerging Health Threats Journal* 4:7159.

Last Week Tonight. 2021. "The Next Pandemic: *Last Week Tonight* with John Oliver." YouTube, February 15. https://www.youtube.com/watch?v=_v-U3K1sw9U.

Latour, Bruno. 2010 [1996]. *On the Modern Cult of the Factish Gods*. Durham, NC: Duke University Press.

Lee, Jon D. 2014. "Chronicle of a Health Panic." In *An Epidemic of Rumors: How Stories Shape Our Perception of Disease*, 8–57. Logan: Utah State University Press.

LoneStar CJaye. 2020. "Bat Soup Song." YouTube, April 6. https://www.youtube.com /watch?v=GOg0cvQYcCU.

Macdonald, Norm. 2020. "Norm Macdonald's Bat Song." YouTube, March 29. https:// www.youtube.com/watch?v=rrhux_CZGRE.

Martin, Emily. (1990) 1999. "Toward an Anthropology of Immunology: The Body as Nation State." In *The Science Studies Reader*, edited by Mario Biagioli, 358–71. New York: Routledge.

McKnight, Albert. 2020. "Theatre Onset Recovers from COVID-19 Pandemic with Show of Short Plays, Musical Titled *Bat Soup*." *Bega District News*, September 2. https:// www.begadistrictnews.com.au/story/6905077/theatre-onset-recovers-from-covid-19 -pandemic-with-show-of-short-plays-musical-titled-bat-soup/.

Messenger, Sharon L., Charles E. Rupprecht, and Jean S. Smith. 2003. "Bats, Emerging Virus Infections, and the Rabies Paradigm." In *Bat Ecology*, edited by Thomas H. Kunz and M. Brock Fenton, 622–79. Chicago: University of Chicago Press.

Monson, Sarah. 2017. "Ebola as African: American Media Discourses of Panic and Otherization." *Africa Today* 63 (3): 3–27.

Mullin, Gemma. 2020. "Missing Link: Coronavirus Outbreak Could Be Linked to Bat Soup Say Scientists." *U.S. Sun*, January 24. https://www.the-sun.com/news/304593/how-coronavirus-couldve-jumped-from-bat-soup-to-humans-according-to-science/.

NBC News. 2020. "'I Am Not a Virus': France's Asian Community Pushes Back over Xenophobia." February 4. https://www.nbcnews.com/news/asian-america/i-gram-not-virus-france-s-asian-community-pushes-back-n1129811.

O'Neill, Marnie. 2020. "Chinese Influencer Wang Mengyun, aka 'Bat Soup Girl,' Breaks Silence." *Chronicle*, February 7. https://www.thechronicle.com.au/news/chinese-influencer-wang-mengyun-aka-bat-soup-girl-breaks-silence/news-story/63ef0cec5b6d448d1843e2e1bcadb14d.

Phys.org. 2020. "Peru Saves Bats Blamed for Coronavirus." March 25. https://phys.org/news/2020-03-peru-blamed-coronavirus.html.

Rivera, Michael. 2017. "Music, Media, and the Ethnopoetics of Two Ebola Songs in Liberia." *Africa Today* 63 (3): 62–76.

Shah, Nayan. 2001. *Contagious Divides: Epidemics and Race in San Francisco's Chinatown.* Berkeley: University of California Press.

Shawty Gawd. 2020. "Bat Soup (feat. Nada 5150, BB Sun & Astral Tap)." YouTube, July 30. https://www.youtube.com/watch?v=kvSzHwSvWoE.

Sontag, Susan. 2001. *Illness as Metaphor and AIDS and Its Metaphors.* New York: Doubleday.

Stone, Ruth M. 2017. "'Ebola in Town': Creating Musical Connections in Liberian Communities during the 2014 Crisis in West Africa." *Africa Today* 63 (3): 78–97.

Thomson, Billie. 2020. "Revolting Footage Shows Chinese Woman Eating a Whole Bat at a Fancy Restaurant as Scientists Link the Deadly Coronavirus to the Flying Mammals." *Daily Mail*, January 23. https://www.dailymail.co.uk/news/article-7920573/Revolting-footage-shows-Chinese-woman-eating-bat-scientists-link-coronavirus-animal.html.

Tsang, Yuki. 2020. "Hundreds of Bats Culled in Indonesia to 'Prevent Spread' of the Coronavirus." *South China Morning Post*, March 16. https://www.scmp.com/video/asia/3075441/hundreds-bats-culled-indonesia-prevent-spread-coronavirus.

Tucker, Boima. 2014. "Beats, Rhymes, and Ebola. Fieldsights: Hot Spots." *Cultural Anthropology Online*, October 7. http://www.culanth.org/fieldsights/592-beats-rhymes-and-ebola.

Tuttle, Merlin D. 2017. "Fear of Bats and Its Consequences." *Journal of Bat Research and Conservation* 10 (1). http://secemu.org/journal-of-bat-research-and-conservation/all-issues/journal-of-bat-research-and-conservation-10/.

Tuttle, Merlin. 2020a. "Concerns for COVID-19 Management in North America." Merlin Tuttle's Bat Conservation, April 9. https://www.merlintuttle.org/resources/concerns-for-covid-19-management-in-north-america/.

Tuttle, Merlin. 2020b. "A Viral Witch Hunt." *Issues in Science and Technology*, March 27. https://issues.org/a-viral-witch-hunt-bats/.

Wald, Priscilla. 2008. *Contagious: Cultures, Carriers, and the Outbreak Narrative.* Durham: Duke University Press.

Wang, Lin-Fa, and Bryan T. Eaton. 2007. "Bats, Civets and the Emergence of SARS." *Current Topics in Microbiology and Immunology* 315: 325–44.

Ward, John. 2020. *Bat Soup.* YouTube, July 11. https://www.youtube.com/watch?v=CNDjQ5sjV8M&list=OLAK5uy_kzF0UqPDQWyWNgCvEcQk6375Jr7P3fO6A.

WhirlwindGaming. 2020. *Tasty Bat Soup (Astronomia meme).* YouTube, April 25. https://www.youtube.com/watch?v=No-lc-PwV5I.

Workingman's Committee of California. 1880. "Chinatown Declared a Nuisance!" The Museum of the City of San Francisco, March. http://sfmuseum.org/hist2/nuisance.html.

Zhan, Mei. 2005. "Civet Cats, Fried Grasshoppers, and David Beckham's Pajamas: Unruly Bodies After SARS." *American Anthropologist* 107 (1): 31–42.

Zhang, Lijia. 2020. "Coronavirus Triggers an Ugly Rash of Racism as the Old Ideas of 'Yellow Peril' and 'Sick Man of Asia' Return." *South China Morning Post*, February 16. https://www.scmp.com/comment/opinion/article/3050542/coronavirus-triggers-ugly-rash-racism-old-ideas-yellow-peril-and.

Zhou, Li. 2020. "Trump's Racist References to the Coronavirus Are His Latest Effort to Stoke Xenophobia." *Vox*, June 23. https://www.vox.com/2020/6/23/21300332/trump-coronavirus-racism-asian-americans.

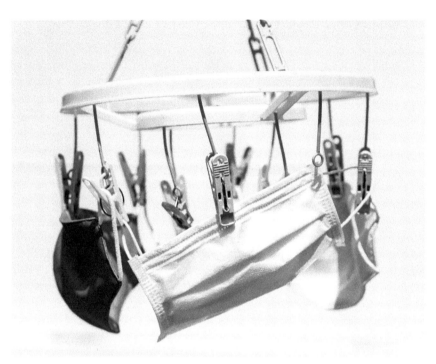

Figure 7.0. Face masks.

Section III
When Vernaculars Meet

THE PARTICULARITY OF SOCIAL DYNAMICS AND PERFORMANCE COMPELLED by the pandemic often necessitated new forms of creative expression and means of being together, particularly as various vernaculars mixed, met, and collided. Throughout the pandemic, some vernaculars met via the positionality of individuals and their communities through a sort of intersectionality. The creative expression of vernacular practices, perhaps normally separated by the performance of different identities, was often altered as space collapsed for many people throughout periods of lockdown, quarantine, and uncertainty and as performance was relegated to a more finite number of mediums. Changes to the ways people inhabited their social worlds also compelled the collision of different vernaculars through space—both physical and virtual—and time. Public space, for example, albeit technically accessible, is often contested in times of protest or crisis. This became abundantly apparent when sharing space was deemed unsafe and against the best interests of public health. Where, how, and why people met in these physical spaces was, then, often framed through the windows of our homes, our televisions and computer screens, and through the lens of safety. Thus, expressions of vernaculars were also negotiated based on these restrictions on space and sociality. In this third section, three chapters explore emergent notions of community and the ways that vernaculars meet in times of pandemics. With an understanding that the dynamic of the pandemic requires investigating preexisting and emergent vernacular forms, these chapters explore how, when, and where vernaculars met—behind the mask.

https://doi.org/10.7330/9781646424818.p003

7

From Risk Semantics to Embodied Practice

Anne Eriksen and Kyrre Kverndokk

NORWAY WENT INTO ITS FIRST CORONA LOCKDOWN on March 12, 2020. At a press conference that day, Prime Minister Erna Solberg announced that the government would implement "the strongest and most comprehensive measures in times of peace" (Norwegian government 2020b). Together with the minister of health, Bent Høie, and the heads of national health authorities, Solberg used a double linguistic register when presenting the radical steps of closing down civil society. Terms like *risk* and *risk groups*, *reproduction rate*, *exponential growth*, and *incidence* all come from the statistical calculations that underlie public health rationality. They are vital to institutional practices of naming potential threats and calculating uncertainties and probabilities with the aim of identifying required measures. This linguistic register represents what Ulrich Beck has called "the semantics of risk" (Beck 2009, 4). The other register that was employed was vernacular language, referring directly to everyday life when calling for solidarity and compliance with the new measures. There are considerable differences between these two registers, the one highly abstract, the other close to common experience. Shifting between them, the prime minister demonstrated the kind of translations that she called on the entire nation to carry out.

The aim of this chapter is to explore how this work of translation was carried out among Norwegians. How were the necessary shifts between professional risk semantics and everyday life and language actually performed? What was needed to transpose terms like *risk group* and *reproduction rate* into meaningful vernacular language and practical everyday social life and work? The level of confidence in the authorities is generally high in Norway (Kleven 2016), and willingness to comply with the infection-control measures presented by the authorities has proved to be strong

https://doi.org/10.7330/9781646424818.c007

(e.g., Klemetzen 2020). There have been no great demonstrations against restrictions or other measures, and polls regularly show that most people in Norway sympathize with the official strategies and are ready to follow recommendations and orders. Nonetheless, the translational work, which was started and demonstrated by the two ministers, had to carry on and be carried out. It takes considerable effort to translate risk vocabulary so that it makes sense in everyday life and to model conduct and social interaction. Our aim is to explore how this was done during spring 2020.

EMPIRICAL MATERIAL AND PERSPECTIVES

Shortly after the lockdown, the Norwegian Museum of Cultural History (Norsk Folkemuseum, https://minner.no/tema/korona), together with the association Memoar, started to collect memories and stories about life during the pandemic. People from all over the country were invited to answer an online questionnaire and to keep diaries. Additionally, a series of digital interviews were conducted. Most of the material is publicly available on the Web (https://minner.no/tema/korona). Of these different genres, diaries, not surprisingly, proved the most demanding to potential authors, and only a small number of such texts was submitted to the museum when the first lockdown gradually ended in May and June. Despite their restricted quantity, however, the diaries have proved a particularly rich source for exploration. Some of them are publicly available (cf. above), but for reasons of privacy protection, all authors have been given fictional names in this article. The diaries describe the experiences of their authors over a period of time, recording the development of the pandemic and the restrictions as well as the writers' responses to these events. The entries often are elaborate, detailed, and thoughtful, presenting the authors' reflections and considerations concerning the changes to their lives brought about by the pandemic. With kind permission from the museum, we will make use of this small collection of nine diaries, written from March to June 2020, to explore how the risk semantics of public health experts and authorities were incorporated, interpreted, rephrased, and remodeled when people tried to adapt to the situation, to make sense of what happened, and to articulate how the lockdown affected their lives, their work, and their neighborhoods.

All the authors are women, ranging in age from mid-twenties to mid-eighties. They belong to what can be called the educated middle class and most have active professional lives. Most of them live with their own families consisting of children and a partner. Some also have elderly parents or other older relatives whom they worry about during the pandemic. A majority live in urban contexts in or just outside the three largest cities in Norway: Oslo, Bergen, and Trondheim. Keeping a diary over time demands effort and dedication, and while all the authors demonstrate literary ambition and skills, some are professional writers. The translations into English have been done by us. To preserve anonymity, we have given all authors fictive names.

The authors and their diaries are not statistically representative of the Norwegian population in general. Nonetheless, due to their detail and richness of expression, we have found these texts to be a good source for exploring how the translational work, or shifts between linguistic registers, that the authorities initiated was then carried out by the authors of the diaries. We will explore this from a double perspective. We will investigate how the vocabulary was integrated in vernacular language and trace some of the semantic shifts that occurred. At the same time, we will study how this work of translation and integration was not merely a linguistic matter, but also implied the production of new habits and practices, turning risk into embodied and habitual memory.

SIGNIFYING THE NATION AS A COMMUNITY

The key word at the press conference on March 12 was *dugnad*. Both ministers emphatically used this term when calling for a common voluntary effort to stop the pandemic (Norwegian government 2020b). The word can be roughly translated as "communal work." Traditionally, the dugnad has been a practical way of getting large or difficult work done through a relatively brief collective effort, normally to enhance the common good and often ending with a celebration. As pointed out by ethnologist Asbjørn Klepp, the traditional dugnad in preindustrial society was based on unwritten, customary rules.[1] A dugnad was often called to carry out large projects that had to be done quickly (for instance, repairing a roof), but it also worked as a security arrangement, ensuring that people got help when it was acutely needed. Knowing the rules of the dugnad and adhering to them meant being part of the community. To set them aside meant to break away from society and to face risk or emergencies without the help of a social network (Klepp 2001, 84). This is still the case. The dugnad is an established communal practice in Norway, referring to different types of voluntary work. You do not shirk the dugnad when your housing cooperative, parents' group, or other local community group calls, even if you hate the work and are not particularly good at it. Everybody is expected to contribute their share, and it is a personal disgrace to refuse (Østberg 1910; Klepp 2001; Simon and

Mobekk 2019). Thus, the dugnad is not merely a practical way of organizing a joint effort; to most present-day Norwegians, dugnad is also a moral issue. It is also frequently referred to as representing typical national values.

By their very conscious use of this term at the press conference on the day the lockdown was declared, the two ministers translated institutional and quantitative risk semantics into the linguistic register of the vernacular. The aim was not only to make abstract language more generally understandable. As a performance, the press conference also demonstrated exactly what the government wanted the entire population to do: to translate risk from mathematical calculations into the relations and obligations of everyday life and practices. This translation could not be done unilaterally by the authorities themselves. The dugnad that was called for did not concern only adherence to the infection-control measures; it referred just as much to the translational work necessary for a practical realization of such adherence.

The first step of this translational work was conducted by Bent Høie, the health minister, the day before the press conference and the start of the lockdown. In an op-ed published in one of the national newspapers, he attempted to prepare the population for the lockdown by explaining the dugnad allegory: "We are good at dugnad in Norway. Many of us have participated in the shared work of our neighborhood or sports association each spring and fall. Before the dugnad, we plan for the major tasks to be done. But new tasks will always turn up as we go along: we do not see them before we have got started. Now we need a dugnad in Norwegian society" (Norwegian government 2020a).[2] By using the term *dugnad*, Høye underscored that Norway is and has to be a community—not an imagined one, but a performed and expressive one. He pointed to the dugnad as a key institution in Norwegian society and appealed to national pride by emphasizing that Norwegians are particularly good at this kind of joint effort. In doing so, he also upscaled the local communal importance of dugnad to a national event: this "dugnad" was necessary to keep the nation going, and the nation, although it would be tested by the pandemic, would be confirmed and even strengthened as a community through this action. In that regard, dugnad represented national qualities.

The values implied are partly those motivating the practice itself, like general participation and unselfish cooperation. Partly, however, what emerges is also a proud belief that the custom represents something distinctly Norwegian, embodied in the relative untranslatability of the word. Choosing this expression, already charged with moral obligations, Høie went one step further and appealed to the nation as an "emotional community."

According to medievalist Barbara Rosenwein, who has coined this term, emotional communities are similar to other social communities such as, for instance, the family, the neighborhood, or the nation. But to understand them, the scholar needs to uncover their "system of feeling" and to focus on "the emotions that they value, devalue, or ignore; the nature of the affective bonds between people that they recognize; and the modes of emotional expression that they expect, encourage, tolerate, and deplore" (2010, 11–12). It will be our argument that by upscaling the term *dugnad* to the national level, Høie correspondingly upscaled the emotions and obligations that people usually have concerning their family, neighborhood, and close relations. In the following section, we will explore how people responded to this appeal and to this way of signifying the nation as a community held together by emotional ties and obligations. This will serve as a means to investigate how the authors experienced and participated in the state of emergency, which the government termed a national dugnad, and what sorts of meaning it produced.

NEW RULES

The term *dugnad* is used in many of the diaries, mostly in self-evident ways that demonstrate the authors' familiarity with the term and its implications. Some of the authors simply repeat the words of the authorities and note that "it is a national 'dugnad' for all of us." However, one of the authors is more ambivalent about the infection-control measures, writing: "I'm glad to see the spirit of dugnad among people. At the same time, I am uncertain whether the Norwegian authorities have made the right decision in being so strict in dealing with the situation" (Strand, 2).[3] The doubts expressed here have not prevented her from adapting the vocabulary. By using the expression "the spirit of dugnad," she underscores that what is at stake is more than the shared responsibility of handling risk. Commonly used in Norwegian, the phrase has a distinctly moral bias, implying a shared will to stand up for the community (Klepp 2001, 82).

This author, Christine Strand, was running a small bar when the pandemic hit. Due to a trip abroad, she started the lockdown period in a legally required quarantine, and her place had to close. Her partner, who was running a restaurant, tried to keep business going by offering takeout service. In isolation at home, she heard stories from him about regular customers taken by the same "spirit of dugnad," thus helping him to keep the business afloat. In using the term, she demonstrates how the dugnad was understood not merely as an implementation of statistically defined risk measures, but as a joint effort of solidarity. Dugnad involves most aspects of social life, and it is a matter of caring for and supporting the community during a societal crisis.

At their most basic, the infection-control measures covered in Norway by the idea of dugnad involved hygiene and distance, as was true everywhere else. In practice, the matter of contagion risk also became a measure of how to relate to other individuals. It meant that new social rules were established and new categories of people emerged.

The diary of Eva Berg gives insight into this shift from statistically based infection risk measures to embodied behavior. She reports having been ill, probably with COVID-19. Test capacity was low in Norway in March and she never was diagnosed. She did not get seriously ill but, living alone, she needed help to get food. Consequently, her experience was more about distance than disease:

> On a freezing afternoon I stand at the parking lot by my home, waiting for supplies. This is Tuesday, 24 March 2020, and I have had mild symptoms for some days. Because of that, I dare not visit the shops. I stand waiting for my good friend, who has done my shopping for me. With the icy wind at my back and the hood well over my head, I wait impatiently to speak to a living human who is not just a face on a screen.[4]

When her friend arrived, he wore gloves "from having visited the shop." They stood one meter apart, for "such are the rules":

> We talk about this and that. We would like to meet soon. In the real way, when this is over. The wind bites. He has to leave, opens his arms and gives me an "air hug." I do the same. That is how things are now. Love in the time of corona. Separated by a microscopically small enemy.[5]

Having been dismissed from her job, Eva decided to visit her parents when she recovered. In their part of the country, contagion was low and she found that life went on very much as usual. She nonetheless observed that the streets were quiet, people stood well apart in the shops, and her mother avoided touching the handrail of the escalators when they went shopping: "So perhaps we are on our way to being well corona educated?"[6]

Margareth Ness writes that as soon as hairdressers were allowed to reopen, people flocked to have their hair done. All of them, however, demonstrated an embodied will to stick to "the rules," and even if very eager for an appointment, people signaled that they would not break with the discipline of the ongoing dugnad:

The phone was chiming and there were people at the door all the time who asked for appointments. The hopeful ones kept a humble distance, as though to say with their entire being that here is someone who is ready to cooperate to get their hair cut.[7]

These two authors both demonstrate how the physical distance required by the infection-control measures was transformed into bodily practices that initially had to be learned. Slowly they were internalized and became embedded in the ways that bodies related to other bodies as well as to their material physical surroundings. In the narratives quoted above, handrails, hugs, and hairdressers' waiting rooms appear as instantiations of new ways to behave, to move about, and to navigate in everyday life—socially as well as physically. The development of new bodily habits was part of the translational work. It was done to serve the community, even if it meant internalizing antisocial practices of separation and distance.

May Foss describes how she went for a walk in her neighborhood and was approached by some youths who showed great interest in her historical knowledge and the stories she could tell about the area where they all lived. After the pleasurable conversation, however, she suddenly stopped herself: "Had I remembered to keep my distance? Luckily it is down to one meter now."[8] At the start of lockdown, the authorities recommended that people keep two meters apart when meeting. As the infection rate decreased, this was cut down to one meter, justified by the reduced statistical risk of infection. This also enabled businesses such as restaurants, movie theaters, and theaters to reopen. However, in everyday life, at least before the pandemic, people did not measure their spatial distance from others in meters. Suddenly remembering the restrictions, May Foss discovered the necessity of actively translating the physical distance occurring in a conversation into the metrical scale demanded by the infection-control regulations. To the author, the distance of one or two meters was not a matter of evaluating rates of risk, but of adhering to the rules established by the authorities and more or less internalized by herself. The doubts expressed by the question reflects a distrust in herself rather than in the health authorities. More important, her doubts demonstrate how she is not yet fully habituated to these roles, although they are clearly on their way to becoming habit.

Social habits are embodied social behavior. When the habits are internalized, people behave more or less automatically, as though by impulse. While Christine Strand refers to "the spirit of dugnad" to characterize a new social mode, the implementation of specific measures is a matter of transformation rather than translation. The downscaling of infection-control

measures and risks from statistics to the practices of everyday life is not
just a matter of translating a terminology from a medical linguistic register
to a vernacular linguistic register. It is also a matter of embodiment. The
linguistically expressed semantics of risk must be transformed into embodied practices, ideally as new habits. This requires at once both cognitive
and embodied work. When we train new habits—for instance, the habit of
walking or biking—we have to repeat it over the course of repeated failures.
We interrupt ourselves, stop and think over what we did right or wrong
(Connerton 1989, 94). Slowly, the new ways of behaving become embodied
as habitual memory. This is certainly also the case for implementing a new
set of social roles.

EMBODIED RISKS

The authors describe how the virus and the infection-control measures
shape the way that they interact with others. These interactions involve not
only distance and masks, but also confidence and trust. Charlotte Aas writes:

> I do not trust strangers at all at the moment. And it seems that I am not
> alone, for when I stood in line to pay in the grocery store and suddenly
> had to sneeze (in my elbow, as I have practiced doing), the cashier gave me
> a terrified glance.[9]

Marianne Fjell reports a similar experience:

> I notice that people keep a good distance when shopping. Steering well
> clear of others is quite natural now. One month ago, people would have
> looked at you if you moved about like that. One to two meters are perfect
> these days.[10]

A couple of months later, in May, Marianne notes that people are becoming
wearier and easily irritated. To illustrate, she relates a recent experience she
had in a shop.

> An older lady scolded another because the one who should pay had to take
> a step back to draw her card. Actually, it was the one who scolded who was
> standing too close, but as I said, in this case it was she who rebuked the
> one in front. I had to turn around and look at something else. I get a bit
> embarrassed in such situations.[11]

The infection-control measures—distancing and sneezing in the elbow—had
become both social norms and bodily habits.

Elizabeth Stein was not aware of this new set of norms for social behavior. Seriously infected with the virus in early March, she was in the hospital while the outside world changed. By early May, when she was finally able to socialize again, the new set of norms had been internalized by others as social behavior, but she was not yet familiar with them:

> The learning curve was steep. I knew that I was free of corona, but it was not written on the forehead! . . . There were some grim looks and some comments before we learned to behave like everyone else: to avoid people like the plague, but by no means, do not forget to smile![12]

The experiences described in these quotations demonstrate how habits that had been normal have turned illegitimate within a short period of time, placing those less experienced suddenly out of step with the new set of social rules. This habitual shift illuminates an important aspect of the translation of a quantitative risk semantics to vernacular notions of risk. The downscaling from statistics to everyday-life practices also transforms the notion of risk from a matter of probability to a social concern. The risk of being infected depends on the relation between oneself and others. Thus, as a social concern, both the risk of infection and the control measures are closely bound up with trusting others. In this perspective, risk becomes the uncontrollable aspect of social relations, which implies that the fear of infection is transformed into anxiety and fear of fellow humans. Hence, the language of skepticism, fear, and even hostile behavior that can be found in these quotations can be seen as the result of this translational work. The terminology demonstrates how the notion of risk had become embodied as part of an affective register. Most of this runs counter to the normal meaning of dugnad, which basically is about doing things *together* in an intimate joint effort. The apparent success with which the dugnad was upscaled to a national context most likely depended on the experience of the nation as an emotional community. Within such a context, distance, even skepticism of others, could be ways to serve the community, while smiles and avoidance could be understood as two sides of the same coin.

CARING THROUGH DISTANCING

The translation, downscaling, and hence transformation of infection-control measures from a statistical regime to everyday-life practices also put the emotional community on trial. With the new infection-control regime, emotionally rooted ways of behaving suddenly became socially illegitimate. What used to be ways of expressing care, such as in-person presence and physical intimacy, suddenly implied careless and risky behavior. This became evident in the collective effort to protect people at risk of being hospitalized or even dying.

The shared responsibility for protecting the groups most at risk was a core argument justifying the lockdown. Prime Minister Solberg explicitly explained that "we do [the national dugnad] in solidarity with the elderly, the chronically ill, and others who are particularly vulnerable to developing serious disease" (Norwegian government 2020b).[13] This was, according to Solberg, a matter not only of solidarity but of caring: "The virus is so contagious that we cannot touch each other, but we must still take care of each other" (Norwegian government 2020b).[14] This paradox of care without physical contact supplied the prime minister with an elegant, albeit untranslatable, phrase for her speech. In our authors' narratives the same paradox is fleshed out as painful experience. The diaries describe how this new kind of caring through physical distancing affected their everyday life, family relations, and emotions.

Marianne Fjell describes how emotionally challenging it was for her to show care through social distancing and isolation. In her case this meant losing contact with her mother, who suffered from dementia and lived in a nursing home. Health institutions did not allow visits during lockdown, not even from family members. As her mother had lost her ability to speak, Marianne could not even reach her by phone. After more than two months, they were finally allowed to meet again, but due to the infection-control measures, the visit needed to happen outdoors:

> We called them and were told to walk around the building and into the garden behind. After a while she came rolling out in the wheelchair. She looks at us, but does not know who we are. I sit down next to her and tell her who I am. Then her tears roll, and mine. Incredibly painful not being able to give her a good and long hug. Have not seen her since the end of February. A nurse comes by and comments that I have to keep my distance. This "rule" of keeping one's distance does not work in practice. When I and my daughter are alone with Mom, and no nurses are present. Who will fold the blanket around her when it falls to the ground? Check if Mom is cold or too warm? When there are no nurses present, I am the one that takes care of her. Mom does not have any language and cannot express herself, so it is important that we who are there pay attention.[15]

This excerpt is written with an extensive use of incomplete sentences. The grammatical subject is often left out and sometimes even the verb. Marianne Fjell employs the same technique elsewhere in her diary, but not as consistently as in this case. The style adds an emotional mood of intensity and sensitivity. The emotional and moral dilemmas the author faces while trying to balance different ways of caring are striking. In this case, the "caring without touching" referred to by the prime minister simply does not work. Caring through distancing is in direct conflict with internalized and affectively embedded notions of care. It becomes obvious in this situation, where her mother lacks the power to communicate. It also profoundly conflicts with being a responsible caregiving daughter.

Another author describes a similar tension between conventional and affectively rooted notions of care and the new regime of care through keeping distance. In this case, however, that tension takes on quite the opposite social significance. While Marianne Fjell describes how she strives to submit herself to the new social norms of caring through distancing, she remains aware that the distancing is a matter of care. For Mari Bakke, it is not a matter of caring but of protecting herself. She lives on a farm next to her son, daughter-in-law, and three grandchildren, who usually run freely in and out of her house. Suddenly everything changes. As an elderly person, she is the one in need of protection, while as an affectionate grandmother she is normally the one who is supposed to show love and care for her family. The conflicting roles are expressed in her diary:

> I am careful in these corona times. One is affected by fear, no matter how rational one tries to be. I would rather not have the children inside my house, and at least not closer than one meter. It is not easy for a grandmother who has been used to having grandchildren on her lap at any time of the day. Nor is it easy for children to understand that the grandmother's lap is no longer a free zone for comfort and joy. I do not know if I am in the risk group. But with some underlying diseases that I usually am comfortable with, one becomes skeptical. Nobody knows everything about this virus which is ravaging the world at the present.[16]

The emotional conflict between showing love and care for her grandchildren and protecting herself from the risk of infection leads to a rhetorical strategy that externalizes the author's fear. The sentences that directly address the fear are written in the third person, making the sense of fear and uncertainty not strictly personal. It is presented as a general state instead—as something that has simply appeared as part of the world in which we live and which in this case threatens to invade both the body and the personal identity of the author. Her uncertainty about whether or not she belongs to the risk group underscores how she conceives of her fear and insecurity as external factors interfering with her everyday life. To belong to a risk group is an ascribed, not a chosen, identity; in her case, it seems to be an identity given to her by the pandemic itself.

IN THE RISK GROUP

Several of the authors address the risks and understand themselves as "in the risk group."

> My husband and I decided to practice voluntary quarantine. After all, we belong to an "endangered species," considering our age (above eighty) and some ailments.[17]

> I have asthma and my blood pressure is a bit too high and I am probably in the risk group.[18]

> Because I am in the risk group, I dare not visit anybody or have anybody come to me at home. But meeting people outside feels much safer.[19]

Advanced age and underlying diseases or issues like high blood pressure, diabetes, and obesity are among the factors known to increase the risk of severe or fatal cases of COVID-19. When using the term *risk group*, the authors refer to information that has been communicated by the health authorities—the term is one that has not been translated from a medical linguistic register to a vernacular one by the authorities. It has nonetheless been rapidly incorporated into the vernacular language, though with a significant semantic shift. Perhaps most conspicuous is the definite singular form that is used by the authors, which serves to gather a number of different health conditions into one large unit to which a person then can be said to belong. In this way, the involved risks are transferred from various preexisting health challenges to one single issue: the risk that defines the group, that is, the (increased) risk of dying from COVID-19.

Equally important is the word *group*. In both medical and vernacular language this term is used for defining risk, but in different ways. In the linguistic register of health experts, a risk group is a statistical category. It refers to the number of individuals who share some common factor that places them at risk, a factor that, iin turn, can be quantitatively calculated. It does not mean that these persons interact or communicate in the way that "group" usually implies in the social sciences. Nor does it mean that they share anything else, or that the calculated risk defines them as persons. Consequently, a risk group is more or less the opposite of an emotional community. In the vernacular, however, the word carries exactly such connotations of coherence, interaction, and personal identity: a group to which you belong says something about who you are, what you do, and to whom you relate. The point here is not to argue that the authors have misunderstood, but that the term they use inevitably changes its meaning when it is transferred from the bird's-eye view of statistics and calculation to the lived experiences of individuals and the emotional community to which they belong. A person who perceives herself to be at risk according to a statistical category cannot go on acting in relation to this category alone if she is to protect herself and fend off the risk. She must translate the abstract category that defines the risk in its own context to the concrete experience of her own life and its specific acts—to the way that she relates to other people and perhaps even to how she understands herself.

LOSS OF IDENTITY

Throughout the spring of 2020, it became clear that the infection-control regime in Norway succeeded in the sense that the reproduction number of infections soon dropped to less than one. For a period during the summer of that year, the daily infection rate was down to a handful of cases. Yet, on a social level, the measures not only kept the disease at a distance, they also affected, challenged, and to some extent even transformed familial relations. In this chapter, we have described how the physical distance from others that was required by the infection-control regime caused emotional dilemmas for Fjell and Bakke when they were not able to fulfill their caregiving roles as a daughter and a grandmother. Other authors describe similar experiences.

Christine Strand had not seen her father for some time when the lockdown started. Like many other Scandinavian senior citizens, he lives in Spain. Christine was planning to visit him to celebrate his sixty-fifth birthday, but this became impossible due to travel restrictions. Instead, she called to congratulate him. She was standing on the platform at the main train station in Oslo when she made the call. While talking to her father, she was approached by someone selling the magazine =*Oslo*, an initiative that helps the homeless earn a small income. "I smile, shake my head, and indicate with my hand that I'm not interested as I continue to talk to Dad" (Strand, 6).[20] The seller gets a similar response from others and, as he passes her again, he spits on her shoes and snarls at her. "I'm so surprised by his rage,"[21] she writes, because she understands herself as "one of the good ones."[22] She mentions that she has volunteered at a local soup kitchen as well as at social gatherings for homeless people. At the bar she was running, the homeless were also always welcome:

> But he does not see that version of me; he sees a privileged young girl
> who can afford to take the train far away on holiday, who is always on the
> phone and does not have time for people like him. I want to scream at him
> that my bar closed to protect the elderly and disadvantaged in society. That
> I have been unemployed for nearly two months and have only received
> 16,000 [Norwegian] kroner as welfare support because the case-processing
> time takes so long. That I will not see Dad on his birthday because we are
> stuck in different countries. That I have lost my job and my everyday life
> because of him.[23]

This is far more than just an uncomfortable incident to her. Her self-
understanding as a "kind person," a socially responsible citizen, and a caring
daughter is contested by this situation. So is her self-image as a hardwork-
ing, self-employed person who is economically independent. Thus, this incident leads to a fundamental identity crisis: her understanding of herself
as a community member in an emotional, caretaking, moral, and economic
sense is fundamentally challenged. Christine Strand, although she is not the
only one of the authors to lose her job and her income, is the one who most
directly questions the official infection-control regime. She refers to a couple of newspaper articles that have questioned if the social and economic
costs of the strict infection-control policies are necessary and appropriate.
She quotes a text by controversial Norwegian philosopher Aksel Braanen
Sterri, who asks whether "we can defend prioritizing saving people who
might die from the virus now over saving people who will die later."[24] The
quote is part of a discussion about whether it is right, from a philosophical
utilitarian perspective, to take care of the risk groups instead of prioritizing
young and healthy persons. Referring to such questions, the author makes
them her own in order to voice her own criticism of the authorities. She
had invested much work and great pride in the bar she was running, and
the place was closed permanently due to the lockdown. Her frustration is
related to the loss of a job and a place she loved. But more fundamentally,
it seems to be related to her loss of identity, her transformation into the
character seen by the homeless magazine seller instead of the person she
used to be both in her own estimation and that of others.

CONCLUSION

These case studies show how "the semantics of risk" involves both professional and lay practices of identifying, describing, and handling risks. The professional practices are characterized by numerical calculations and scientific
modeling of probable infection scenarios, while our material demonstrates

how vernacular infection-control measures and notions of risk are experienced and embodied as social and relational practices. The empirical basis of this study is not by any means representative of the Norwegian population as a whole or any particular social group, but the richness of the diaries has enabled us to point out some cultural dynamics of the translation process from an infection-control regime imposed by health authorities to vernacular understandings and practices. In our explorations of the translation from calculations and statistics to social concerns, we have wished to stress that this is not merely a matter of dutiful adaptation. The translational work that goes on involves rescaling, rephrasing, and personally experiencing. We have also tried to show that these processes do not reflect a poor understanding of scientific information among the population in general—they represent actions and measures necessary to turn abstractions into social realities. The success of the dugnad that was called for in Norway depended on the development of this kind of vernacular pandemic expertise.

We have argued that the transfer of statistically based infection-control measures to everyday-life practices is not simply a matter of translating the terms and recommendations of experts into a more understandable language, nor does it involve a more or less successful one-way communication from the health authorities to the population. What has taken place instead is a collaborative process of translating and enacting notions of risk and infection-control practices. This co-production can be said to work at three different levels. First, on a semantic level, the authorities mediated between a strictly statistically based medical register and that of vernacular language. This included the appeal to the nation as an emotional community, communicated by the upscaling of the meaning of dugnad. Second, the prescribed measures had to be incorporated into everyday life as new social practices, while new terms and phrases found their way into everyday speech. Finally, to fully become social habits, the measures had to be transformed into bodily habits.

The collaborative adoption of infection-control measures and practices that we have explored in this essay was of course intended to keep the pandemic under control. What it also did, however, and what is an important element of the strategy's comparative success, was to collaboratively produce Norwegian social protocols in terms of the ethics, notions of care, and social consciousness that affectively bound people together as an emotional community, and also demonstrated trust in fellow humans and confidence in the political and bureaucratic authorities. These two aspects are firmly connected. A well-functioning welfare system is presumably an important aspect of the production of confidence in the authorities in a situation where people lose jobs and income due to the implementation of an infection-control regime. However, the analysis also points to another aspect of this co-production of trust and confidence that so far has attracted less attention. An effective infection-control regime needs to be embodied as social habits in ways that do not challenge how people understand themselves as responsible citizens and as caring and emotional social beings, but rather appeals to this understanding and builds on it.

NOTES

1. Etymologically, the word *dugnad* comes from Old Norse *dugnaðr*, meaning good work, help, or force. It is related to the modern Norwegian verb "duge," which means to be good or fit for doing something.

2. "Vi er gode på dugnad i Norge. Mange av oss har vært med på jobben som nabolaget og idrettslaget gjør i fellesskap hver vår og hver høst. Før dugnaden planlegger vi de store arbeidsoppgavene. Men det dukker alltid opp nye oppgaver underveis, som vi først ser når vi er i gang med jobben. Nå trenger vi en dugnad i det norske samfunnet." "Bent Høie, Innkalling til dugnad."

3. "Jeg blir glad av å se dugnadsånden blant folk. Samtidig er jeg usikker på hvorvidt norske myndigheter har tatt det riktige valget ved å være såpass strenge i håndteringen av situasjonen."

4. "En iskald ettermiddag på parkeringsplassen utenfor borettslaget mitt på Holmlia står jeg og venter på matforsyninger. Det i er tirsdag 24. mars 2020 og jeg har hatt milde symptomer noen dager. Derfor tør jeg ikke å gå på butikken. Nå står jeg og venter på min gode venn som har vært og handlet for meg. Med isvinden i ryggen og hetta trukket nedover hodet venter jeg utålmodig på endelig å få snakke med et levende menneske som ikke bare er et ansikt på en skjerm."

5. "Vi snakker om løst og fast. Vi må jo møtes snart. Sånn på ordentlig, når dette er over. Vinden biter. Han må dra, strekker ut armene og gir meg en 'luftklem', stadig en meter unna. Jeg gjør det samme. Sånn er det blitt. Kjærlighet i koronaens tid. Adskilt av en mikroskopisk liten fiende."

6. "Så kanskje vi nå er i ferd med å bli godt korona-oppdratt?"

7. "Telefonen ringde og det kom folk på døra i eit jamt sig for å spørja etter time. Dei håpefulle stod audmjukt på avstand, som om dei ville visa med heile seg at her er ein som vil samarbeida for å få håret klipt."

8. "Hadde jeg husket å holde avstand. Heldigvis holdt det nå med en meters avstand."

9. "Jeg stoler ikke på fremmede i det hele tatt for tiden. Og det er jeg visst ikke alene om, for da jeg sto i kassakø og plutselig måtte nyse (i albuekroken, som jeg har øvd meg sånn på) så kassadama på meg med et skrekkslagent blikk."

10. "Merker at folk tar god avstand når vi handler. Det å gå i bue forbi folk er helt naturlig nå. For en måned siden ville folk sett rart om du gikk på den måten. 1–2 meter er perfekt i disse dager."

11. "Eldre dame som kjeftet på ei annen dame, da hun som skulle betale måtte gå tilbake for å dra kortet. Egentlig var det hun som kjeftet som kom for nærme, men her var det altså hun som kjeftet på henne som stod foran. Jeg måtte bare snu meg og se en annen vei. Blir litt flau i slike situasjoner."

12. "Det ble en rask læringskurve for oss. Jeg visste jo at jeg var Coronafri, men det sto jo ikke skrevet på panna! . . . Det ble en del stygge blikk og noen kommentarer, før vi lærte oss å oppføre som alle andre: Å sky folk som pesten, men for all del, ikke glem å smile!"

13. "Vi gjøre i solidaritet med eldre, kronisk syke og andre som er spesielt utsatt for å utvikle alvorlig sykdom."

14. The original phrase has an untranslatable pun. The idioms for "taking care" and "to touch" use the same verb in Norwegian, *å ta*. Solberg used this pun to say that we need to take care of (*ta vare på*) each other now, even if we cannot touch (*ta på*) each other. "Viruset er så smitsomt at vi ikke kan ta på hverandre, men vi skal altså ta vare på hverandre."

15. "Vi ringte dem og fikk beskjed om å gå rundt bygget og inn i hagen bak. Etter en stund kom hun trillende ut i rullestolen. Hun ser oss, men vet ikke hvem vi er. Jeg setter meg ned ved siden av henne og sier hvem jeg er. Da triller tårene hennes, og mine. Utrolig vondt å ikke kunne gi henne en god og lang klem. Har ikke sett henne siden slutten av februar. En pleier kommer forbi, og kommenterer at jeg må holde avstand. Det fungerer ikke i praksis denne 'regelen' om å holde avstand. Når jeg og min datter er alene med mamma, og ingen pleiere er tilstede. Hvem skal ta teppet rundt henne når det faller på bakken? Sjekke om mamma fryser, eller er for varm? Når det ikke er pleiere til stede, så må jeg passe på. Mamma har ikke språk og kan ikke forklare seg, så det er viktig at vi som er der, følger med."

16. "eg er forsiktig i disse koronatider. Man blir påvirket av frykten, uansett hvor rasjonell man prøver å være. Jeg vil helst ikke ha barna inne hos meg, og i alle fall ikke nærmere enn en meter. Det er ikke lett for en bestemor som har vært vant til å ha barnebarn på fanget både tidlig og sent. Og heller ikke lett for barn å forstå at bestemorfanget ikke lenger er fri sone for trøst og kos. Jeg vet ikke om jeg er i risikogruppa. Men med noen underliggende sykdommer som jeg lever godt med i hverdagen, blir man jo skeptisk."

17. "Min mann og jeg bestemte oss for å praktisere frivillig karantene. Vi tilhører jo 'en truet art' tatt alder (over 80 år) og noen helseplager i betraktning."

18. "Jeg har astma og litt høyt blodtrykk og er vel således i risikogruppen."

19. "Sidan eg er i risikogruppa, går eg ikkje på besøk til nokon eller har nokon heime her. Men å møta kvarandre ute kjennest mykje tryggare."

20. "Jeg smiler, rister på hodet, og indikerer med hånden at jeg ikke er interessert mens jeg fortsetter å prate med far."

21. "Jeg blir så overrasket over raseriet hans."

22. "Jeg ser på meg selv som en av de snille."

23. "Men han ser ikke den versjonen av meg; han ser en privilegert ung jente som har råd til å ta toget langt av gårde på ferie, som alltid er på telefonen og ikke har tid til sånne som ham. Jeg har lyst til å skrike etter ham at baren min stengte for å beskytte de eldre, svakere i samfunnet. At jeg etter å ha vært arbeidsløs i snart 2 måneder kun har mottatt 16.000 kroner fra NAV fordi behandlingstiden er så lang. At jeg ikke får se pappa på dagen hans fordi vi sitter fast i hvert vårt land. At jeg har mistet jobben og hverdagen på grunn av ham."

24. "Kan vi forsvare at vi prioriterer å redde mennesker som kan dø av viruset nå, istedenfor å redde mennesker som dør senere?"

REFERENCES

Beck, Ulrich. 2009. *World at Risk*. London: Polity.

Connerton, Paul. 1989. *How Societies Remember*. Cambridge: Cambridge University Press.

Klemetzen, Kristian Havnes. 2020. "Oslofolk Vil Ikke Stenge Skolene.—Kan være Eneste Måten å Stoppe Smitten På, sier Raymond Johansen." *Aftenposten*, November 19. https://www.aftenposten.no/oslo/i/Gar59m/oslofolk-vil-ikke-stenge-skolene-kan -vaere-eneste-maaten-aa-stoppe-smi.

Klepp, Asbjørn. 2001. "From Neighbourly Duty to National Rhetoric: An Analysis of the Shifting Meanings of Norwegian Dugnad." *Ethnologia Scandinavica* 31:82–98.

Kleven, Øyvind. 2016. "Tillit til politiske institusjoner: Nordmenn på tillitstoppen iEuropa." *Samfunnsspeilet* 2: 13–18.

Norwegian government. 2020a. "Bent Høie. Innkalling til dugnad." *Kronikk i VG*, November 3. https://www.regjeringen.no/no/aktuelt/innkalling-til-dugnad/id269 3216/.

Norwegian government. 2020b. "Koronasituasjonen: Pressekonferanse om nye tiltak for å bekjempe koronaviruset." December 3. https://www.regjeringen.no/no/aktuelt /pressekonferanse-om-nye-tiltak-for-a-bekjempe-koronaviruset/id2693286/.

Østberg, Kristian. 1925. *Dugnad*. Oslo: Grøndahl & Søns bogtrykkeri.

Rosenwein, Barbara H. 2010. "Problems and Methods in the History of Emotions." *Passions in Context* 1 (1): 1–32.

Simon, Carsta, and Hilde Mobekk. 2019. "Dugnad: A Fact and a Narrative of Norwegian Prosocial Behavior." *Perspectives on Behavior Science* 42 (1): 815–83. https://doi.org/10 .1007/s40614-019-00227-w.

SOURCES

The Norwegian Ethnological Research at the Norwegian Museum of Cultural History: Diaries from March to June 2020, written by Charlotte Aas, Mari Bakke, Eva Berg, Marianne Fjell, May Foss, Margareth Ness, Elizabeth Stein, Christine Strand, Ellen Vik.

8

Zoom, Zoom, Zoom
The Creation of Virtual Space, Culture, and Community
during the Pandemic through Digitized Platforms

Kinsey Brooke

INTRODUCTION

THE CONSEQUENCES OF THE COVID-19 PANDEMIC consisted of not only the public health threat caused by the actual virus but also a forced shift in practice to most transactions of business and daily living. As society was prompted to seek adaptations to many social settings, practices that have generally been conducted in the public arena were now corralled into the private sphere, where people could maintain a safe social distance, ranging from minimal face-to-face interaction to quarantine. As a result of these unprecedented spatial, social, and interactive guidelines and mandates, professional entities and non-corporate individuals who once relied on in-person components now had to seek modifications to their practices and routines. For example, gatherings such as office parties and baby showers switched to online formats in an attempt to mirror "normal" happenings. As a substitution for people's ability to physically walk around a living room or multipurpose space to socialize with peers or coworkers over drinks, platforms such as Zoom and Gathering enabled similar activities by providing "breakout" spaces—people could join and switch from room to room in order to be a part of smaller group conversations. Ultimately, this produced the simulated effect of someone being able to work their way around a room, chatting with people as they go, just as they would at an in-person party.

Instead of allowing everyday traditions, art forms, and habits, or what I refer to as vernacular culture, to be placed on an elongated pause, many people and organizations in both the public and private sectors sought

https://doi.org/10.7330/9781646424818.c008

and found virtual means to continue to conduct their various expressions
of culture despite the ongoing pandemic conditions. The obvious reason
for this is twofold: first, organizations that rely on patron income could
not afford to lose the interest and participation of the public; and second,
people now confined to personal dwellings experienced an urgent need
for social outlets and public engagement. In an attempt to satisfy both of
these needs, virtual spaces were created to accommodate the COVID-19
safety requirements and virtual practices and experiences quickly became
the norm. Educational institutions at every level, from Ivy League universities to local preschools, transitioned to online classes; healthcare professionals saw patients through telemedicine outlets when possible; attorneys
and financial advisors met with their clients either virtually or by phone
consultations; religious organizations held worship services through online
streaming; and other miscellaneous businesses and social organizations,
such as dance studios, book clubs, lecture series, conferences, festivals, and
concerts, were also conducted through various virtual platforms.

Transitioning activities from an in-person model to a virtual system
brought an array of challenges, with both positive and negative results.
Instead of facing total cancellation or closure, numerous entities advanced
through the virtual obstacles and found ways to perform their purposes
online. There are existing studies surrounding technology's impact on
socialization habits and customs, and I am not aiming to analyze the lengthy,
multifaceted, and complicated relationship between humans and channels
of technology. Rather, I seek to hone in on the individual and communal
pursuit of virtual opportunities in place of in-person offerings due to pandemic restrictions. To that end, this chapter discusses how the use of virtual space promotes outlets for folklife and public arts programming, and
how such space can provide a framework for community and be utilized
for modes of expression, practice, and learning. The arguments cited and
made within this chapter do not assert that virtual platforms or engagement are ideal. Instead, the virtual systems which provide an answer to the
pandemic's question are analyzed from the angles of socialization, community, and cultural expression. First, I establish the elements of digitized
space, including the sensorial and temporal dimensions for experiencing
such virtual space; then I move into advertising and marketing strategies
for online events and explore how the shift to virtual events engenders a
sense of community that serves in place of physical interaction. Following
this, I examine as case studies two public-facing folklore organizations,
the Newfoundland and Labrador Folk Arts Society and the Smithsonian
Folklife Festival, both of which have, during and as a direct result of the

COVID-19 pandemic, made the transition to virtual platforms in order to maintain expert and audience participation.

VIRTUAL SPACE: THE EXPERIENCE

Virtual technology, electronic communication, social media platforms, and remote working and learning environments were by no means new phenomena when the COVID-19 pandemic struck. Personal and professional communication via email took off in 1980s and 1990s, online collegiate curriculum and work-at-home employment options have developed significantly over the last two decades, and social media outlets took the 2000s by storm. However, there is one significant difference in the progression and use of these facets before and after the COVID-19 pandemic: before, users elected to participate in these virtual channels, whereas during the COVID-19 pandemic, there was often no other option. In March 2020, almost everything shifted to an online format, with the exception of specific critical services, and if people wanted to attend or participate, they had no other choice but to do so virtually. In response to this massive shift, increasingly more virtual outlets became available, creating virtual spaces in place of physical ones. To understand this viable system, it is useful to examine the confines of virtual space and how it is widely applied and engaged.

Steven Jones examines the experience of virtual space in terms of communication and points out that during times of crisis, when our normal routines are interrupted, "we are struck by the sudden intensity of the local, the immediate apprehension that we are in the here, and now, and unable to attend to matters beyond our physical reach" (1997, 19). He defines a type of quasi-space that is perceived in these instances: "Space is at that moment something we inhabit rather than something through which we move. To put it colloquially, we feel it 'close in' around us. And what startles is that very physical presence of space, that feeling of something, or some absence, pressing against you when the lights go out" (19). From this explanation, I draw a broad definition of virtual space as a digitized channel through which we experience. The specifics of what we experience and when we experience it may differ, but in the words of Jones, virtual space is "something we inhabit rather than something through which we move" (19).

While we may not literally *move through* virtual space as we do physical space, by visiting virtual sites and participating in virtual events, we are in essence "transported" to that place and time through the use of virtual space, a process that carries significant implications for the expression and participation in cultural activities. As Nick Couldry explicates regarding virtually mediated sites and their relationship to niche enthusiasts, there is a "hierarchical relationship between the 'media world' and the non-media, or 'ordinary,' world" (2005, 70), and such sites often "involve a sense of 'being there'" (66). Virtual realities are employed to fill in the gaps when people cannot physically access a certain place or people and must view or participate from a distance. In keeping with this paradigm, it follows that during the threat of COVID-19, numerous cultural activities and pursuits transitioned to online formats.

Prior to the pandemic, virtual space was generally additive, not always necessary, and applied widely for nonessential purposes. However, for virtual space to encompass both private and public settings and operations is not a new phenomenon. Jan Fernback notes, "Cyberspace is public space; at the same time, cyberspace is private space where, via e-mail, two users can argue politics or fall in love, or several users on a private listserver can strategize a meeting or discuss the finer points of a classroom lecture" (2002, 3). The experiences realized through cyberspace can be intimate in nature, such as a digital conversation, or public, such as a festival that is virtually attended by thousands of people, the event enhanced by high-occupant breakout rooms and discussion sections.

This public-private dichotomy can be kaleidoscopic in that from a certain perspective, "public" events might be seen as more private due to individuals being able to attend from the privacy of their own homes, and specific "public" events, which prior to the pandemic might generally have only consisted of a few people, could now be broadcasted on global virtual networks, exponentially increasing accessibility and viewership. This is worth noting in relation to vernacular culture in that the potential audience for culturally based events has, in theory, broadened due to virtual access. When in-person participation was the default orientation, people had the burden of adjusting their schedules and the potential expense of traveling to the physical location. With the adaptation of virtual platforms, participants only need the required device, internet connectivity, and, in some cases, to be granted access to the event through prior registration, potentially rendering an event more feasible and economical as well as enabling more widespread attendance.

During the pandemic, as people were distanced from conventional forms of activity and interaction, it became crucial to engender a new intentionality for approaching virtual space and enabling the public to virtually engage. The internet, which is the medium through which most virtual space is enacted, is often understood "mainly in spatial terms" as we comprehend "its ability to 'take us places'" (Jones 1997, 22). Physical borders—or in this case, virtual borders—are not the only dimensions of consideration. Time is also a critical agent. Virtual space not only affects the physicality of experiences, it also has the potential to "capture" experiences—an event, conference, or performance can be recorded and thus made available regardless of time constraints, such that the live action time is no longer of importance.

Now that people are able to *experience* events that happened in the past by logging into virtual space, generic references to time become increasingly obsolete. Jones writes, "The Internet's insertion into modern life represents a further displacement, or divergence, between our sense of 'lived time' (the time that passes according to our senses, the time of 'being') and our sense of 'social' or 'functional' time (the time that we sense as a form of obligation, or as time for 'doing,' for 'capturing')" (1997, 23). As I assert that space happens in correlation with experience, then, as Jones illustrates, "the Internet itself can, of course, provide some semblance of a place for 'being'" (23). Experiencing, observing, participating in, and essentially *being* within virtual space creates not only the means for virtual expression but also leaves an experiential impression on the participants. Unsurprisingly, visiting virtual places and holding events in virtual spaces have both positive and negative aspects.

Fernback notes, "Virtual space is socially constructed and re-constructed space" (2002, 1), and Tim Cresswell argues that place, and perhaps a sense of place, is "not just a thing in the world, but a way of understanding the world" (2004, 11). Therefore, audience demographics, aesthetics, and other designs and simulations are taken into consideration, and the virtual event is formulated just as any physical event might be marketed—to a certain crowd for a specific function. In an interview, Matt Homann, who runs a company that works with both virtual and nonvirtual event planning, elucidates, "If you know that people are coming to an event and engaging virtually, it is less about managing the tools and more about managing their attention" (Kaplan 2020). He continues, "We had become collaborative creatures online before this crisis in bits and pieces. Now, it requires more intention because for so many conferences and meetings, that connection happened accidentally. It happened in the hallways" (Kaplan 2020).

Throughout COVID-19, the spontaneous social and professional communications that before happened "in passing" were prevented by quarantines and social distancing requirements, fueling the need to create new spaces and strategies that might allow for similar interactions, and consequently opened the discussion surrounding the challenges of virtual events. Homann explains, "The real question is: How might you be far more intentional about building the hallway or the engagement time? Sometimes that happens in small breakout groups or by collaborating asynchronously after the event ends" (Kaplan 2020). Whether these measures are effective or not, and regardless of whether people would prefer in-person events to events held online, these strategies and challenges are all components that many entities had to face and try to negotiate in the wake of the pandemic.

Obvious benefits of an online format include mitigating transportation costs for participants and employees—taking the traveling, lodging, and dining expenses out of the equation for attendance. The website vFairs published an article that assists readers in navigating through the unknowns of online event hosting. The author praises the capacity of virtual formats because they possess the ability to "reach a wider audience, [and] invite keynote speakers from across the globe" (Zaman 2022). With the advent of virtual platforms for hosting virtual events, potential participants who previously could not afford to travel to the occasion no longer encountered financial restrictions as an obstacle. Similarly, people who could maybe not take an entire week off from work to give a onetime lecture or host an afternoon workshop no longer face time constraints that would limit their involvement, since virtual formats eliminate the added travel time. Moreover, virtual formats, provided that participants have the necessary tools, frequently establish a more widely accessible platform.

Advertising the benefits of online trade shows and expos, the article on vFairs instructs its readership, "Drop all that disappointment arising from the thought of a canceled event and take your event where your users are currently spending most of their time—their laptops and phone screens" (Zaman 2022). Judging by this communication, the new virtual terrain has become the portal to the world, and people and places are now accessed simply through a device. As a result, physio-sensorial intentions and perceptions have been transferred from a networking handshake to a touch screen. The implications for the interrelationship between virtual space and vernacular culture are numerous. A *CNN Style* article states, "There are countless cultural experiences at your fingertips to make your time indoors more artful and imaginative" (Willingham 2020). Virtual space may continue to be a primary avenue through which to express and partake in vernacular culture, reconfiguring virtual space to become a type of vernacular space.

VIRTUAL EVENTS AND ADVERTISING

Due to such massive demand, several websites, newspapers, and blogs have created lists and databases compiling various museums, orchestras, art galleries, and performing arts centers that are offering virtual events.

But how exactly do you design a virtual event that matches the tenets, outcomes, involvement, and interest strategies that standard in-person events do? According to Jillian Ryan (2020), "Marketers need to remember the fundamentals of good marketing and devise next steps that account for the target audience and what the event's goals were." Ryan expand on this procedure: "The challenge for companies will be being nimble enough to move away from their event strategy—often months in the making and fully paid for—and pivot to produce digital content or engagements that can still influence the intended audience." Highlighting that there is an "intended" or "target" audience for virtual events provides evidence that such events cater to a certain community of people, whether that be a group of business executives, high school athletes, or heavy metal music fans.

Online festivals, concerts, lectures, and classes are best found and promoted through the indexes that are designed for such purposes. One of the top databases that viewers can consult is the Google Arts & Culture database, which acts as a gateway to a plethora of online experiences. The website's slogan is "Bringing the world's art and culture online for everyone" (Google Arts & Culture 2021). The creators and staff members of this initiative note that the program works with "cultural institutions and artists around the world" to create the virtual offering. The mission statement outlines that the aim is "to preserve and bring the world's art and culture online so it's accessible to anyone, anywhere." This database is massive, listing virtual experiences from over two thousand cultural entities. With virtual selections and activities ranging from museum collections, performances, and other cultural resources, the assortment of activities is almost overwhelming. One emphasized feature is called "Zoom into a masterpiece," iin which by the click of a button, observers can view a famous work of art with informative narration. The website advertises, "Discover hidden details in the world's greatest treasures with ultra high-resolution images, and enjoy in-painting tours curated by experts."

An additional efficacious feature is the "Street View" program, which takes you virtually to famous destinations. The website markets this activity by advertising that the experience will be "as if you were there in person" (Google Arts & Culture 2021). At the time of this writing, the thumbnail picture for this feature is the Great Sphinx in Egypt. When viewers clicks on this option, they are taken to an encompassing menu offering further options allowing them to "visit" diverse popular locations, such as the Australian National Surfing Museum, the Taj Mahal, the Museo Frida Kahlo, and the British Museum, to name just a few. Among the copious options are virtual visits to locations, landmarks and, of course, museums.

Links to different outlets spotlight assorted experiences with striking phrases such as "10 Museums You Can Explore Right Here, Right Now," "Explore Iconic Monuments from Every Angle," "10 Incredible Libraries from around the World," "10 Incredible Locations of Street Art around the Globe," "11 Dramatic Virtual Tours of Stages around the World," and "Take a Tour of Virginia Woolfe's Life in London" (Google Arts & Culture 2021). These options are only a small number of the extensive activities that can be accessed through this database.

Another noteworthy database is the Colorado Business Committee for the Art's "Virtual Arts & Cultural Experiences during COVID-19 Archive." The compilers stress the importance of finding ways to view and partake in various forms of art, asserting, "It is now that we need the arts most as a society to unite us, provide comfort, inspire creativity and ease stress in troubling times" (CBCA 2021). The website consists of pages, arranged by category, containing links to virtual offerings from sources such as museums, various performing arts entities, and ecological organizations. Other virtual opportunities include film festival screenings, literary festivals, and poetry groups, in addition to a number of online classes for activities such as musical theater and dance, and a series of virtual "First Friday" art walks. On the homepage of this archive, the creators announce: "There are numerous ways we can ensure that the arts remain a part of our lives despite the need for social distancing to slow the spread of the coronavirus. CBCA will continue to compile and share virtual arts and cultural experiences, such as online dance classes, live streamed concerts, recorded theatre performances, creative activities for kids, and virtual gallery tours."

Each of these databases lists an assortment of compelling and stimulating cultural opportunities for interested parties. By merely sampling each website, the viewer can understand the momentous concern and care that has been taken by these (and many other) organizations to continue their normal output and maintain public interest in what they have to offer.

In accordance with social distancing, the average foot traffic was curbed, so virtual traffic was substituted. Because acts of socialization, networking, and learning moved to online formats, communities involved with such efforts also had to make a shift from being physical communities to online ones. Virtual events tap into the themes, motivations, goals and, most important, objectives and interests of these communities. To further explore this connection between an online event and a community, we must first understand the principles of community and the formation of virtual communities as a result of the pandemic.

VIRTUAL SPACE AS A CONDUIT FOR COMMUNITY

The absence of face-to-face contact engenders a void in the social channels that generally foster communal interaction. A virtual community may function in place of in-person interaction. Through this everyday substitution, virtual travel, learning, and socialization become vernacular, taking the place of previously normal modes of ordinary patterns of living. What draws people to participate virtually may be the same motivation that inspires them to participate in face-to-face activities—their personal interests, hobbies, and competencies. Someone who is interested in the painter Andy Warhol and would plan to visit his exhibition at an art museum might be inclined to attend a virtual viewing and tour at the art gallery. Someone who wanted to learn to play the harp, as in the case of a friend of mine, is motivated to seek out virtual harp lessons just as they would in-person music lessons. The individual leanings and pursuits that draw people to in-person events also prompt them to seek virtual replacements, especially when in-person activities are not possible.[1]

Community, companionship, and camaraderie are three facets that were affected by the social limitations of the pandemic, and therefore all three pillars were sought through digitized participation. The forced transference from inhabiting the in-person social world to negotiating the virtual one has thus caused an intermixing of personal and cultural identities with virtual identities and communities. Evelyn Osborne contends that "identity is used to categorize and associate a person with a set of values or habits" (2015, 84). The relationship between values and practice—or, as she states, "habits"—is naturally manifested in a vernacular sense within virtual space. Radoslav Baltezarevic et al. note that "virtual identity consists of two entities in both [the] real world and the virtual world" (2019, 12).[2] This virtual identity is a building block in forming and experiencing a virtual community.

Space and sense of place foster community and a shared identity through what is valued and enacted within that space. A shared connection to place connects "those things that add up to a feeling that a community is a special place, distinct from anywhere else" (Stokes et al. 1997, 192). In terms of adopting a sense of community as associated with virtual space, it is the process of forming a relationship to space that a community inhabits that is of concern. Moreover, a community must find ways to mitigate the lack of a physical connection to "space" and instead find ways to adapt digitally. Osborne notes that "although the concept of place is not necessarily agreed upon between [scholarly] disciplines, in general, the idea of place has moved from a simple geographical location towards a socio-cultural process and experiential concept" (2015, 84). This construction relies on socio-evolutionary shifts, of which the pandemic is a prime example.

Baltezarevic et al. wrote: "The Internet restructured the way of organizing social and interest communities and enabled the emergence of new media that combine the potentials of previous media with the intention of creating hybrid social and cultural forms. . . . However, these new, technologically mediated, forms of social interaction have changed the very way people form groups and the way they exist within them. Communication within virtual community creates new opportunities for people to interact and communicate, facilitating the development of new social relations" (2019, 7). Holding these foundational concepts at the forefront, to flesh out these constructs through tangible illustrations, we will explore two virtual examples that feature folk culture, organizational practices, and virtual participation.

VIRTUAL VERNACULAR CULTURE: TWO CASE STUDIES

Since physical travel was intermittently curbed during the height of the pandemic due to either travel restrictions or personal concerns, people were frequently dealing with two antipodal ends of existing—on the one hand, they were confined to their homes, only seeing occupants of their immediate household, whereas on the other hand, through the use of computers, they were able to travel, experience, and meet other people who might be thousands of miles away and experience folklife, traditions, and places while never leaving their homes. Folkloristic experiences were put on a global platform that could be accessed from any location with the internet. Thus, ethnographic features and presentations were moved from a solely physical space to a virtual one. Accessing these avenues required traversing virtual space, which, although not confined by location, is still a constructed platform with social designs and aesthetics.

The Newfoundland and Labrador Folk Arts Society (NLFAS) began producing a weekly virtual show titled *The Broadside* featuring local musicians and storytellers. Monday nights from 8:00 to 9:15 p.m., NLFAS begins a live-stream webcast on YouTube. The series is hosted by John Clarke, an event coordinator for the society, and is broadcasted each week out of St. John's, Newfoundland. The YouTube channel for *The Broadside* explains that during the pandemic NLFAS desired to continue to provide the local community, and those interested further afield, with programming showcasing the folk arts of the region. "After our very first online Newfoundland and Labrador Folk Festival this summer, we're bringing you live music via the interwebs every Monday night" (NLFAS 2021a).

The episodes generally begin with an introduction to the society and the Web series by Clarke, followed by musical sets performed by local musicians. Acts have included Anita Best, Quote the Raven, Kyle Gryphon and Kady Meaney, and Fergus O'Byrne, among many others. The musicians will often play a variety of cover tunes and original compositions. In between sets, Clarke usually conducts an informal interview with the performers, so the audience learns a little bit about their background and musical heritage. Often references are made to Newfoundland culture, and the history of certain songs and other prominent traditions are discussed.

While most of the performers are musicians, sometimes the entertainment features storytelling and recitations or jokes, often of regional significance. These performances express vernacular life and language. A live-chat feature is enabled during the stream in which viewers make comments and NLFAS posts pertinent information. Viewers frequently chime in with their location, and it is easy to discern that this series has a global audience. The efforts of the performers, NLFAS employees, and the regular, dedicated audience members who participate in the live chat can be seen as "public expressions of identity" (Couldry 2005, 63) in relation to these vernacular traditions. In this sense, as Couldry discerns, "the community of fans connects people who do not know each other, across different regions and classes . . . [to] a temporary sense of that community, what the French sociologist Michel Maffesoli . . . has called the 'empathetic sociality' we feel when we find 'those who think and feel as we do'" (64).

One of their thematic episodes was titled the "Jiggs Dinner Special." Jiggs Dinner is a local traditional meal consisting of boiled vegetables and salted meat—usually beef. The band that performed in this episode, the Salt Beef Junkies, paid homage to a main staple of the dinner. Clarke and his co-producer and technical assistant, Gracie Reid, began the episode with a brief discussion of Jiggs Dinner and later returned to the conversation during the intermission. They spoke casually of the tradition, noting the components and variations of the recipe, and telling viewers it is a meal routinely eaten on Sundays. Additionally, they shared personal memories of how their grandparents used to make it.

Clarke encouraged viewers to put comments in the live chat about their experiences with Jiggs Dinner, and people communicated back and forth regarding the meal and the tradition's history. It was a virtual conversation about this aspect of vernacular culture. They shared interesting cooking advice about how to make salted meat and included links to favorite recipes in the live chat. Finally, a virtual raffle was conducted in which they gave away two free Jiggs Dinner meals provided by a local grocery store/deli. In this way, they invited the public to participate in this tradition and fostered learning about this customary meal, all without any corporeal face-to-face interaction. This back-and-forth mimicked in-person meeting. People participated in this vernacular culture through their device screens, interacting with each other and these tradition bearers the best that they could, virtually. The emcee team would highlight certain items in the live chat, putting them on the main screen and personally commenting on them, so viewers were interacting with each other and the hosts, simulating an in-person gathering.

A second thematic episode, titled "International Accordion Day Squeezefest," celebrated the accordion music tradition of Newfoundland. Once again, Clarke and Reid discussed the instrument and musical tradition with each other and with a number of accordionists. Detailed conversations were conducted with Dave Penny and Fergus O'Byrne, two of the performers. Penny chatted with Clarke about the so-called Accordion Revolution, a campaign produced for the 2005 Newfoundland Folk Festival devised to attract accordionists to participate in the festival in an attempt to win inclusion in the *Guinness Book of World Records* for most accordions playing a song in unison. This effort was discussed in great detail, and it was revealed that they were successful in breaking the record.

In addition, Fergus O'Byrne was interviewed regarding the differences between accordions and concertinas. He discussed the history of the concertina and gave basic musical demonstrations, talking through the finger/hand movements required for playing and showing the scales. This was a virtual show-and-tell. O'Byrne provided specifics about his musical background, spoke about his instrument's provenance, age, and history of repairs, and discussed general upkeep tasks such as tuning. As they had in the "Jiggs Dinner Special," the emcee team conducted a raffle featuring accordion CD giveaways from O'Brien's music store, a local independent music store in downtown St. John's that supports traditional music, selling instruments, songbooks, and CDs.

Through this webcast, virtual vernacular culture is expressed and promoted through a number of approaches. These episodes are interactive and informative for people who are either outsiders to or beginners in the subject matter, and they provide a sense of community and stimulation for parties who are already interested in and familiar with the topics. Local artists are supported by their participation in the webcast, the series operates as an advertisement for NLFAS and their other events, and the episodes and viewership promote local businesses that support this culture through the giveaway items in the virtual raffles. Most important, however, vernacular culture and traditions are highlighted, endorsed, and maintained. In this way, both local and global audiences experience the expression of folklore simply by watching the episodes and participating in the chat, some benefiting from a more tangible experience if they win one of the giveaway items.

In moving the meetings to this online platform, the participation is virtual but still significant. Fernback explains, "Cyberspace is a repository for collective cultural memory—it is popular culture, it is narratives created by its inhabitants that remind us who we are, it is life as lived and reproduced in pixels and virtual texts" (2002, 2). This paradigm is the summation of these webcast episodes. Through cyberspace, culture and cultural memory are expressed, deposited, and put on display for others to see and partake in.

Prior to COVID-19, NLFAS held a well-attended annual folk festival and offered weekly "folk nights" at a local pub in addition to hosting a number of other special events. The society's community participation and programming would have been missed if they had not found a means to operate despite pandemic conditions. The NLFAS website advertises that the yearly festival and the folk nights that are usually held in person at the Ship pub are considered "rites of passage for up and coming folk and traditional musicians, and beloved by seasoned performers" (NLFAS 2021b). Both performers and local enthusiasts generally view these events as avenues to engage their craft and develop camaraderie with like-minded people. Desiring to maintain participant interest and involvement, NLFAS took the initiative to broadcast these events in a digitized modality.

Another outstanding example is the 2021 Smithsonian Folklife Festival. An extension of the world-renowned Smithsonian Institution, the annual festival is one of the largest such events dedicated to the celebration of folklore and folklife. Tthe festival website advertises, "The Smithsonian Folklife Festival is an international exposition of living cultural heritage annually produced outdoors on the National Mall of the United States in Washington, DC, by the Smithsonian Institution's Center for Folklife and Cultural Heritage," (Smithsonian Institution 2021). As a result of COVID-19, the Smithsonian Folklife Festival transitioned its programming, featuring expositions, demonstrations, and artisan interviews, to an online format. The 2021 festival, Beyond the Mall: Making Matters, was conducted virtually on June 25–27, 2021. The festival theme reflects the experience of the pandemic, as is noted on the website: "This year's Smithsonian Folklife Festival was born from conversations about the ways artisans, cooks, and musicians—as individuals and communities of practice—have responded to the pandemic" (Smithsonian Institution 2021).

Also included is a statement highlighting the resiliency of the participants of the festival, their practices, and the festival effort as a whole:

"*Beyond the Mall* acknowledges that the vibrant spirit of our physical event is not bound by time or location. This weekend is a future-facing reflection of the Festival's legacy of making community no matter the circumstance" (Smithsonian Institution 2021). Fernback discusses community in terms of shared interests and values, noting that "community is a bounded territory of sorts (whether physical or ideological)" (2002, 4). In this vein, a virtual community could be one that is formed by attending the same events that were initially created physically for a niche community. In contrast to communities that were composed of people in your immediate surroundings who perhaps shared similar skills and traits, pandemic-responsive events have supported virtual communities, which have become a temporary norm, holding true to Fernback's assertion that "the term 'community' encompasses both material and symbolic dimensions" (4). To this end, a virtual identity maintains a symbiotic relationship with the status of virtual communities in that one often informs the other. Activities of the festival included virtual story circles, workshops, and demonstrations, each showcasing aspects of culture and, in doing so, also nurturing an existing community surrounding the practitioners and viewer-enthusiasts.

The story circles, which were narrated sessions, consisted of one or more participants discussing their art form or type of craftsmanship. "Languages of Home and Diaspora: Nourishing Palestine in Food and Verse" was one such session that was virtually accessed via live stream. This was a multifaceted session in that written and verbal art such as storytelling and poetry recitations were featured, but a cooking demonstration was also showcased. The hosting participants were Reem Kassis, a writer and chef, and Zeina Azzam, a poet and activist. Their session centered on the interconnectivity between family, history, food, and sense of place. The content was an interesting blend of cooking presentations and poetry reading, with thematic conversations between the two hosts peppered throughout the session. Azzam would often read one of her original poems while Kassis was demonstrating her cooking. The camera view would be split, with one host on each side of the viewer's screen, exhibiting both of their actions in unison. The camera angle would often show a close-up of Kassis completing her cooking tasks, his allowing viewers to see her movements exactly, as if they were watching her in person.

At regular intervals, each host discussed her personal connections to her culture and to food, telling of her lived experiences and sharing stories about her family. These two hosts were showcasing different skills—one food culture and the other poetry, but both paid homage to the roots of their heritage, and their interaction with each other while offering their respective demonstrations gave viewers a diverse and well-rounded experience of these two art forms.

Another narrative session was comprised of three stone masons, Joe Alonso, Nick Benson, and Sebastian Martorana. Their slot, "Stories in Stone: Master Artisans on Tools, Technique, and Meaning," consisted of a discussion surrounding this type of craftsmanship and their professional experiences of masonry, carving, and sculpting. Each conversed about major projects he had worked on, such as the Martin Luther King Jr. Memorial, the Washington National Cathedral, and the Eisenhower Memorial in Washington, DC. Throughout the virtual conversation, pictures of these projects were put on the screen, displaying vivid examples of the results of this craft form. Relevant tools, such as different types of trowels, mallets, and hammers, were displayed in a show-and-tell-like manner as the participants discussed the pros and cons of using each type of tool, how they progressed to master them, and which type of tool worked best for particular situations and different types of stone. This allowed the audience to see the instruments up close as they learned about them. In addition, each participant discussed how he came to learn masonry skills and how he hoped to pass on that knowledge to the next generation. Occasionally views of their workshops were given, and photos of worksites showed the entire process: from the workshop to the work in progress to the finished result.

Both of these sessions were streamed virtually and provided closed captioning and a sign language interpreter, which was generally the case for the virtual forums, making the experience more accessible. Though the festival programming was online, the quality and distinct nature of the sessions maintained continuity with the festival's history. The website describes: "Initiated in 1967, the Festival has become a national and international model of a research-based presentation of contemporary living cultural traditions. Over the years, it has brought more than twenty-three thousand musicians, artists, performers, craftspeople, workers, cooks, storytellers, and others to the National Mall to demonstrate the skills, knowledge, and aesthetics that embody the creative vitality of community-based traditions" (Smithsonian Institution 2021).

As demonstrated by these examples, such diverse traditions were not totally paused during the pandemic. Via the virtual world and virtual space, showcasing, practicing, and learning vernacular traditions still took place. Asa Briggs describes culture as "the creative expression of a particular society through its symbols, literature, art, and music, and for some, its institutions and the values and experiences that shaped them" (1992, 4). It naturally follows that virtual outlets used for cultural expression, and for participants to find inclusion and community in culture, succeed when face-to-face outlets are suppressed. The Smithsonian Folklife Festival is a major example of an entity that has achieved this feat.

In previous years the festival showcased vernacular traditions and artistry, and now a virtual medium allows this to continue under unprecedented circumstances. Highlighting the innovation of this new COVID-19 reaction, the website details, "For the first time, the Folklife Festival is providing visitors with the opportunity to participate in hands-on workshops from home. Together we'll learn about Zapotec textile dyeing, Senegalese metalsmithing, Korean home cooking, and much more" (Smithsonian Institution 2021). The creation of virtual space and the resiliency of community propelled the festival forward, maintaining the communities of practitioners and viewers alike.

CONCLUSION

Despite a perhaps stereotypical view that virtual representations of people and places are of lesser quality than physical reality, Couldry argues that "media representations of the social world make certain places more important" (2005, 60). This elevated status inevitably affects the social world and mainstream modes of communication and interaction. According to Baltezarevic et al., "Since a virtual community allows individuals to break social barriers and facilitates contacts with heterogeneous individuals, it allows for the formation of a virtual group identity. Members of a virtual community establish a group identity and a sense of belonging on the interactive network platform . . . Further, through consecutive communication and information exchange among members, a bridged social capital is formed" (2019, 8). Continuing in this vein, Charles Withers deems the socio-evolutionary structure of space and sense of place a "social practice" and "process" (2009, 638). Relation to place generates a sense of individual and communal identity that is often linked to the manifestation and safeguarding of culture. Consequently, when these events had to shift to online-only interaction, the virtual experience worked to engender and feed the cultural identities and communities of the participants.

Dominic Strinati posits, "Through virtual interaction with others, the individual gradually builds personal identity based on these experiences, while the media serve only as an accessible reference framework for the building of collective and personal identities" (1995, 239). Mirjana Ule contends, "Who or what we are, is not so much a matter of personal essence (beliefs, feelings, etc.), but of how we are constructed through a variety of relationships, interactions, etc." (2000, 249). Many efforts made as a direct result of the pandemic have worked to maintain the expressions and values of specific communities, making events, celebrations, and informative content virtually accessible to the community members and a wider audience.

Though there are differing opinions on the components of culture, the formation of culture, the preservation of culture, and the commodification of culture, Briggs conveys a unifying theme: "All anthropological approaches to culture center . . . on regularities within cultural patterns, explicit or implicit. Culture is seen as being transmitted from one generation to the next through symbols and through artifacts, through records and through living traditions" (1992, 9). He makes interdisciplinary connections, stating, "Whatever the standpoint of the writer, the history of culture in the twentieth century has always been directly related to the history of communications" (6). To this end, ultimately, all types of interaction, and therefore communication, almost fully shifted to virtual communities, which found ways to express and participate in culture, and virtual expressions of personal and communal identities found pathways to nurture personal and communal values and interests.

Virtual space affords a sense of unboundedness. David Crouch, Rhona Jackson, and Felix Thompson assert that "unboundedness gains its meaning from a promise, but nothing more than a promise, that boundedness can be transcended" (2005, 3). The pandemic, in causing massive shutdowns to our real-world practices, prompted the creation of numerous virtual outlets. In their vernacular response, cultural entities resisted total closure and isolation, instead forging routes onto the virtual landscape to allow cultural expression and transmission. In the process, existing communities and identities were supported, potentially new ones were formed, and interested individuals from diverse locations, time zones, and backgrounds could log on and participate.

NOTES

1. This is, of course, dependent on internet and device access and individuals having the technological skills necessary to participate in online activities.

2. Baltezarevic et al. (2019) note that they draw this definition from the work of Ruth Halperin and James Backhouse (2008).

REFERENCES

Baltezarevic, Radoslav, Borivoje Baltezarevic, Piotr Kwiatek, and Vesna Baltezarevic. 2019. "The Impact of Virtual Communities on Cultural Identity." *Symposion* 6 (1): 7–22.

Briggs, Asa. 1992. "Culture." In *Folklore, Cultural Performances, and Popular Entertainments: A Communications-Centered Handbook*, edited by Richard Bauman, 3–11. New York: Oxford University Press.

CBCA. 2021. "Virtual Arts & Cultural Experiences during COVID-19 Archive." Colorado Business Committee for the Arts, Online Archive. https://cbca.org/virtualart expereincescovid19archive/.

Couldry, Nick. 2005. "On the Actual Street." In *The Media and the Tourist Imagination: Converging Cultures*, edited by David Crouch, Rhona Jackson, and Felix Thompson, 60–75. London: Routledge.

Cresswell, Tim. 2004. *Place: A Short Introduction*. Oxford: Blackwell.

Crouch, David, Rhona Jackson, and Felix Thompson. 2005. "Introduction: The Media and the Tourist Imagination." In *The Media and the Tourist Imagination: Converging Cultures*, edited by David Crouch, Rhona Jackson, and Felix Thompson, 1–13. London: Routledge.

Fernback, Jan. 2002. "The Individual within the Collective: Virtual Ideology and the Realization of Collective Principles." In *Virtual Culture: Identity and Communication in Cybersociety*, edited by Steven G. Jones, 42–57. London: SAGE.

Google Arts & Culture. Online Database. https://artsandculture.google.com/.

Halperin, Ruth, and James Backhouse. 2008. "A Road Map for Research on Identity in the Information Society." *Identity of the Information Society Journal* 1 (1): 71–87.

Kaplan, Ari. 2020. "Navigating a New Era of Virtual Events during the COVID-19 Pandemic." *ABA Journal*, May 22. https://www.abajournal.com/news/article/navigating-a-new-era-of-virtual-events-during-the-coronavirus-crisis.

Jones, Steven G., ed. 1997. *Virtual Culture: Identity and Communication in Cybersociety*. London: SAGE.

NLFAS (Newfoundland and Labrador Folk Arts Society). 2021a. *The Broadside*. YouTube channel. https://www.youtube.com/channel/UCNrgcMuJeGJLkz_c6KOtrmg/featured.

NLFAS. 2021b. "Living Our Traditions." *Newfoundland and Labrador Folk Arts Society*. https://nlfolk.com/.

Osborne, Evelyn. 2015. "The Most Irish Place in the World? 'Irishness' in the Recorded Folk Music of Newfoundland and Labrador." *MUSICultures* 42 (2): 79–102.

Ryan, Jillian. 2020. "How Marketers Can Adapt to Event Cancellations Brought on by Coronavirus." *eMarketer*, March 5. https://www.emarketer.com/content/coronavirus-event-cancellation-b2b-marketers.

Smithsonian Institution. 2021. "Smithsonian Folklife Festival." *Smithsonian*, https://festival.si.edu/.

Stokes, Samuel N., A. Elizabeth Watson, and Shelley S. Mastran. 1997. *Saving America's Countryside: A Guide to Rural Conservation*, 2nd ed. Baltimore: Johns Hopkins University Press.

Strinati, Dominic. 1995. *An Introduction to Theories of Popular Culture*. New York: Routledge.

Ule, Mirjana. 2000. *Sodobneidentitete: V vrtincudiskurzov (Modern Identities: In the Whirl of Discourse)*. Ljubljana: Znanstveno in publicističnosredišče.

Willingham, A. J. 2020. "All the Virtual Concerts, Plays, Museums and Other Culture You Can Enjoy from Home." *CNN Style*, March 27. https://www.cnn.com/style/article/what-to-do-at-home-streaming-art-museums-concerts-coronavirus-trnd/index.html.

Withers, Charles W. J. 2009. "Place and the 'Spatial Turn' in Geography and History." *Journal of the History of Ideas* 70 (4): 637–58.

Zaman, Huda. 2022. "7 Types of Events You Can Take Online during a Pandemic." *vFairs*, August 29. https://www.vfairs.com/7-types-of-events-you-can-take-online-during-a-pandemic/.

9

Virtual Tarantella Folk Music and Dances
Local Resilience, Global Spectacle, and Digital Communities

Incoronata Inserra

SINCE THE COVID-19 LOCKDOWN BEGAN in March 2020, several examples of music-centered vernacular creativity have been reported in Italy, such as balcony music performances. In this chapter, I look at the pandemic circulation and representation of tarantella, a southern Italian genre of folk music and dances, by considering not only balcony performances but also virtual concerts and music videos, remote classes, and special music and dance projects circulating on social media. My goal is to map out major trends in this emerging phenomenon as a way to explore the cultural and artistic resilience of southern Italian communities, performers' and cultural brokers' appeal to ancient tarantella music and dance rituals as an antidote to the pandemic, as well as expressions of collective grief and community support through music and dance. I argue that while this strong virtual presence of tarantella is a direct product of the 2020 pandemic, its emergence reflects a much longer process of globalization and digitization of this folk tradition. Indeed, since the 1990s, tarantella has been at the center of a strong revitalization movement that has brought several changes to the tarantella tradition—ranging from innovation to commercialization (Inserra 2017)—and also spurred the growth of online tarantella communities. Read within this larger context, the pandemic tarantella phenomenon represents the latest step in a thirty-year transformation process, as it reflects not only the growing presence of tarantella online but also current debates surrounding in-person tarantella gatherings and performances. Such debates focus on changing notions of tradition, place, and community. More generally, this case study allows us to reflect on circulation and representation dynamics related to traditional music and dance traditions within the COVID-19 pandemic context.

https://doi.org/10.7330/9781646424818.c009

TARANTELLA'S HISTORICAL AND
SOCIOCULTURAL CONTEXT

Most readers outside of Italy associate the term *tarantella* with "Neapolitan tarantella" (*tarantella napoletana*), a specific music and dance form that became famous worldwide through nineteenth-century classical music and also through nineteenth- and twentieth-century Italian migration (Paliotti 1992; Rauche 1990). Beyond Neapolitan tarantella, the term describes a complex genre of folk music and dances exhibiting major geographical and historical differences within the southern Italian context (Gala 1999, 22). Elements common to the whole genre are the use of a frame drum to beat time—even as several types of drum are used—extensive motion of the arms, and the couple-dance format.[1]

Historically, the term *tarantella* is associated with pre-Christian rites and rural healing practices most prevalent in the Apulia region of southern Italy, but also present in other parts of southern Italy and the Mediterranean coasts at least until the eighteenth century. Starting in the seventeenth century, scholars wrote about tarantella as a "spider's bite syndrome," explaining that people bitten by tarantulas would engage in a frenetic dance that helped them enter a state of trance and expel the spider's poison, thus accelerating the healing process (Sigerist 2003). This medical interpretation remained prevalent until 1959, when Italian anthropologist Ernesto De Martino conducted fieldwork research about the "tarantism" phenomenon in the Apulia region and concluded that this ritual was better understood within the larger socioeconomic, cultural, and religious structure of the Italian south (De Martino 2005).[2] De Martino was tracing what he considered to be the last remnants of a music and dance ritual that was dying out due to the increasing economic and social involvement of the Catholic Church. The 1950s–60s call for industrialization and modernization in the south, which sought to purge those aspects of southern culture deemed unfit for a modernized Italy, further contributed to the dismissal of these rituals over time. By the early 1960s, tarantella music and dance rituals had become mostly a symbol of the social and economic degradation and backwardness of those regions (Apolito 2000).[3]

The post-1990s revitalization of tarantella has led to the unprecedented popularity of this genre throughout Italy and internationally, from northern Italian cities to major European ones and from New York City to Honolulu.[4] This is evident from the extensive organization of festivals,[5] concerts, and workshops; the proliferation of folk music groups and album production—from local to national and international distribution via the world music label—the production of feature films and documentaries;

the increasing presence of tarantella performances within mainstream music events; a strong tourism boost, especially in the Apulia region; and the wide circulation of tarantella music and dance on social media. This revitalization has contributed to transforming tarantella from a rural, religious, and rooted tradition into an urban, secular, migrant, and global one. For example, it has commercialized the local festivals, extended the festival time beyond the Catholic calendar, consolidated a concert stage format, and introduced new dancing styles and a dance workshop format that allows students to learn in a class rather than from old-timers at the local festivals (Inserra 2017). Scholars and practitioners, both in Italy and internationally, have widely debated the current changes to the tarantella tradition (Inserra 2017, 47–57), particularly the loss of what local drummer Raffaele Inserra calls "'o spirito d' 'a festa," or the essence of the (traditional) festival (60). In their view, these new festival and performance formats do not favor the kind of organic community gathering that is typical of traditional festivals. At the same time, this process of revitalization has favored innovative and socially engaged music projects, as southern musicians like Eugenio Bennato employ tarantella rhythms to narrate the peculiar history of southern Italy as an internal colony, referred to as the "Southern Question" (Gramsci 1995; Bennato 2010). Today, these southern regions struggle with the highest rates of unemployment, pushing younger generations to migrate to the north or internationally, and poor economic, social, and health infrastructures (Inserra 2017, 19). Within this scenario, musicians and scholars often appeal to the healing power of tarantella to help southern Italians make sense of their present condition (47–54)[6] and also help musicians from the south who moved elsewhere reconnect to their roots (84–95). This reclaiming of tarantella's ritual aspects ranges from a genuine desire to employ its rhythms as therapy to appreciation of the genre as an artistic concept to cultural sensationalism (143–52), and it often takes place through the reenactment of the tarantism ritual (6–7, 46).

The two main tarantella forms that I mention here are the *pizzica* from the Apulia region and the *tammurriata* from the Campania region. Pizzica has become especially popular as a result of the post-1990s revival, given its direct link to tarantism even in its name (from the Italian *pizzicare*, or "to bite") as well as its frenetic and trance-inducing rhythm and dancing steps. However, the revival has also helped popularize various other tarantella forms, including the tammurriata, which I am familiar with through personal connection and fieldwork research.[7] Tammurriata performances bear no direct link to the tarantism rituals but have developed within a similar Catholic festival context and as an expression of the local peasant culture

(Inserra 2017, 12–16). Tammurriata takes its name from the large frame drum used to beat the time, called *tammorra*, and is often accompanied by other instruments and by the use of *castagnette* (castanets); it is also characterized by a slower tempo than other tarantella forms (Gala 1993). The increasing popularity of tammurriata has followed a trajectory very similar to that of pizzica, moving from local to national and international festivals and performances; for this reason, Italian scholars often include the revitalization of tammurriata within the larger tarantella revival phenomenon.

LOCKDOWN TARANTELLA

As a tarantella scholar and aficionada living outside of Italy, I consistently follow tarantella fan groups and musicians on Facebook. I especially did so during the spring 2020 lockdown, as most in-person tarantella events were canceled and music sharing and conversations happened remotely. What initially sparked my interest in the virtual tarantella phenomenon was a video that circulated on Facebook at the time and became viral in a few hours. The video shows a woman dancing at the center of St. Oronzo Square in the southern Italian city of Lecce; she is wearing the long flowing skirt and large scarf typical of southern Italian pizzica dance performances, but unlike most performances, which feature white and red, the ritual colors of pizzica, she is dressed entirely in black to reflect the moment of collective grief that Italy is going through (Puricella 2020). What especially made this performance go viral was a heated debate on social media about whether the dancer was violating lockdown regulations (Agnello 2020). As a result, local filmmaker Roberto Leone decided to speak up and publicly justify the legitimacy of the video, explaining that this was an impromptu performance he had stumbled upon as he was walking in the area; he emphasized that he suddenly heard loud pizzica music coming from the square nearby, and there he found the dancer. He also clarified that the dancer lives within two hundred meters (656 feet) of the square, so she was technically within her allowed "workout space" and therefore did not violate the Italian safety protocol (Agnello 2020). Whether Leone's account is real or orchestrated, the debate generated by this video clearly reflects the collective trauma caused by the pandemic in Italy and ways that online communities helped Italian residents share both grief and hope. As Leone himself put it, "Here's to believing that tomorrow all will be over and that we will all hug again, with the warmth that characterizes the Salentine people" (Leone 2020a). In addition, this story illustrates how both media and cultural industries often appealed to the tarantella healing rituals to convey a sensationalist story of lockdown. In his official account, Leone comments that the dancer's movements are precisely calculated as she steps over the square's well-known mosaic of the she wolf, which reproduces the city's coat of arms and therefore represents the city itself, as if "she wants to wake everybody up from their [pandemic] sleep" (Puricella 2020). According to local news source *Lecce prima*, "In a period in which we are all 'bitten' by the virus and trapped by this powerful poison, with our bodies shaken by acute pain and uncontrollable spasms, some strive to free themselves and the city with an increasingly accelerated rhythm" (Agnello 2020).

It is worth noting that on the one hand, this sensationalist use of the tarantella rituals confirms scholar Giovanni Pizza's observation that within the current revival, the tarantism ritual is "decontextualized, reified, and projected onto an ill-defined universal dimension" (2004, 205); on the other hand, the pandemic seems to have inspired tarantella artists and practitioners to look for similarities between the suffering involved in historical tarantism and the one perceived by Italian residents as a result of the pandemic, unlike most revivalist interpretations, which have transformed tarantism "into a positive symbol, freed of its connection to suffering" (205). As such, this recent music and dance production offers tarantella scholars the opportunity to reflect on the role of ancient tarantella rituals within a pandemic context and examine the ways these in-person and community-engaged rituals are replicated in a virtual context.

Moreover, this example reflects Leone's willingness to turn a social media debate into an opportunity for both artistic production and local advertising, while also showcasing the resilience of the local tarantella communities. In fact, even after he highlighted the spontaneous nature of this event in the local and national media, Leone released a curated video of the performance titled *D'incanto la pizzica* (Pizzica Charm), featuring music by internationally renowned pizzica group Canzoniere Grecanico Salentino (Leone 2020a)[8]; he later used this short segment as part of a longer lockdown documentary on the city of Lecce (Leone 2020b). Given the important role of the tarantella revival as a tourism catalyst in the region in the last thirty years, it is not surprising to see tarantella appear in local initiatives to revitalize the local tourist industry during the pandemic.

As I illustrate in the following pages, collective trauma and support online, local resilience, and the attempt to replicate virtually tarantella's embodied communities resurfaced in different ways throughout the Italian lockdown experience. The virtual tarantella phenomenon is therefore important for understanding not only the tarantella revival as a whole but also the larger pandemic context from a vernacular perspective. An analysis of this phenomenon in its entirety would go beyond the scope of this chapter, especially given the increasing presence of tarantella on social media sites; here I focus my analysis on music and dance production circulating on Facebook and on local and national news media in the spring of 2020.[9]

BALCONY PERFORMANCES

The emergence of a balcony performance trend in Italy during the spring 2020 lockdown has been widely reported both nationally and internationally (Barcellona 2020; Taylor 2020). An integral component of the Italian urban landscape, the balcony space soon became the main social and cultural hub, as also confirmed by several balcony events such as the displaying of Italian flags and banners with the ubiquitous "Andrá tutto bene" or "All will be well" slogan (Barcellona 2020; see also Robinson, this volume). Both the close proximity of condominium balconies in larger urban areas and the absence of a home backyard or garden in these areas must have contributed to this phenomenon.

My focus here is on balcony performances as they reflect local reactions to lockdown, not only among residents but especially among folk music practitioners and aficionados. Since the pandemic hit, the "Italian music industry's live-sector losses surpassed over 100 million euros, with an added 60 percent drop in physical record sales, a 70 percent drop in synch revenue and a 70 percent drop in background music revenue collected from shopping establishments" (Worden and Cantor-Navas 2020, 1). The emergency measures passed in March 2020 by the Italian government to respond to the situation included a grant of €130 million to be shared between the film and live-music industries and a further €10 million euros for all authors and visual artists (Worden and Cantor-Navas 2020, 1). However, many did not deem these measures sufficient to help sustain these drowning industries, which led not only to a nationwide protest by media and cultural industry workers on May 30, 2020, in twelve Italian cities (*Sky Tg24* 2020), but also to the proposal of an amendment to the government's decree on the matter and several nationwide campaigns to support the proposal in the following months (*La repubblica* 2020). As a niche market, Italian folk music is especially vulnerable to the costs of canceled live events, so much so that in May 2020 a collective of artists across Italy, including several practitioners of southern Italian folk music and dances, created a support network aiming at "preserving the extraordinary cultural heritage of Italian folk music nation-wide, while respecting local cultural traditions."[10] The collective, called Musicapopolarenuntefermare ("Traditional Music, Do Not Stop"), organized several initiatives throughout 2020–21, including a crowdfunding campaign and virtual conferences and performances circulating mainly through social media.[11]

The first reported balcony performance took place soon after Prime Minister Giuseppe Conte declared full lockdown on March 9, 2020. As an immediate response to the prime minister's decision, a group of musicians from Rome, the twenty-piece street band Fanfaroma, organized a sound flash mob (*Flashmob sonoro*), a "countrywide event to alleviate the frustrations of a national ban on public gatherings" (Fanfaroma 2020).[12] At 6:00 p.m. on Friday, March 13, and from north to south, Italy resounded with loud singing and musical instruments, ranging from the Italian national anthem and other national icons like the World War II partisan resistance song "Bella ciao" to pop, classic, jazz, rock, and folk music—tarantella included. In contrast to the silence experienced within the urban landscape at the time both in Italy and internationally (Ward 2021), "many came out on their balconies . . . to bring back a bit of life in the almost deserted urban streets" (Barcellona 2020). This sound flash mob ended up becoming a "moment of release [that] spurred more organic musical celebrations in the following day" (Worden and Cantor-Navas 2020, 1). As the balcony gatherings continued in the following days and weeks, their social media presence also increased, highlighting a variety of voices and musical perspectives.

The recurring presence of the national anthem in these lockdown balcony performances suggests that participants were able to conjure up Benedict Anderson's (2006) image of a nation-centered "imagined community"—something usually limited to soccer matches in Italy. At the same time, the presence of tarantella and other traditional music genres reminds us that Italy's music-based imagined communities are embedded in very localized musical expressions that are at least as important as nationalized ones, in line with Italy's campanilistic social formation. For example, a video uploaded to YouTube on March 12, 2020 and shared on Facebook by user Marina Bocchino features a group of women performing on their balcony—one playing the tammorra frame drum and the other two playing castanets or filming the other performer—and also a man on another balcony, singing and playing the tammorra drum accompanied by a small child holding a tambourine (*bMagazine* 2020). Together, they perform a tammurriata song titled "Vesuvio" by Neapolitan folk group E Zézi, among the first to bring back the tammurriata rhythm on both local and national stages in the 1970s.[13] This is a song that most tammurriata practitioners will know how to play or sing along to and whose lyrics express the important role of Mount Vesuvius in defining Neapolitans' collective identity (Inserra

2017, 116–17), thus well suited for such a locally based communal effort. The video was filmed in the province of Benevento in the Campania region, where all tammurriata events, including major seasonal festivals attracting thousands of participants, were canceled throughout the spring 2020. By performing tammurriata on the balcony and choosing a regional music repertoire, local folk music practitioners and aficionados were able to make up for the lack of live music events while also expressing their shared interest in tammurriata as an important expression of local culture.

Another example of this focus on local culture and resilience comes from a video uploaded to YouTube on March 14 featuring a woman on her balcony playing a tarantella tambourine next to a small child. A man joins in, playing a larger frame drum from a window on another floor, while another man is playing the accordion from another building (Roberts 2020). They are all tuning their instruments to a recorded folk music song that is heard over speaker phones throughout the neighborhood. Two people from the balcony above the accordion player are filming the performance, while the maker of the video is able to film the whole scene from what is safe to assume is a balcony or window on the opposite corner (*Corriere della sera* 2020). Advertised as a flash mob performance, the video was shot in the Agrigento province of the Sicilian region of southern Italy, which reflects the group's choice to perform the well-known Sicilian traditional song "Ciuri ciuri."

Even as they convey the local resilience of local music traditions and southern Italian dialects, however, these examples also reveal an effort to focus on songs that are popular enough to resonate throughout Italy (and abroad through the Italian diaspora). This is an important aspect to consider because it reminds us that in tarantella's passage from the local to the global and the digital, local culture circulates more easily when codified as mainstream (Inserra 2017, 175–76). Another noteworthy aspect related to globalization and digitization relates to the idea that local performances are now made available to social media users both in Italy and internationally. For example, the second video was reported by Italian national newspaper *Corriere della sera* as a Facebook post shared by user Lillo Fioretto and also published by London-based music magazine *Classic FM*, which in turn reported that the video was shared on Facebook by Spanish politician Íñigo Errejón (2020). In his post, Errejón comments in both Italian and Spanish: "Italy, we all love you! All together we will make it!" As of July 26, 2021, the post shared by Errejón received 14 million views and was liked by over one hundred thousand people; in the comment section, one can find people writing from all over the world, including many Italian expatriates. This ultimately suggests that this lockdown tarantella experience has the potential to help consolidate the place of southern Italian folk music and dance on the global stage by helping tarantella performances circulate online in an unprecedented way.

The idea of community expressed in both videos has to do not so much with the local community as with immediate family and condominium units. For example, the child's recurring presence reflects how immediate family members were confined within the same apartment space, therefore constituting the performing unit of the single balcony performance. Moreover, Bocchino titles her video *Musica, amicizia e riunioni di condominio ai tempi del coronavirus* (*Music, Friendship, and Condominial Gatherings in the Time of Covid*), which clearly highlights the *condominio* (neighborhood) as the core of community sharing during lockdown. To the extent that balcony and condominium spaces provided a sense of community, they also offered the opportunity for an organic gathering that resembled, on a much smaller scale, the traditional festival. At the same time, the communities emerging from these spaces combine virtual and real-life elements, since these events were often "advertised on the web, happened within a non-digital space, and then returned to the web through live streaming and video uploads, and news reports" (Noce 2020). In other words, at least in the case of lockdown balcony performances, it was still possible for tarantella gatherings to resemble the kind of grassroots assembly that is associated with the traditional festivals, but the national and international diffusion of this phenomenon became possible within a digital framework.

Tammurriata practitioner Antonio Quartuccio, who has been attending the local tammurriata festivals for several years, organized a balcony tammurriata performance and uploaded the video to his YouTube channel on May 6, 2020, also sharing it on Facebook (Quartuccio 2020). The video, shot by Quartuccio himself on an amateur device, shows him playing the tammorra drum from his balcony, but one can hear the voices of the neighbors coming from the nearby balconies. As Quartuccio announces at the beginning of the video, this is a community performance by residents of the San Michele quarter (from the name of the nearby church devoted to Saint Michael) in the town of Torre del Greco, near the city of Naples, and with the help of the WhatsApp group chat. The performance showcases Quartuccio's desire to share his passion for tammurriata.[14] This example shows that although the event was planned online, the performance still reflects group participation dynamics that are typical of in-person tammurriata gatherings and festivals. In fact, as Quartuccio sings "Tammurriata nera" (Black Tammurriata)—a popular post–World War II song to which the whole neighborhood is able to sing along[15]—the neighbors are ready to join in, re-creating a call-and-response dynamic typical of traditional tammurriata songs that is still performed at local festivals. Far from dying out, then, these in-person group dynamics continued through the balcony gatherings. In addition, this example suggests a newly found sense of community that went beyond the balcony performances and spurred the grassroots organization of local cultural events beyond the pandemic. As Quartuccio explains, "Since then, now we all know each other in the streets and we're also thinking about creating a citizen association that helps organize events in our quarter, especially in time for the next San Michele festival." Moreover, the whole neighborhood is now involved in a crowdfunding initiative, which has extended to other neighborhoods, in support of a local hospital. "We want to show that Torre del Greco is not silent," Quartuccio explains, "and even if we are confined to our homes, we are socially engaged."[16] This balcony performance phenomenon, therefore, reflects ways that traditional notions of community and place can both endure through collective and traumatic change and are at the same time transformed by it.

VIRTUAL CONCERTS AND MUSIC VIDEOS

Throughout the pandemic several tarantella music groups, especially major groups such as Alla Bua and Canzoniere Grecanico Salentino, organized virtual concerts using live streaming and then uploaded the video recording on social media and YouTube to give everyone the opportunity to watch the event. While this type of event is the closest to in-person music performances, its organization was not possible during the spring 2020 lockdown, since musicians were confined to their own homes and were not able to get together in person to rehearse or perform. Many instead decided to meet through the Zoom call, which allowed them to jam together via the computer screen. However, in most cases the Zoom call was recorded and edited into a music video before being released, which in turn created a hybrid performance genre that has continued throughout the pandemic, probably also because it is easier for most people to watch recorded content in their own time. The audience's ability to participate in a musical event in the very moment in which it happens is certainly lost in this music video structure; yet, to the extent that they still look like Zoom calls, these videos give off the vibe of a live performance. Regardless, the significance of these videos lies less in the relationship between the performers and the audience and more in the relationships of the performers themselves. In fact, their main goal is to provide the impression of a group performance "by layering individually recorded videos of musicians performing in isolation." In doing so, they "present a spirit of communitas and fortitude, invoking the power of music to 'bring people together'" (Datta 2020, 249). A noteworthy example is offered by Apulian practitioner Cosimo Pastore, who shared his solo tarantella performance video as a Facebook post on April 23, 2020. Confined to his own apartment space, Pastore responded to artistic isolation by creating a composite performance in which he appears on nine different cameras at the same time, playing a different instrument in each instance—from classic to electric guitar and ukulele to more traditional folk instruments such as the mandolin, accordion, and tammorra frame drum (Pastore 2020). As Anita Datta notes in relation to virtual choirs, these lockdown performers, then, "remind audiences of [their] continued existence and respond to an urge to seek continuity for abandoned projects and routines" (2020, 249). A second example is offered by Apulian pizzica dancer Veronica Calati (2020) in her description of a tarantella ensemble concert video that was uploaded to her Facebook page on March 18, 2020, and featured three folk musicians and herself as a dancer, all joined by a Zoom call. Calati highlights the importance of these performances to fight the artist's isolation, even if it simply means to sing or dance to break the silence of home confinement.[17] Borrowing again from Anderson's idea of an imagined community, one could argue that these virtual performances help build imagined artist communities beyond the walls of one's lockdown home.

One way that these recorded performances are able to affirm the artists' online presence in the absence of real-life music events is by narrating salient moments in the local festival calendar as well as the Italian holiday calendar; in doing so, these artists are also able to demonstrate their active participation in the life of the community and its shared struggles. On March 18, 2020, on the occasion of the *fanoje* celebration in Monte Sant'Angelo sul Gargano in the Apulia region, local group Rione Junno released a video featuring their solo concert accompanied by images of previous celebrations when people would gather in the streets. Following the fanoje ritual tradition, in which peasants would start a big fire to propitiate the gods to ensure a good harvest, every year locals celebrate with a big fire in the public square as well as music and dancing. In the absence of real-life gatherings, the video offers a way for locals and tarantella aficionados to participate, albeit virtually, in a ritual moment of purification and propitiation by igniting the ritual fire through one's "voice and heart," giving thanks to the "fire of art, which does not die but continues to resist" (Rione Junno and Niro 2020). As they strive to reenact a collective ritual experience that is especially necessary during a time of pandemic, these musicians are not alone, as the video was co-sponsored by the Apulia regional government in an effort to advertise arts and culture during the pandemic. This in turn reflects Italian anthropologist Omerita Ranalli's (2021) observation that "small and big communities have responded in several ways to the impossibility of living their ritual and festive events in order to keep these events alive, often using internet and especially social media networks, therefore offering a space, albeit virtual, for the celebration of the local festivals." Within this new scenario, the internet and social media can actually help preserve these traditional festivals by functioning as "mediation among all the institutional entities devoted to safekeeping the [local] heritage and its communities."[18]

On April 13, 2020 (Easter Monday celebration), the Milan-based pizzica group Ascanti uploaded a music video with the hashtag #iorestoacasa ("I stay home"). Developed out of the group's lockdown experience, the video features individual performances by three musicians and a dancer, each performing from a private apartment or outdoor space (Ascanti 2020b). Given the importance of Easter Monday in Italian culture as the first collective outdoor celebration of the year, the video offers a moment of virtual celebration, especially for urban residents confined to windows or balconies as their only outdoor outlets. The hashtag works as a reminder that celebrating from your home is the right thing to do, given the circumstances, therefore directly contributing to the many social initiatives aimed at communicating the importance of social distancing at the time.

Ascanti's second lockdown video, uploaded on YouTube on May 3, 2020, was titled "Music in the Time of Coronavirus"; this video is also structured as a collage of live performances, but the backdrop for each performance is a tropical beach paradise as a way to inaugurate the Italian summer season; the sound of a Hawaiian ukulele further reiterates the idea of the exotic vacation vibe (Ascanti 2020a). In the second part of the video, the musicians are filmed again in their own private home space, while the TV voice-over reiterates personal hygiene recommendations dictated by COVID-19 safety protocol. The video hashtags—#iosuonodacasa ("I perform from home") and #quasiliberi ("Almost free")—remind us that this is an especially important moment in the pandemic. On April 26, the Italian government declared that May 4 would inaugurate the beginning of phase 2, in which most citizens were authorized to leave their homes for work, exercise, or family visits, as long as they stayed within the geographic limits of their region of residence. Once again, Ascanti's video acts as a musical commentary on this particular moment in the pandemic while also reiterating the importance of respecting safety measures.

On the occasion of International Workers' Day on May 1, a national holiday in Italy, the folk group Malicanti, which specializes in southern Italian music from the Apulia region, released a video titled *Malidettu lu '50*. Malicanti proposes an original folk song that draws inspiration from local workers' songs from the fields to the factory (Malicanti 2020).[19] The video starts with a brief introduction by tarantella scholar Vincenzo Santoro, who points out that "singing about worker's struggles seems an appropriate way to celebrate this peculiar May 1 holiday, knowing that the fight for worker's rights and for a better world never ends." Santoro is clearly referring to the devastating effects of the pandemic on the Italian workforce. The most striking feature of this performance is that each individual screen shows the location from which the musician is connecting—across Italy, Europe, and Latin America—and where the group members were traveling for work and stuck when the pandemic hit. This choice reminds us, once again, that, while providing communication and support among local musicians during the pandemic, these virtual performances also contribute to the continued global circulation of the tarantella tradition by amplifying these local voices on a digital screen.

Another element emerging from these music videos is both musicians' and dancers' own reflection on the lockdown experience and the role played by tarantella within this context.[20] Special mention here goes to internationally renowned pizzica group Canzoniere Grecanico Salentino and their lockdown music video project titled, in English, "We're All in the Same Dance." Conceived by Mauro Durante and his wife and dancer Silvia Perrone and directed and edited by Gabriele Surdo, the video was released on YouTube on April 20, 2020, and features an original composition by Mauro Durante to the frenetic rhythm of pizzica and a collage of over one hundred dancers performing pizzica steps, each from their own lockdown space across the world (Durante 2020; Protopapa 2020). By juxtaposing three dancing segments in one composite image and then adding new segments as the song continues, the video showcases a variety of lockdown perspectives: many wear the long flowing skirt typical of pizzica performances, but others wear leggings or other informal clothing that reminds us of their home confinement; many dance barefoot to re-create the feeling of a tarantella ritual, but others wear heels or even use skateboards. Moreover, although most of them re-create the steps of a pizzica dance performance, others try different types of dances or even aerial acrobatics. More important, each segment shows the dancer's feet, focusing on the dancing steps, or her torso; the segments are combined to form the image of one person, which reiterates the idea of being united through dance, as suggested by the title.

In addition, the video alternates the dancers' segments with brief segments showing the Italian urban scenario of lockdown balconies and houses, contrasting these scenes with images of fields, animals, and plants to highlight the struggle of home confinement during the first phase of lockdown. The two final segments feature an image of a fetus in between two dancers' videos and a small child playing in the fields, as the background moves away from the lockdown cities to serene skies and summer flowers in bloom—a clear message of hope and rebirth at the end of the pandemic tunnel. As Durante points out in his introduction, "Not so long ago, in southern Italy, music and dance were used to exorcise the poison of the Taranta spider demon. Today, in the midst of the coronavirus emergency, a music comes out the walls of a house in Puglia and crosses the world. The dance goes global: hymn to life, antidote to the privations of the lockdown" (quoted in *Songlines* 2020). Once again, Durante's words reflect not only a willingness to reenact tarantella rituals to exorcize the pandemic, but also the spectacularization of the ritual on the global world music scene, which is confirmed by their choice of an English title for the project.[21]

The recorded performance *Quarantella* (a word play on quarantine and tarantella) offers a similar commentary on tarantella's role within the Italian lockdown experience. The video was released on April 9, 2020, by the nationally recognized Orchestra Popolare La Notte della Taranta (2020) and presents performances by fifteen musicians and ten dancers, including well-known tarantella dancer Lucia Scarabino. While sharing the multitrack video structure of most virtual performances at the time, this video also contains an original music composition by Daniele Durante and narrates, in southern Italian dialect and humoristic tones, the Italian quarantine experience and the therapeutic help of tarantella:

> If your head gets foggy
> don't pay attention to it
> instead play, sing, and dance
> this beautiful quarantella
> . . . the drum, tambourine, and this pounding rhythm
> the pressure rises/with the blood that boils.

In the first half, the video employs various rhythms, melodies, and performing styles, while in the second half it shows a unifying, collective performance of a traditional pizzica tune, with dancers following along, each from their own lockdown space—yet another way to represent the idea of social and cultural unity during a particularly difficult moment. What's more, through the catchy refrain "You gotta stay home!" ("T'hai stare a casa!")—

an exhortative version of the popular lockdown hashtag #iorestoacasa ("I stay home") that is made even stronger by the use of dialect—the video becomes an explicit invitation to follow social distancing regulations, southern Italian style.

ONLINE TARANTELLA CLASSES AND COMMUNITIES

The concerns widely shared by scholars and practitioners regarding the post-1990s tarantella revival include the pedagogical aspects embedded in the transmission of these traditions outside of the traditional calendric festivals. As scholar Roberto De Simone, a leading voice in the 1970s tarantella revival, points out, "A traditional festival combines celebratory and didactic elements, and here the role of the maestro, through his own examples and authority, makes it possible for the tradition to continue" (2005). Local musicians, then, often struggle to find ways to make sense of these changes.[22] Giuseppe Gala also observes that the revival has "reinvented several ways of dancing that have no direct connection with their traditional forms and are not based on a constructive dialogue with older generations," thus lacking the "collective memory" that is at the center of every tradition and allows it to live on (2002, 133).

When the Italian government announced full lockdown, such concerns about tradition must have seemed less important, especially since "intimacy, hugs, hands and handouts [had] become toxic. Physical distance, on the other hand, [was] sound, healthy and a sign of solidarity" (Ulfstjerne 2020, 83). The flash mob organized on March 21, 2020, by Milan-based music group Briganti Musiche dal Sud, one of the main promoters of the tarantella revival in northern Italy, clearly reflects such a shift. Advertised with the hashtag #ballatecidacasa ("Dance for us from home"), the flash mob was geared toward students enrolled in Briganti's tarantella courses, which were canceled during lockdown. The Facebook event page announced a "flashmob to anchor ourselves to dancing. . . . It is not a demonstration of your [dancing] skills or a competition and neither is this part of the tradition: dance as you like! Alone or, if you manage to convince someone in your family, you can dance with a partner or as a group" (Briganti Musiche dal Sud 2020). This explicit call to ditch the tradition altogether reflects an important moment within the larger tarantella revival: upholding the tradition might not be the main priority as musicians struggle to keep their classes going, and students need mostly an emotional release and bonding with fellow classmates. Briganti's focus, therefore, shifted from teaching the tradition to providing a communal space in which students could keep practicing what they had learned up to that moment. This choice also helped Briganti cultivate a feeling of nostalgia that would keep their students' interest alive and help them feel like an integral part of the tarantella dancing community. In fact, Briganti asked all participants to record themselves while dancing from home, collected the videos, and edited them all into short video clips that were regularly posted on their event discussion page and also on Briganti's main Facebook page. Moreover, Briganti posted videos of their music and dance shows and past workshops as a "learning aid." The first event was successful enough to justify more flash mob events in the following weeks, sometimes focusing on specific dance genres such as tammurriata, pizzica, and so on.

As an immediate reaction to the pandemic, then, these dance flash mobs reflect a mix of improvisation, adaptation, and innovation. For example, the flash mob organized by the students of the Milan-based dance school Mediterranea Danza E Arti was uploaded as a YouTube video on March 9, 2020 (Panera 2020). The video shows a group of women, each performing pizzica dance steps alone from her own home space; they all dance to the song "Ritmo di Contrabbando" ("A Rhythm on the Sly"), an original composition by musician Eugenio Bennato, among the first to rediscover the tarantella rhythms in the 1970s and still one of the leading voices of the revival today. Well known within the revival context, this song carries the frenetic rhythm of tarantella healing rituals while also describing a folk music genre that reflects the continuing subaltern role of southern Italy within the Italian national context (Bennato 2010). While encouraging the dancers to think of southern Italian culture and traditions, Bennato's modern take on tarantella music in this song allows for more freedom on the part of the dancers, who are able to dance to this song without necessarily adopting traditional couple dancing or a specific dancing style.[23] This type of adaptation was already visible in nontraditional festivals and performances before the pandemic. While such choices seem to be more justified during lockdown, they also contribute to the continued transformation of tarantella traditions in the long run.

Throughout 2020 and leading up to the spring of 2021, many tarantella music and dance cultural associations and schools stayed shut,[24] while several strove to stay alive by familiarizing themselves with the Zoom platform and devising teaching strategies that would allow them to continue their courses online. However, a shared concern was how to teach tarantella dancing in the online format while respecting its cultural significance and traditions. After a few months of feeling personally and professionally stuck, Apulian dancer and teacher Veronica Calati decided to give online classes a try. She created a remote class setting in her living room, including a large TV screen and all the music set up used for in-person classes, so much so that "it almost, almost seemed like [she] had those people standing in the room in front of [her]."[25] The course featured various tarantella traditions and attracted sixty students, who connected from Italy and abroad, including not only Italian-speaking expatriates but also English-, French-, and Spanish-speaking participants.[26] This was a revelation for Calati, as she had never imagined that a tarantella dance class online could be possible. One way that she dealt with this new format was to make sure that each class was divided into smaller sections of twenty students, so she could see all their body movements well on screen and also make sure to group together students with the same skill level. Another strategy was to invite tarantella musicians from across Italy to play "live" for the class on Zoom while her students danced, which helped students feel the energy of live tarantella music even from their home space. In addition, Calati used linguistic instruction to guide her students, employing her voice as the main teaching tool in the absence of her bodily presence. She left choreography for last, paying attention to each student's body relationship with rhythm and music, while also helping students who participated in couples improve their dynamics. Notwithstanding all the technical difficulties and pedagogical struggles, this experience was a very positive one, not only professionally but also personally, as it helped Calati "take a break, even briefly, from pandemic life and go back to my old life, knowing that once the TV screen was turned off the room returned to emptiness."

In response to my question about teaching tarantella dance online, Calati states that it all depends on how you do it: "If you manage to light that fire . . . to reach students through the screen through music . . . through communication . . . it's a very positive thing for all." At the same time, she acknowledges, it remains a very different experience than in-person classes, especially since you don't get to socialize with your students outside of class and solidify your relationship with them that way. I find this last point especially significant, as it reminds us that the element of socialization and bonding comes not only from the act of dancing but also from spending time together before and after dancing, which was not possible within the lockdown context. Moreover, Calati's experience shows her ongoing effort to find "proximity and intimacy" with her students through the screen, but also that the proximity she is able to reach remains "mediated by digital means" (Ulfstjerne 2020, 83), which makes these virtual dance gatherings all the more complex.

Others responded to the situation very differently. When asked why she would not teach dancing online, Campanian musician and dancer Maria

Piscopo replied, "It makes no sense teaching traditional dance online, since folk dancing is born out of the [physical] relationship between the dancers; in a remote context this relationship disappears."[27] Instead, Piscopo's goal was to "maintain an authentic relationship and emotional bond with her students and also limit the inauthenticity that comes from the lack of human contact, the lack of a hug." Therefore, she decided to organize a seminar on the historical, cultural, and ritual aspects of the tarantella genre, while her partner Francesco Salvadore was able to teach the tammorra drum on Zoom. Using the WhatsApp application as a way to communicate with course participants and also manage course enrollments, Piscopo was able to teach the course throughout the winter and spring of 2020–21, with over eighty participants tuning in from all over the world. Reflecting on this experience, Piscopo was positively surprised by "the strong emotional involvement of the participants and also their active participation during class discussions," but has no doubt that "once the pandemic is over, we will all return to more conventional gatherings where we can reestablish our bodies' legitimate right to meet [physically]."

Piscopo's words echo those of my longtime festival companion and tammurriata enthusiast Letizia Scote, who explains, "I'm not interested in taking virtual classes because it makes no sense. Tammurriata is closely linked to being present in the moment, to the local community . . . how do you manage to re-create the energy that happens inside the [tammurriata] dancing circle if you cannot re-create the circle virtually? You cannot describe the circle, you need to try it."[28] During our conversation about the virtual tarantella, renowned tarantella scholar Vincenzo Santoro also reiterated the difference between dancing with a partner in person and dancing alone onscreen, since tarantella is essentially a couple dance that is hard to replicate in the absence of physical contact with the dancing partner.[29] Therefore, he warned, re-creating the kind of organic couple dance dynamics found on festival grounds, or even at the dancing school, is very hard onscreen.

Such concerns are not limited to the Italian border; Tullia Conte, Italian artist and scholar whose Paris-based association Sudanzare organizes shows and workshops for French-speaking participants, also shared her concerns about the online dancing classes advertised in Italy.[30] Conte explains that "even though such moments offer social interactions among participants, they lack critical awareness and willingness to safeguard the values that are embedded in body interactions" during the dance. Sudanzare decided instead to offer a seminar focused on "training body and mind to help improve the psychophysical conditions of the participants during their mandated home confinement" using a variety of musical traditions, including tarantella, and also a mix of yoga, shiatsu, and Chinese medicine. While illustrating Conte's deep reflection on the tarantella tradition, this act of adaptation also reflects the irony of respecting the cultural specificity of tarantella while employing and combining several other cultural traditions from around the world. Similar to the act of exporting tarantella for a global market, then, the main issue at stake within a virtual pedagogical context is what can be easily and successfully replicated virtually and what cannot, how one goes about replicating, and what the effects of this replication are.

As these examples show, an important innovation emerging from these remote class experiments is their ability to open up the tarantella music and dance experience to aficionados residing both in different parts of Italy and abroad, thanks not only to Zoom but also to social media advertising and applications. My conversations with some of Piscopo's students confirmed that several of those connecting from abroad are in fact Italian expatriates like myself, who would have not been able to participate in in-person classes and therefore saw this moment as an unexpected opportunity. Southern Italian–born and resident in the central Italian city of Pisa, where she moved because of her job, Piscopo herself is one of many southerners who learned to play the drum and dance in the southern festivals and is now contributing to spreading southern Italian folk traditions throughout Italy and abroad.

One would be remiss not to mention the important role played by Facebook groups such as Amici Pizzicati, Pizzica e Dintorni, Popolo e Tammorra, or Pizzica e Tarantella in the online circulation and advertisement of tarantella events throughout the pandemic. Such online communities have existed for several years and they provide information about upcoming events, especially in bigger cities like Milan, Rome, or Florence and outside the context of the Catholic-based traditional festivals in the south. When the pandemic hit, these groups provided a natural space for sharing communal grief and support as well as for helping tarantella aficionados feel less isolated, while also fueling their passion for music and dancing. Even a quick look at posts and memes shared in the spring of 2020 on the Amici Pizzicati page, one of the leading groups for tarantella practitioners in the Milan area, shows a sense of nostalgia toward previous dancing gatherings conveyed through the sharing of old event posts and photos. In addition, the page was used to deliver messages of hope and unity, similarly to the balcony performances and virtual music events. In providing a space for community sharing during such a difficult time, these online groups ended up taking on new social roles and also helped cement the place of tarantella within a digital framework.

Finally, in reflecting on the virtual tarantella phenomenon it is important to acknowledge the absence of many performers, students, and festival participants who have remained offscreen throughout the pandemic and have been waiting patiently for local events to return. Even though most tarantella musicians and practitioners, both old and young, operate a Facebook page and keep some kind of social media presence, for many of them, especially those belonging to older generations, lack of familiarity with computer technology must have constituted a major obstacle. Much like the urbanized and globalized performances spurred by the tarantella revival, these online communities are "reinvented" communities that attract different groups of participants than do the rural and religious festivals in the south. Considering the transformations that tarantella as a whole has gone through since the revival, one wonders if the changes brought by this pandemic will further impact the tradition in the future.

CONCLUSIONS

My analysis of the pandemic tarantella phenomenon—specifically balcony performances, virtual music and dance performances, music videos, virtual music and dance classes, and online tarantella communities—illustrates recurring themes that have to do with working through collective trauma, sharing one's personal and cultural connections to southern Italian traditions, and reflecting on the role of ancient tarantella rituals within a pandemic context. Spurred by the 2020 pandemic, artists' and practitioners' reinterpretation of southern Italian "communities," "traditions," and "places" especially suggests continuity between the global and the digital tarantella, therefore inviting further reflection on the reinvention of tarantella music and dance traditions since the 1990s, as well as the social and cultural significance of these traditions within both globalized and digitized scenarios.

ACKNOWLEDGMENTS

I am grateful to tarantella scholar Vincenzo Santoro for his invaluable research assistance and advice as I put together this chapter. I am also indebted to fellow tarantella aficionado and scholar Ahmed Daoud for sharing music video material and providing an Italy-based perspective on the topic.

NOTES

1. While most repertories feature couple dances (not necessarily man-woman), four-dancer, circle, and processional choreographies are also possible, depending on geographical context. Adding to such complexity, in the case of couple dancing, the dancers' movements can symbolize rites of fertility, initiation, and courtship, especially if the dancers are of opposite sexes. As for the drum-based rhythm, different types of tarantella feature rather different rhythmic patterns, such as 2/4, 6/8, 4/4, and 12/8, and various instruments, such as drum, bagpipe, accordion, violin, mandolin, and flute (Gala 1999).

2. De Martino argued that psychological factors, such as unrequited love, feelings of depression connected to puberty, or the economic and social status of *tarantati* (victims), must have all contributed to this phenomenon.

3. In the 1970s, tarantella music and dances became again the object of interest on the part of both scholars and musicians; however, it remained a niche genre mostly known among southern Italian left-wing intellectuals, especially given its connection with Italian student and feminist movements and with the American folk music revival (Inserra 2017, 32–39).

4. Here I draw on my own published research (2017) as the first extensive study in English of the post-1990s revival and its global circulation.

5. The most important example is the annual Notte della Taranta (Night of the Taranta) festival, held in the town of Melpignano in the Apulia region since 1998 and devoted to southern Italian rhythms. Following its large success, the festival has contributed to popularizing the tarantella genre both nationally and internationally, while also boosting tourism in the region. Over time, the festival's scope has also become increasingly international, thanks to the presence of many artists from around the world, including artists from world music, rock, and pop music scenes.

6. Following this trend, cultural broker and scholar Anna Nacci uses the term *neotarantismo*, or "neotarantism" to describe this revitalization phenomenon (2001, 11).

7. My fieldwork research focused on the tammurriata festival scene in Campania as well as the larger tarantella revival in the northern Italian city of Milan, where many southerners migrate for work, often bringing tarantella traditions with them.

8. The song chosen for the video, "Taranta," also helps Leone draw similarities between the feeling of being on lockdown and that of being a *tarantato*, that is, possessed by the tarantella "dancing mania"—from "having a torment in [your] chest / that consumes you and does not stop" to the need to dance to stop this madness: "If it's taranta let it dance / if it's melancholy leave it outside."

9. While in-person events started happening again in summer 2020 (though on a much smaller scale and under strict safety regulations), a new wave of infections in fall 2020 drove Italian residents back to their home spaces, thereby spurring a new season of virtual events. In spring 2021, the slow circulation of vaccines in Italy, together with still-strict gathering regulations, contributed to the continuation of remote events. As for online classes, most of them did not start until a few months later and continued throughout the winter 2020 and spring 2021.

10. This is the description of the June 4, 2020, streaming conference and performance event that was shared on their Facebook page.

11. Their video manifesto, released on June 21, 2020, is a collective spoken-word performance focusing on the folk musician's role in collecting the wealth of Italian local traditions and making them available to a global audience. "I collect this [local] memory as

a treasure returned from the sea and I offer it to the unknown faces of the multicultural city. . . . I am a testimony to a plural identity. It is here that I exist. It is here that I want to go. It is here that I unveil myself. . . . I AM TRADITIONAL MUSIC" (PizzicArte Cultura e Musica del Sud 2020).

12. Their Facebook event page advertised the flash mob as "an experiment in distant socializing" whose goal was to "break the silence" and encourage Italian residents to participate widely regardless of their musical skills (even beating pots and pans would do), since the main goal was to "to be heard, as music is the best medicine to cure the soul and in this moment we need it" (Fanfaroma 2020). As a matter of fact, several nationally recognized musicians participated in the event. Fanfaroma also asked participants to upload their performance videos to the event discussion page, which was populated with video documentation in the following days and weeks. The event page shows that over twelve thousand people were either interested or participated, while the discussion page shows over fifty uploaded videos.

13. In 2000, the song was released in the world music scene as a cover by Neapolitan group Spaccanapoli and as such it was featured in the American TV show *The Sopranos*.

14. Antonio Quartuccio, Facebook Messenger conversation with the author, July 21, 2021. As he puts it, "With other neighbors we decided to make this video and create activities that helped tone things down a bit . . . We wanted to show how my neighborhood was reacting to these difficult time . . . Making that video [also] helped others get interested in this type of culture, hoping that it won't die out as these are our roots."

15. The song is representative of the internationally renowned Neapolitan song tradition and characterized by the tammurriata rhythm and singing style as well as local folk culture imagery.

16. As a reward for his planning initiative, Quartuccio was asked to decorate the neighborhood balconies on the occasion of the celebration for the local soccer team Turri and now plays a more active role in the local community. "The neighbors now greet me in the streets like I did something beautiful," he concludes proudly.

17. "Do we sing and dance for you? Do we sing and dance for us? We sing and dance to satisfy a need, to send away frustration, melancholy, and solitude among these four walls than cannot reply back. Music and Dance, then, will be the means to express ourselves beyond every wall, to listen, to listen to each other" (Calati 2020).

18. This effort was clearly visible in the organization of the twenty-third iteration of the internationally renowned Notte della Taranta festival, which spanned the last week of August 2020 and employed streaming technology to showcase, on national TV, live concerts from several parts of the Apulia region. With over four hundred artists, nineteen itinerary points, and no live audience, the organizers were able to keep the annual media broadcasting while also guaranteeing public safety, all the while providing advertisement for the Apulian tourist industry (*Leccesette* 2020).

19. It's a politically engaged song whose lyrics include excerpts from the Apulia fieldwork notes collected by American ethnomusicologist Alan Lomax and his Italian colleague Diego Carpitella in 1954 as well as from 1970s Apulian musical group Ucci (Santoro).

20. This has been a common trend throughout the pandemic, as also suggested by the group Sette Bocche's 2021 video performance #*vaccinatour* (Sette Bocche 2021).

21. As confirmed by their lockdown album *Meridiana*, the group is very much aware of their role in diffusing localized southern Italian rhythms internationally, "offer[ing] a lesson in how to turn local music into a global brand" (Spencer 2021).

22. Neapolitan singer Marcello Colasurdo, who has famously performed tammurriata both within and outside the local context as well as nationally and internationally, describes this duality: "It is exactly there, from the old–timers, that I learn new tammurriata texts, that is, the traditional ones, which have been passed on orally and vary according to each geographical area. What you sing on the festival site you don't sing on the stage: real tammurriata is danced, played, and sung at the local festa, for hours and hours, without a microphone. It is there that you can measure everyone's performing skills: musicians, singers, and dancers" (Mauro 2004, 219).

23. As Giovanni Pizza puts it, this " 'popular dance' with an indefinite trance meaning" is a watered-down version of tarantella's unique history and cultural values (2004, 201).

24. These often included major names such as Milan-based Briganti and Canto Antico (Inserra 2017).

25. Veronica Calati, WhatsApp conversation with the author, July 27, 2021.

26. While the tarantella revival has certainly encouraged the increasing participation of Italian expatriates and tourists from all over the world in the local festivals, the shift to online classes and performances during lockdown created a new space for Italian expatriates like myself to participate while being physically far from home. Tarantella artists like Calati, Maria Piscopo, and Tullia Conte all confirmed this shift during our conversations.

27. Maria Piscopo, WhatsApp conversation with the author, July 27, 2021.

28. Letizia Scote, email to the author, July 19, 2021.

29. Vincenzo Santoro, Zoom conversation with the author, June 15, 2021.

30. Tullia Conte, email to the author, July 25–28, 2021. While not Italy-based, Sudanzare's classes had an average of thirty students, of whom four to five were Italian expatriates living in France and two were French-speaking students connecting from Italy.

REFERENCES

Agnello, Fabiana. 2020. "A Lecce si esorcizzano i 'morsi' del coronavirus a passo di pizzica." *Lecce prima*, April 19. https://www.lecceprima.it/attualita/coronavirus -esibizione-pizzica-sant-oronzo-lecce.html.

Anderson, Benedict R. O. 2006. *Imagined Communities: Reflections on the Origin and Spread of Nationalism*. Rev. ed. London: Verso.

Apolito, Paolo. 2000. "Tarantismo, identità locale, postmodernità." In *Quarant'anni dopo De Martino: Atti del convegno internazionale di studi sul tarantismo*, edited by Gino L. Di Mitri, 1:137–46. Nardò, Italy: Besa.

Ascanti. 2020a. *Musica ai tempi del coronavirus*. Pizzica con ukulele. YouTube, May 3. https:// www.youtube.com/watch?v=qoCgsgj8HPc.

Ascanti. 2020b. Pizzica Rhoggy #pasquettaimperfetta. YouTube, April 13. https://www .youtube.com/watch?v=tjrt6_8N9UY.

Barcellona, Gaia Scorza. 2020. "Coronavirus, l'Italia sul balcone: Canzoni contro la paura." *La repubblica*, March 13. https://www.repubblica.it/cronaca/2020/03/13/news /coronavirus_italia_al_balcone_canzoni_contro_la_paura-251221289/.

Bennato, Eugenio. 2010. *Brigante se more: Viaggio nella musica del sud*. Rome: Coniglio Editore.

bMagazine. 2020. "La musica ai tempi del Coronavirus. A benevento si suona dai balconi." March 12. http://www.bmagazine.it/la-musica-ai-tempi-del-coronavirus-a-bene vento-si-suona-dai-balconi/.

Briganti Musiche dal Sud. 2020. "#Ballatecidacasa: flash mob in differita." Facebook event, March 21. https://www.facebook.com/events/505143913467095.

Calati, Veronica. 2020. *Cantico degli emarginati.* Facebook post, March 18. https://www.facebook.com/watch/?ref=search&v=21084294005552&external_log_id=e7d0c737-078f-4236-9d52-679a392d0d0a&q=veronica%20calati.

Corriere della sera. 2020. "Agrigento, tra fisarmoniche e tamburelli si canta 'Ciuri, ciuri' dai balcony." March 14. https://video.corriere.it/cronaca/agrigento-fisarmoniche-tamburelli-si-canta-ciuri-ciuri-balconi/a048e32e-660d-11ea-a287-bbde7409af03.

Datta, Anita. 2020. "'Virtual Choirs' and the Simulation of Live Performance under Lockdown." *Social Anthropology/Anthropologie sociale* 28 (2): 249–50. https://doi.org/10.1111/1469-8676.12862.

De Martino, Ernesto. 2005. *The Land of Remorse: A Study of Southern Italian Tarantism.* Translated by Dorothy Louise Zinn. London: Free Association Books.

De Simone, Roberto. 2005. "Tammurriata: Così scompare la tradizione." *Il mattino,* December 27.

Durante, Mauro. 2020. *We're All in the Same Dance.* YouTube, April 20. https://www.youtube.com/watch?v=2MxRG0Jpdak&t=1s.

Errejón, Íñigo. 2020. "Italia, ti vogliamo bene! Tutti insieme ce la faremo. Italia, te queremos! Todos juntos saldremos adelante." Facebook post, March 13. https://www.facebook.com/watch/?ref=external&v=676005459809026.

Fanfaroma. 2020. Flashmob Sonoro! Facebook event, March 13. https://www.facebook.com/events/4167551866603698.

Gala, Giuseppe. 1993. "Ballo sul tamburo della Campania." In "'Io non so se ballo bene': Canzoni a ballo e balli cantati nella tradizione popolare ttaliana." Special issue, *Choreola* 9 (3): 196–202.

Gala, Giuseppe. 1999. *La tarantella dei pastori.* Florence: Ed. Taranta.

Gala, Giuseppe. 2002. "'La pizzica ce l'ho nel sangue': Riflessioni a margine sul ballo tradizionale e sulla nuova pizzicomania del salento." In *Il ritmo meridiano: La pizzica e le identità danzanti del salento,* edited by Vincenzo Santoro and Sergio Torsello, 109–53. Lecce, Italy: Edizioni Aramirè.

Gramsci, Antonio. 1995. *The Southern Question.* Translated by Pasquale Verdicchio. West Lafayette, IN: Bordighera.

Inserra, Incoronata. 2017. *Global Tarantella: Reinventing Southern Italian Folk Music and Dances.* Chicago: University of Illinois Press.

La repubblica. 2020. "L'appello dei musicisti per i lavoratori del settore: 21 Giugno, non sia una festa #SenzaMusica." June 13. https://www.repubblica.it/spettacoli/musica/2020/06/13/news/iolavoroconlamusica-259120800/.

Leccesette. 2020. "Notte della taranta. Domani il concertone su Rai 2." August 27. https://www.leccesette.it/eventi/72510/notte-della-taranta-domani-il-concertone-su-rai-2.html.

Leone, Roberto. 2020a. "D'incanto la pizzica." YouTube, April 20. https://www.youtube.com/watch?v=k3e5IcAjrdA.

Leone, Roberto. 2020b. *Lockdown Lecce 2020.* YouTube, June 17. https://www.youtube.com/watch?v=J6MhpHG4k_w.

Malicanti. 2020. *Malidettu lu '50.* YouTube, May 1. https://www.youtube.com/watch?v=FLkx_zuXQoo.

Mauro, Giuseppe. 2004. "La tammurriata: Intervista con Vicidomini, 'O Lione e Colasurdo." In *Tammurriate: Canti, musiche e devozioni in Campania,* edited by Antonello Lamanna, 212–25. Rome: Adnkronos.

Nacci, Anna, ed. 2001. *Tarantismo e neotarantismo: Musica, dance, transe; bisogni di oggi, bisogni di sempre.* Nardò, Italy: Besa.

Noce, Tiziana. 2020. "Un 25 Aprile nuovo: Isolato ma connesso." In *Studiare la pandemia. Diseguaglianze e resilienza ai tempi del COVID-19*, edited by Domenico Cersosimo, Felice Cimatti and Francesco Raniolo. Rome: Donzelli.

Orchestra Popolare La Notte della Taranta. 2020. *Quarantella*. YouTube, April 9. https://www.youtube.com/watch?v=uW6Q0CvXeFc.

Paliotti, Vittorio. 1992. *Storia della canzone napoletana*. Rome: Newton Compton.

Panera, Valentina. 2020. "Corona virus. Si danza nelle case." YouTube, March 9. https://www.youtube.com/watch?v=gBtMmgAR0GY.

Pastore, Cosimo. 2020. *Cosimo x 9 . . . Una tarantella suonata in compagnia di altri 8 me!* Facebook, April 23. https://m.facebook.com/story.php?story_fbid=2984943868261917&id=100002389990974.

Pizza, Giovanni. 2004. "Tarantism and the Politics of Tradition in Contemporary Salento." In *Memory, Politics and Religion: The Past Meets the Present in Europe*, edited by Frances Pine, Deema Kaneff, and Haldis Haukanes, 199–223. Münster: LIT.

PizzicArte Cultura e Musica del Sud. 2020. *Video manifesto #musicapopolarenuntermare*. YouTube, June 21. https://www.youtube.com/watch?v=aKPMYuGmPp4.

Protopapa, Titina. 2020. "Pizzica di speranza: 'We're All in the Same Dance': Il violino di Mauro Durante fa ballare tutti #NessunoEscluso." *LecceNews24.it*, April 24. https://www.leccenews24.it/attualita/we-are-all-in-the-same-dance-mauro-durante-silvia-perrone-gabriele-surdo-amnesty-international.htm.

Puricella. 2020. "A Lecce si esorcizza il coronavirus: Una ballerina nella piazza deserta a passo di pizzica." *La Repubblica*, April 20. https://video.repubblica.it/edizione/bari/a-lecce-si-esorcizza-il-coronavirus-ballerina-nella-piazza-deserta-a-passo-di-pizzica/358554/359110.

Quartuccio, Antonio. 2020. "Tammurriata dai balconi." YouTube, May 6. https://www.youtube.com/watch?v=Mgw8n4IygKw.

Ranalli, Omerita. 2021. "Comunità patrimoniali ai tempi del Covid: La rete per la salvaguardia delle feste di Sant'Antonio Abate." *Dialoghi mediterranei*, July 1. http://www.istitutoeuroarabo.it/DM/comunita-patrimoniali-ai-tempi-del-covid-la-rete-per-la-salvaguardia-delle-feste-di-santantonio-abate/.

Rauche, Anthony. 1990. "The Tarantella: Musical and Ethnic Identity for Italian Americans." In *Italian Americans in Transition: Proceedings of the XXI Annual Conference of the American Italian Historical Association*, edited by Joseph Vincent Scelsa, Salvatore John LaGumina, and Lydio F. Tomasi, 189–97. Staten Island: John D. Calandra Italian American Institute.

Rione Junno and Raffaele Niro. 2020. *Notte di fuochi*. Facebook, March 18. https://www.facebook.com/officialrionejunno/videos/2864923680416778.

Roberts, Maddy Shaw. 2020. "Quarantined Musicians Play and Sing from Balconies in Locked-Down Italy." *Classic FM*, March 16. https://www.classicfm.com/music-news/videos/quarantined-italy-musicians-play-sing-balconies/.

Sette Bocche. 2021. *#vaccinatour*. YouTube, July 6. https://www.youtube.com/watch?v=cSOuPV9B2L4.

Sigerist, Henry E. 2003. *Breve storia del tarantismo*. Nardò, Italy: Besa.

Sky Tg24. 2020. "Coronavirus, scendono in piazza i lavoratori dello spettacolo." May 31. https://tg24.sky.it/spettacolo/2020/05/30/coronavirus-fase-2-manifestazione-lavoratori-spettacolo/amp.

Songlines. 2020. "We're All in the Same Dance Video." May 7, 2020. https://www.songlines.co.uk/news/we-re-all-in-the-same-dance-video.

Spencer, Neil. 2021. "Canzoniere Grecanico Salentino: Meridiana review—Where Puglia Meets bhangra." *Guardian*, May 22. https://www.theguardian.com/music/2021/may/22/canzoniere-grecanico-salentino-meridiana-review.

Taylor, Ana. 2020. "Music and Encouragement from Balconies around the World." *Atlantic*, March 24. https://www.theatlantic.com/photo/2020/03/music-and -encouragement-from-balconies-around-world/608668/.

Ulfstjerne, Michael Alexander. 2020. "Songs of the Pandemic." *Anthropology in Action* 27 (2): 82–86.

Ward, Meredith C. 2021. "Sounds of Lockdown: Virtual Connection, Online Listening, and the Emotional Weight of COVID-19." *SoundEffects* 10 (1): 7–26.

Worden, Mark, and Judy Cantor-Navas. 2020. "Fighting the Lockdown Blues." *Billboard* 132 (7): 20. http://search.ebscohost.com.proxy.library.vcu.edu/login.aspx?direct =true&AuthType=ip,url,cookie,uid&db=f5h&AN=142466045&site=ehost-live& scope=sit.

Index

About the Authors

Pieper Bloomquist, an oncology nurse from Grand Forks, North Dakota, is a traditional artist specializing in Swedish bonadsmålning and a participant in the Art for Life Program. She is an American Scandinavian Foundation fellowship recipient, an instructor at the American Swedish Institute, and a member of the community of professional bonadspainters with the Unnaryds Bonadsmuseum, Unnaryd, Sweden. Her work is shown regionally, including a fall 2022 exhibit at the Swedish American Museum in Chicago.

Sheila Bock is associate professor in the Department of Interdisciplinary, Gender, and Ethnic Studies at the University of Nevada, Las Vegas. Much of her research approaches storytelling as a mode of meaning-making that works powerfully to shape how individuals and communities respond to experiences of marginalization, particularly in contexts of illness. Her work in this area has been published in the *Journal of Folklore Research*, the *Journal of Medical Humanities*, the *Western Journal of Black Studies*, *Health, Culture, and Society*, and multiple edited volumes.

Ben Bridges is a dual PhD candidate in folklore and anthropology at Indiana University. His research focuses on traditional Southeast Alaska Native arts involving red and yellow cedar, examining contemporary practices of harvesting and art-making in the context of the logging industry and climate change. This work ties into some of his other ongoing projects on vernacular responses to global environmental phenomena and the intersections between landscapes and memory. He has published in *SAPIENS* and the *Oxford Research Encyclopedia of Anthropology* and regularly presents at American Folklore Society meetings.

Ross Brillhart is the program manager at the Divided Sky Foundation in Ludlow, Vermont. His research investigates the intersections of music, sound, and health with a concentration on developing and implementing humanistic applications for healthcare and public health based on ethnographic data. His current project is an ethnography of sober concertgoers in the jam band music scene, focusing on their creation of sober spaces and cultures of recovery at concerts and their sonic understandings of sobriety and recovery. Brillhart also has ongoing projects centering on religion, sound, healing, and the natural world in the Blue Mountains of Jamaica; music and sound in hospice care; and music, sound, and Parkinson's disease.

Kinsey Brooke is a graduate student at Indiana University in the folklore and ethnomusicology department and an Erasmus Mundus Scholar. Her research centers on diaspora studies, labor literature, protest texts, narratives of trauma, women's socioeconomic development of the nineteenth and twentieth centuries, factory labor conditions, and the intangible cultural heritage of Atlantic Canada and the Southern Appalachian region of the United States.

James I. Deutsch is a curator and editor at the Smithsonian Institution's Center for Folklife and Cultural Heritage, where he has helped plan and develop numerous public programs on subjects ranging from China, Hungary, and the Peace Corps to the National Aeronautics and Space Administration, the Mekong River, World War II, and the Silk Road. In addition, he is an adjunct professor in the American studies department at George Washington University. Deutsch has taught at universities in Armenia, Belarus, Bulgaria, Germany, Kyrgyzstan, Norway, Poland, and Turkey.

Anne Eriksen is professor of cultural history at the University of Oslo and professor of cultural studies at the University of Bergen. She has published widely on collective memory, the notions of tradition and history, and examples and exemplarity. She is an expert on early modern medical history and is currently doing work in environmental history.

Troyd Geist is the state folklorist with the North Dakota Council on the Arts, director of the Folk and Traditional Arts Apprenticeship Program, and creator and director of the Art for Life Program. He co-authored with Dr. Timothy J. Kloberdanz the book *Sundogs and Sunflowers: Folklore and Folk Art of the Northern Great Plains* and authored *Sundogs and Sunflowers: An Art for Life Program Guide for Creative Aging, Health, and Wellness*. Other work and interests include traditional culture in relation to Alzheimer's, Bell's palsy, guided imagery, and fetal alcohol syndrome.

Diane E. Goldstein is emeritus professor and former chair of the Department of Folklore and Ethnomusicology at Indiana University. She is the author of *Once upon a Virus: AIDS Legends and Vernacular Risk Perception* (2004), co-author of *Haunting Experiences: Ghosts in Contemporary Folklore* (2008), co-editor of *The Stigmatized Vernacular: Where Reflexivity Meets Untellability* (2016) and *Reckless Vectors: The Infecting Other in HIV/AIDS Law* (2005), and editor of one of the earliest interdisciplinary HIV/AIDS anthologies, *Talking AIDS: Interdisciplinary Perspectives on Acquired Immune Deficiency Syndrome* (1991). Goldstein's specialties include folk medicine, cultural issues in healthcare, risk perception, HIV/AIDS, stigmatized illnesses, legend and rumor surrounding health, narrative, ethnography of communications, folklore and violence, folklore and trauma, and applied folklore. She is past president of the American Folklore Society and the International Society for Contemporary Legend Research.

Julianne Graper is an assistant professor at Indiana University, Bloomington, whose work focuses on sound and bat-human relationality in Austin, Texas. Her work has appeared in *Sound Studies*, *MUSICultures*, and the volumes *Sounds, Music, Ecologies* (2023, edited by Jeff Todd Titon and Aaron Allen) and *Songs of Social Protest* (2018, edited by Aileen Dillane et al.). Her translation of Alejandro Vera's *The Sweet*

Penance of Music (2020) won the Robert M. Stevenson Award from the American Musicology Society. She has presented her research at the annual meetings of the Society for Ethnomusicology, the British Forum for Ethnomusicology, and the Society for American Music. She holds a PhD from the University of Texas at Austin.

Incoronata (Nadia) Inserra is an assistant professor at Virginia Commonwealth University; she received a PhD in English from the University of Hawai'i at Mānoa with a focus on folklore and cultural studies. Her research interests include the intersections of folklore, globalization, and digitization as well as folklore as community engagement. She is the author of *Global Tarantella: Reinventing Southern Italian Folk Music and Dances* (2017).

Andrea Kitta is a folklorist and professor at East Carolina University, where she studies vaccination, belief, contemporary legends, and the supernatural. She is the author of *Vaccinations and Public Concern in History: Legend, Rumor, and Risk Perception*, which won the Brian McConnell Book Award in 2012. Her monograph *The Kiss of Death: Contagion, Contamination, and Folklore* won the Chicago Folklore Prize and the Brian McConnell Book Award in 2020. Dr. Kitta is the recipient of the Teacher/ Scholar Award from ECU (2016) and the Board of Governors Distinguished Professor for Teaching Award (2019).

Kyrre Kverndokk is professor of cultural studies at the University of Bergen, Norway. He has published on the practice and politics of Second World War memories, the history of folklore studies, and the cultural history of natural disaster and climate change temporalities. He is the leader of the research project Gardening the Globe: Historicizing the Anthropocene through the production of Socio-nature in Scandinavia, 1750–2020.

Lucy M. Long directs the independent nonprofit Center for Food and Culture (www.foodandculture.org) and teaches folklore, American studies, ethnic studies, nutrition, and tourism at Bowling Green State University in Ohio. With degrees in folklore and folklife (PhD, University of Pennsylvania) and ethnomusicology (MA, University of Maryland), she has been involved since the 1980s in humanities-based research on food, music, and dance as mediums for meaning, identity, community, and power. She has conducted ethnographies in Northern Ireland, Ireland, Spain, ethnic American communities, southern Appalachia, and the eastern Midwest. She has produced numerous documentaries and community education programs and has worked extensively in interpretation in public humanities. Among her publications are *Culinary Tourism* (2004), *Regional American Food Culture* (2009), *Ethnic American Food Today: A Cultural Encyclopedia* (2015), *The Food and Folklore Reader* (2015), *Ethnic American Cooking: Recipes for Living in a New World* (2016), *Honey: A Global History* (2017), and *Comfort Food Meanings and Memories* (2017). During 2020, she conducted a virtual oral history, *Finding Comfort/Discomfort through Foodways during the COVID-19 Pandemic*.

Andrew Robinson is a photographer, artist, and senior lecturer in photography at Sheffield Hallam University, where he co-founded the Centre for Contemporary Legend with Dr. David Clarke and Diane Rodgers. His practice investigates expressions of identity and material culture through a visual anthropology of people, place, and trace, applying creative strategies that integrate still and moving imagery with text, audio, and found materials. His current research interests include the visual representation of vernacular English custom and folklore and the relationship between folklore and national identity in a post-digital, post-Brexit, and post-COVID landscape. Recent publications include a co-edited special edition of *Revenant* (2023) and a chapter in *Folklore and the Nation* (Routledge 2021). Andrew's work has been published and exhibited widely and he has undertaken art commissions and residences in a range of contexts, including art, education, health, and social research.

Theresa A. Vaughan is professor of humanities and assistant dean of the College of Liberal Arts at the University of Central Oklahoma. She received a PhD in folklore from Indiana University. Her research interests have long included gender and foodways, and she is currently the lead editor of *Digest: A Journal of Foodways and Culture*, an open-access journal published by the American Folklore Society's Foodways Section. Her most recent book is *Women, Food, and Diet in the Middle Ages: Balancing the Humours* (2020).